DATE			

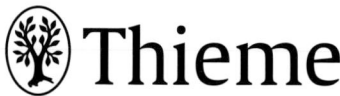

Physical Therapy for the Stroke Patient

Early Stage Rehabilitation

Jan Mehrholz, PhD
Professor, Head of Research Institute
Medical Academy for Rehabilitation
Klinik Bavaria in Kreischa
Kreischa, Germany

With contributions by
Janet H. Carr, Claudia Flaemig, Gert Grellmann,
Jan Mehrholz, Frank Oehmichen, Marcus Pohl,
Ralf Schlosser, Roberta B. Shepherd

139 illustrations

Thieme
Stuttgart · New York

Library of Congress Cataloging-in-Publication Data

Mehrholz, Jan.
  [Fruehphase Schlaganfall. English]
  Physical therapy for the stroke patient : early stage reha-
bilitation / Jan Mehrholz ; with contributions by Janet H.
Carr ... [et al.].
    p. ; cm.
  Includes bibliographical references and index.
  ISBN 978-3-13-154721-7 (hardback)
  I. Carr, Janet H. II. Title.
  [DNLM: 1. Stroke–rehabilitation. 2. Physical Therapy
Modalities. 3. Rehabilitation–methods. WL 356]
  616.8'1062–dc23   2012006777

This book is an authorized translation of the German edition published and copyrighted 2008 by Georg Thieme Verlag, Stuttgart. Title of the German edition: Frühphase
Schlaganfall: Physiotherapie und medizinische Versorgung.

Translator: Alexandra Kuhn-Thiel, MD, Wachenheim,
Germany

Illustrator: Christine Lackner, Ittlingen, Germany

Important note: Medicine is an ever-changing science undergoing continual development. Research and clinical experience are continually expanding our knowledge, in particular our knowledge of proper treatment and drug therapy. Insofar as this book mentions any dosage or application, readers may rest assured that the authors, editors, and publishers have made every effort to ensure that such references are in accordance with **the state of knowledge at the time of production of the book.**

Nevertheless, this does not involve, imply, or express any guarantee or responsibility on the part of the publishers in respect to any dosage instructions and forms of applications stated in the book. **Every user is requested to examine carefully** the manufacturers' leaflets accompanying each drug and to check, if necessary in consultation with a physician or specialist, whether the dosage schedules mentioned therein or the contraindications stated by the manufacturers differ from the statements made in the present book. Such examination is particularly important with drugs that are either rarely used or have been newly released on the market. Every dosage schedule or every form of application used is entirely at the user's own risk and responsibility. The authors and publishers request every user to report to the publishers any discrepancies or inaccuracies noticed. If errors in this work are found after publication, errata will be posted at www.thieme.com on the product description page.

© 2012 Georg Thieme Verlag KG
Rüdigerstrasse 14, 70469 Stuttgart, Germany
http://www.thieme.de
Thieme Medical Publishers, Inc., 333 Seventh Avenue,
New York, NY 10001, USA
http://www.thieme.com

Cover design: Thieme Publishing Group
Typesetting by Druckhaus Götz GmbH,
  Ludwigsburg, Germany
Printed in China by Everbest Printing Ltd

ISBN 978-3-13-154721-7
eISBN 978-3-13-166481-5

For my two girls, Sofie and Katja
For Katharina and Gerhard

List of Contributors

Janet H. Carr, EdD (Colombia), MA, DipPhty, FACP
Associate Professor
Faculty of Health Sciences
The University of Sydney
Sydney, Australia

Claudia Flaemig
Qualified Assistant in Health and Social Care
Klinik Bavaria in Kreischa
Kreischa, Germany

Gert Grellmann, MD
Supervising Physician
Department of Cardiology and Angiology
Klinik Bavaria in Kreischa
Kreischa, Germany

Jan Mehrholz, PhD
Professor, Head of Research Institute
Medical Academy for Rehabilitation
Klinik Bavaria in Kreischa
Kreischa, Germany

Frank Oehmichen, MD
Professor, Director of Cardiology and Angiology
Department
Klinik Bavaria in Kreischa
Kreischa, Germany

Marcus Pohl, MD
Professor, Head of Department of Neurological
Rehabilitation
Klinik Bavaria in Kreischa
Kreischa, Germany

Ralf Schlosser, MD
Department of Neurological Rehabilitation
Klinik Bavaria in Kreischa
Kreischa, Germany

Roberta B. Shepherd, EdD (Colombia), MA,
DipPhty, FACP
Professor
Faculty of Health Sciences
The University of Sydney
Sydney, Australia

Preface

Physical therapy and rehabilitation following stroke: what an exciting and fascinating topic!

Yet—why are we writing an entire book on physical therapy in stroke patients during the early phase after stroke? Quite simply, in order to give answers to the countless questions which have arisen on the subject of the early phase following stroke over the course of the past few years.

This condition carries special significance for many of us, as stroke represents one of the most common causes of physical handicap in the industrialized nations, resulting in limitations in participation and quality of life, not only of the patients, but also of their family members. Another consequence is the considerable burden placed on our health and social systems by this frequently occurring illness.

One of the most important therapeutic options for stroke patients is represented by physical therapeutic methods. It has been demonstrated that as few as 30 extra minutes (this corresponds to approximately 2.2% of a patient's waking hours) of physical therapy a day, specifically aimed at arm and leg exercises, has the favorable effect of bringing about a significant increase in everyday competence in patients who have suffered stroke. There is virtually no medication or neurosurgical therapy which would be able to duplicate such results.

There have been many questions posed recently, among them the following:
- Is physical therapy following stroke effective?
- When, indeed, should this therapy be initiated?
- What scientific studies are available on this topic?
- What practical significance do these studies have?

This book is meant to supply answers to these and many other questions. The scientific substantiation provided by physical therapy is thus taking on increasing importance. A number of studies have confirmed that not only the objective targets, but also the methods employed in physical therapy, are crucial in terms of the optimal recuperation of patients who have suffered stroke.

Besides their own therapeutic experience, and in the sense of an evidence-based approach, physical therapists should principally aim to incorporate not only the individual patient's particular needs and preferences, but also the best available scientific evidence. After all, evidence-based practice supports our ethical–moral obligation to patients and their family members in our endeavors to offer them the best possible therapy.

At this time I would like to thank all therapists for their many questions and ideas, and all participating authors for their professional cooperation, without which it would not have been possible to write this book. Besides the exceptionally professional collaboration with the group of authors, I would also like to bring special attention to Rosi Haarer-Becker, Fritz Koller, Eva-Maria Grünewald from Thieme Verlag, Angelika-M. Findgott, Anne Lamparter from Thieme Publishers, as well as all the others who were directly or indirectly involved —thank you all very much! And thanks also to Roberta and Janet, for this very special opportunity to be able to work with you.

And who is meant to read this book? This book is ultimately directed at anyone and everyone interested in, or working in the field of, rehabilitation in stroke patients.

Jan Mehrholz

Contents

1 Background Information on Stroke—Incidence, Risks, Survival Rates and Chances, Causes, and Related Disorders

Marcus Pohl and Jan Mehrholz

It ain't what you don't know that gets you into trouble. It's what you know for sure that just ain't so.
(Attributed to Mark Twain)

Physical therapists are confronted almost daily with patients who have suffered stroke. But how much do they actually know about the causes, definitions, incidence, and consequences of stroke? This chapter presents a collection of facts on stroke aimed at educating those new to the topic, as well as health-care professionals, about this illness, which affects people all over the world.

■ Definition

The disease pattern of stroke can be defined in clinical as well as diagnostic terms. According to the World Health Organization (WHO), stroke is a condition in which clinical signs of focal or global impairment of cerebral functions develop rapidly, last longer than 24 hours unless interrupted by surgery or death, and exhibit no apparent nonvascular cause. The terms "apoplectic insult," "apoplexia cerebri," and "cerebrovascular accident" (CVA) are synonymous with "stroke."

Clinically speaking, an acute neurological deficit presents as the result of a large area of impaired circulation. Stroke can thus be defined as vessel-related functional impairment of a specific region of the brain. The condition is classified according to the localization and type (Mumenthaler 2002). The types are subdivided as follows (Mumenthaler 2002):
- Ischemic stroke (80%–83% of all strokes)
- Intracerebral hemorrhage (ICH, 10%–12%)
- Subarachnoidal hemorrhage (SAH, 7%–8%)

Steiner et al. (1997) suggested a further subclassification of stroke:
- Ischemic:
  - Originating in the carotid artery
  - Vertebrobasilar
- Hemorrhagic parenchymal:
  - Supratentorial
  - Infratentorial
  - With bleeding into the ventricles
- Subarachnoidal hemorrhage.

Causes of ischemic stroke are:
1. Thrombus (occlusion of an artery in the brain: thrombotic brain infarction).
2. Embolism (a "traveling" thrombus), so-called embolic cerebral infarction or thromboembolic cerebral infarction.
3. Systemic hypoperfusion (reduced circulation, watershed or border infarctions) or venous thrombosis (thrombosis of the sinus veins).

In the case of thrombotic cerebral infarction, a thrombus blocks the arterial lumen, thus hindering blood flow into the distal brain tissue. Thrombi themselves originate mainly in areas of increased deposits on the arterial walls, called atherosclerotic plaques. As the occlusion of the artery takes place over an extended period of time, this type of stroke also occurs very slowly. Thus, the original process can remain undetected for a long time.

A thrombus (**Fig. 1.1**) can cause an embolic stroke, even if it does not block the vessel completely. This happens when the thrombus "travels," that is, when it becomes detached from the vessel wall. This "wandering" thrombus is termed "embolism."

The most common pathological conditions caused by thrombi in large vessels are:

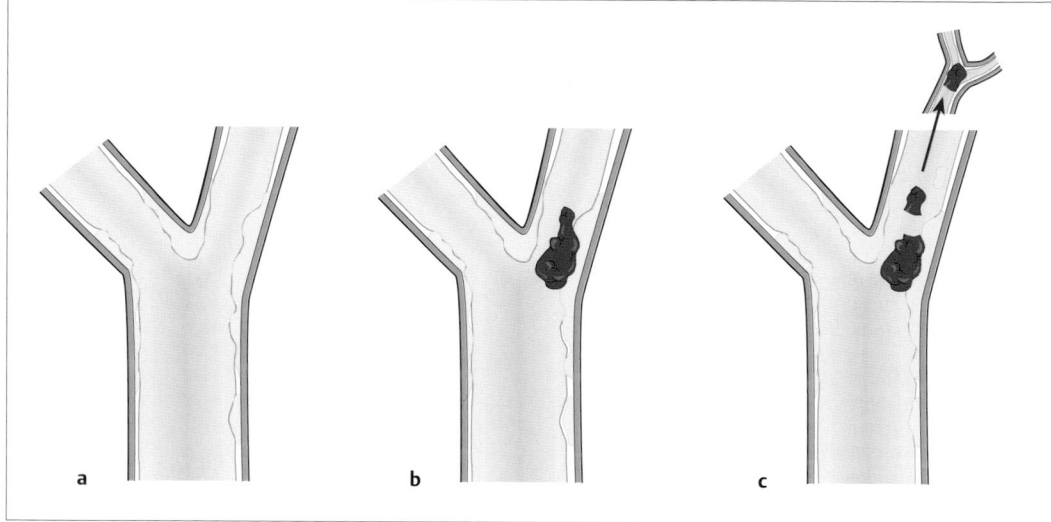

Fig. 1.1 a–c   Atherosclerosis (a), thrombosis (b), embolism (c).

- Atherosclerosis
- Dissection(s)
- Takayasu arteritis
- Giant cell arteritis
- Arteritis/vasculitis, noninflammatory vasculopathy
- Moyamoya syndrome
- Fibromuscular dysplasia

Two-thirds of cases of ischemic stroke take place in the area supplied by the carotid artery and one-third in the region of the vertebrobasilaris arteries (Mumenthaler 2002).

With embolic infarction, arteries become blocked by a thrombus which has detached itself from the wall and traveled to another part of the blood vessel. Here, four categories can be distinguished:

1. Of known origin, that is, the heart (e.g., different types of arrhythmia, inflammatory heart diseases, artificial heart valves, myocardial infarction, open foramen ovale).
2. With the heart as the potential place of origin.
3. Arterial origin, that is, an embolus which has become dislodged from an arteriosclerotic vessel wall (e.g., the aortic arch).
4. Of unknown origin.

Cerebral infarction is characterized by poor oxygen levels in the affected tissue (ischemia). As a result of decreased oxygen flow, the glucose concentration in the affected area also decreases. This lack of substrate triggers a cascade of further reactions of varying types, which further, in the case of an ischemic stroke, cause damage such as excitotoxicity, peri-infarction, depolarization, inflammation, and apoptosis. These will not be discussed here, however; more detailed descriptions are available in the current literature.

With **cerebral hemorrhage**, bleeding of compact areas of various sizes takes place in the brain tissue (**Fig. 1.2**), into the ventricular system, and in some instances also in the subarachnoidal space. The most common causes are bleeding associated with high blood pressure due to the tearing of blood vessels (rhexis), bleeding from vessel abnormalities (such as aneurisms or angiomas), or clotting disorders of various origin. By far the most common cause (around 80%) of intracerebral hemorrhage is spontaneous rhexis bleeding from the end branches of the lenticulostriatal artery.

Ischemic stroke is further classified according to etiology, anatomy, course of illness, and severity:

- Lacunary cerebral infarction
- Terminal vascular bed infarction
- Marginal zone infarction
- Space-occupying infarction (e.g., malignant middle cerebral artery infarction)
- Cerebral micro- or macroangiopathy

An older classification, no longer generally accepted, is made according to chronological course

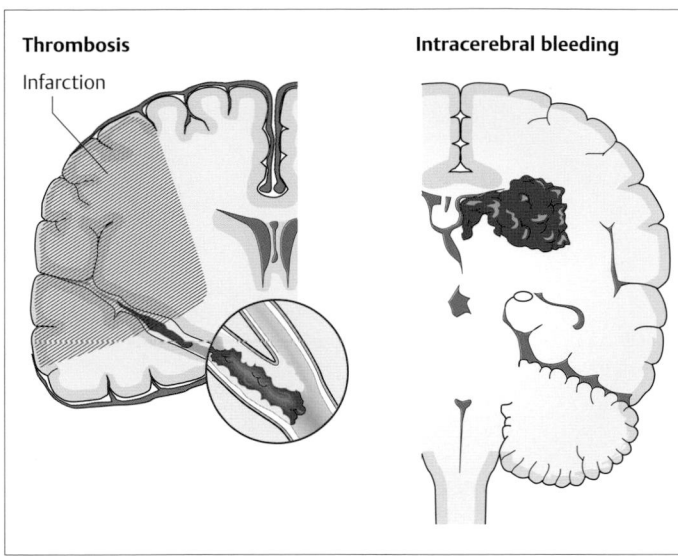

Thrombosis   **Intracerebral bleeding**

Infarction

Fig. 1.2 Distinction between infarction and cerebral hemorrhage.

of illness and severity of the stroke symptoms, on the basis of the length of time neurological symptoms are displayed:

- Transitory ischemic attack (TIA), termed a "ministroke." According to the traditional WHO definition cited above, this is actually *not* a stroke. The division of stroke and TIA into different clinical entities is considered impractical and is of little clinical importance. Strokes and TIAs are caused by the same pathological processes, according to the definition introduced above; patients who have already suffered a stroke or TIA are at increased risk of suffering another stroke.
- Reversible ischemic neurological deficit (RIND): symptoms disappear completely within 24 hours.
- Partial reversible ischemic neurological deficit (PRIND), with a favorable prognosis in terms of reversal of symptoms.
- Definitive stroke: Reversal of symptoms does not take place within the first 24 hours.

Improved imaging techniques detect a definitive stroke even in cases of TIA, RIND, and PRIND, so these clinical syndromes cannot always be distinguished from a definitive stroke.

The clinically most significant physiological parameters in the early or acute phase following stroke are:

- **Blood pressure.** Following a stroke, the cerebral autoregulation of blood pressure is impaired. Higher blood pressure improves perfusion; lower values reduce perfusion. Thus, a higher than normal blood pressure value is actually desirable in the acute phase (e.g., with the help of medication). Spontaneous values of up to 220 mmHg (systolic) can be tolerated.
- **Glucose.** Patients who have suffered stroke should have normal blood glucose levels. A high blood glucose level must always be treated to prevent secondary damage caused by this condition (anaerobic glycolysis and accumulation of lactate, with ensuing tissue acidosis).
- **Oxygen.** It is assumed that hypoxia and an excessively high concentration of CO_2 cause further damage to the tissues which have already been damaged by ischemia. Stroke patients are therefore generally given oxygen immediately or are intubated as soon as possible and put on a respirator.
- **Temperature.** Body temperature influences the extent and course of cerebral infarction. Low body temperatures (hypothermia) are desirable in this case; an increase in body temperature (fever), on the other hand, yields unfavorable results. Therefore, an increase in body temperature should always be avoided; instead, the aim should be to *reduce* body temperature.

■ Incidence and Distribution

Incidence of Stroke

Stroke is one of the most common illnesses today worldwide. It is a condition that affects the older members of the population. The average age of stroke victims is 75 years for women and 70 years for men, and the lifetime risk of stroke for people over 65 years of age is one in six (Seshadri et al. 2006). More than 50% of all cases of stroke occur in individuals over 75 years of age. Because of their higher life expectancy, more women are affected than men.

In the United States stroke is the leading cause of mortality and the most common cause of neurological disability in older persons. However, a study published by Carandang and coworkers indicates that the number of cases of stroke in the United States has actually been *decreasing* slightly in the last few decades, due to improved diagnostic techniques and acute care, as well as treatment of risk factors (such as high blood pressure), and that this trend may well continue in the future (Carandang et al. 2006).

In the European Union, more than 1 million people suffer stroke every year (Jørgensen et al. 1995). Of all the European countries, the incidence of stroke is lowest in France; nevertheless, the number of new cases registered is still considered to be too high (101 per 100 000 inhabitants). The incidence in the total population of Germany, based on the data index, is 182 per 100 000 inhabitants per year (Kolominsky-Rabas and Heuschmann 2002). According to mathematical scenario calculations by Lierse and coworkers, the incidence is 219 per 100 000 inhabitants per year (Lierse et al. 2005).

Calculations made by the Erlangen Stroke Project support the assumption that in Germany the annual rate of stroke could increase from the current number of 200 000 to up to 290 000 (projected increase of patients over 60 to ca. 38% of the total population) (Kolominsky-Rabas et al. 2006). In comparison to other European countries there is a higher percentage of cases of cerebral hemorrhage causing stroke; this is explained by the higher rate of patients with elevated blood pressure. It is not yet completely foreseeable, however, how demographic developments will influence the number of cases of stroke in Germany. In particular, the phenomenon of compression of morbidity (people are living longer, but they are also staying healthy longer) has not been included in this prognostic equation, due in part to its complexity.

Prevalence of Stroke

International sources list the prevalence of stroke as 500–800 per 100 000 inhabitants (Thom et al. 2006). According to Lloyd-Jones and colleagues, the prevalence in the United States is 2.9% in the total population (Lloyd-Jones et al. 2010).

In 2001, the US Congress entrusted the Centers for Disease Control and Prevention (CDC) with the task of implementing state-based registries to develop and implement systems for collecting data on acute stroke care provided to patients, analyzing the collected data, and using the results of those analyses to guide quality improvement interventions at the hospital level through partnerships with hospital doctors, stroke care teams, and administrators. The Paul Coverdell National Acute Stroke Registry includes, to date, health department programs in six states: Georgia, Massachusetts, Michigan, Minnesota, North Carolina, and Ohio.

Survival

Stroke can often be fatal. Cerebrovascular illnesses are the third most common cause of death in industrialized nations (Truelsen et al. 2003). Mortality due to stroke is strongly dependent upon the age of the patient and the etiology of the stroke.

In the United States, among individuals 45–64 years of age, 8%–12% of ischemic strokes and 37%–38% of hemorrhagic strokes result in death within 30 days, according to the Atherosclerosis Risk in Communities (ARIC) study of the National Heart, Lung, and Blood Institute (Rosamond et al. 1999). In a study of individuals 65 years of age recruited from a random sample of Health Care Financing Administration Medicare Part B eligibility lists in four US communities, the 1-month case fatality rate was 12.6% for all strokes, 8.1% for ischemic strokes, and 44.6% for hemorrhagic strokes (El-Saed et al. 2006).

In the United States, stroke accounted for approximately 1 in every 18 deaths in 2006. Stroke mortality in 2006 was 137 119; any-mention mortality in 2006 was approximately 232 000 (National Center for Health Statistics, Health Data Interactive File, 1981–2006). When considered separately from other cardiovascular disease, stroke ranks third among all causes of death, behind diseases of the heart and cancer (National Center for Health Statistics).

According to a census performed under the auspices of the Erlangen Stroke Project, around 66 000 patients die in Germany every year as a result of stroke complications. This means that more people die of stroke and related complications than of lung cancer. The 10-year death rate is 76% or 87%, depending on whether or not the patients have been treated in stroke units (specialized wards designed to treat patients in the acute phases of stroke) (Stroke Unit Trialists' Collaboration 2007). The significantly reduced life expectancy of stroke patients can thus be realistically compared with that for patients with malignant neoplasias.

A more recent study has demonstrated that death rates following stroke have declined significantly in the last few decades (Carandang et al. 2006). The introduction of stroke units, lysis therapy during the acute phases, and improvements in in-patient and outpatient follow-up care (rehabilitation, nursing care, and physical therapy) may be responsible for this trend. However, it is important to mention that an increase in survival rate (more patients surviving the stroke) does not necessarily lead to an improvement in activities of daily living or quality of life for the affected patients and their families. In the worst case, an improved survival rate can mean an increased prevalence of patients with a large number of restrictions. This not only limits the patients' quality of life, but also has an impact in terms of health science, ethical, and politico-economic aspects.

The estimated direct and indirect cost of stroke in the United States in 2010 is US$73.7 billion. The mean lifetime cost of ischemic stroke in the United States is estimated at US$140 048. This includes in-patient care, rehabilitation, and the follow-up care necessary for lasting deficits (Taylor et al. 1996). Kolominsky-Rabas and colleagues calculated costs of €7.1 billion for Germany in 2004 for all treatment for all patients who have had a first stroke. The cost of stroke treatment in the next 20 years in Germany is expected to total €108.6 billion (Kolominsky-Rabas et al. 2006). It is thus clear that the economic burden worldwide on national health care systems is extremely heavy and on the increase. Spieler and coworkers concluded in this context that every early intervention aiming at reducing motor impairment will drastically reduce the economic burden weighing down the health-care system by affording proper care of stroke patients (Spieler and Amarenco 2004, Spieler et al. 2004).

■ Risks and Causes

A wide range of factors that can cause stroke is now known. These risk factors can be classified into modifiable and nonmodifiable. Avoidance of such risk factors is called prevention, further subdivided into primary, secondary, and tertiary prevention.

Nonmodifiable Risk Factors

The most important *nonmodifiable risk factor* is age; gender and genetics are factors of lesser importance.

Modifiable Risk Factors

The most important *modifiable risk factors* for stroke are high blood pressure, heart arrhythmia (especially atrial fibrillation), smoking, diabetes mellitus, high blood lipids and high cholesterol, alcohol consumption, and physical inactivity.

Primary prevention reduces the risk of stroke for persons who have not suffered stroke. Various risk factors have been identified whose modification results in decreased risk of stroke. These include:

Hypertension (High Blood Pressure)

High blood pressure is the most important, and in most cases modifiable, risk factor responsible for stroke. Two out of three individuals over 65 years of age have high blood pressure. In up to 70% of all strokes, hypertension plays a leading role.

Treating high blood pressure alone (reduction to values below 140/95 mmHg) already reduces the risk of stroke considerably. Optimal blood pressure values lie around 120/80 mmHg, according to guidelines set by WHO. High blood pressure in patients increases their risk of stroke six to eight times, compared to those with normal blood pressure. The higher the (elevated) blood pressure, the higher the risk.

High blood pressure can often be treated effectively by changing dietary and other habits; however, many people require medication in addition to these measures.

Arrhythmia and Atrial Fibrillation

According to reports from the Competence Network Stroke (www.Kompetenznetz-schlaganfall. de), atrial fibrillation in particular increases the risk of stroke drastically (approximately five times higher). Each year, approximately 1 in every 20 patients with atrial fibrillation suffers a stroke. In cases of atrial fibrillation in the context of rheumatic heart damage, the risk of stroke is increased 17-fold.

Diabetes Mellitus

The risk of stroke is two to three times higher in patients with diabetes mellitus. Even when this condition is kept well under control to avoid secondary complications, it appears that it is still a significant factor in patients at increased risk for stroke. Whether or not proper management of the illness serves to prevent stroke is still unclear, however. It is known to be important that a diabetic patient's blood pressure should be kept below 130/85.

Hyperlipidemia

The connection between elevated total cholesterol values and disease has been more thoroughly researched for coronary heart disease than for stroke. A diet low in salt and fat and high in fiber, fruit, vegetables, and whole grain products is recommended by the American Heart Association (Lichtenstein et al. 2006).

Cigarette Smoking

Smoking is a risk factor for both sexes; smokers are up to six times more likely to suffer stroke than nonsmokers. Quitting smoking reduces the individual risk; after 2 years of abstinence, the risk is already reduced by one-half (Pearson et al. 2002).

Alcohol Consumption

The American Heart Association recommends moderate alcohol consumption (e.g., a maximum of one glass of wine per day); excessive alcohol consumption is not advised (Lichtenstein et al. 2006).

Physical Inactivity

Regular physical activity (3×30 minutes per week or more) reduces the risk of stroke, probably as a result of favorable effects on body weight, blood pressure, cholesterol level, and glucose tolerance. There is a linear relationship between the extent of exercise and risk reduction for strokes as well as for heart attacks (Lichtenstein et al. 2006).

Hormone Replacement

Hormone replacement therapy in postmenopausal women increases the risk of stroke (Rossouw et al. 2007).

Examples of individual 10-year risks for stroke based on the results of the Framingham Study

Mr. S. is 65 years old and has an average systolic blood pressure value of 140 mmHg. He is not taking medication for high blood pressure, however, as he considers his blood pressure to be only slightly elevated. His heart is in good condition; so far his GP has found no signs of heart muscle hypertrophy, heart arrhythmias, or even atrial fibrillation. He smokes, in spite of the ever-increasing price of tobacco, and does not plan to give up this, his only vice. During a recent routine checkup, signs of arterial occlusive disease and type 2 diabetes were detected.

D'Agostino Score: necessary for the study are age, systolic blood pressure, antihypertensive medication, atrial fibrillation, left ventricular hypertrophy and presence of cardiovascular disease.

Mr. S.'s risk of suffering from stroke within the next 10 years is 22% (his risk is 1 in 5). It is, incidentally, just as likely that he would suffer from dementia later in life. The probability of his *not* having a stroke is 78%.

Mr. S.'s 65-year-old wife, Mrs. M., has always had elevated systolic blood pressure values of around 160 mmHg and for this reason has been taking blood pressure medication for some time, as prescribed by her physician. Mrs. M. also has heart muscle hypertrophy and cardiac arrhythmia, diagnosed several years ago. As a result of these findings, she not only reduced her (already minimal) cigarette smoking, but actually gave it up altogether. Fortunately, as she herself reports, no type 2 diabetes was diagnosed at her latest routine checkup. Mrs. M.'s risk of stroke in the next 10 years is 62% (her risk is 2 in 3). The likelihood of her *not* having a stroke is 1 in 3.

■ Disorders and Their Consequences

Important disorders caused by strokes are paralysis of one or more limbs, usually on one side of the body, but sometimes on both sides. Because of the anatomic crossing of major descending nerve pathways, the side of the body generally affected is contralateral to the location of the brain lesion. Often, language comprehension and speech disorders, impairment of the visual field, sensory impairment and difficulty swallowing, dizziness, cog-

nitive impairment, incontinence, and other deficits occur (Mumenthaler 2002). The type and extent of the symptoms depend on the type of stroke and the area damaged.

Lesion in the Left Cerebral Hemisphere

This may result in the following symptoms:
* Muscle weakness (hemiparesis) or complete muscle paralysis (hemiplegia) or lightheadedness, as well as impairment of the sense of touch (sensory or vibratory)
* Aphasia, speech impairment, especially comprehension and speech production or motor coordination
* Apraxia (often with left-sided brain damage), impairment of the completion of more complex movements such as combing hair or opening a letter; the individual movements or the motor skills themselves, on the other hand, often remain intact.

Lesion in the Right Cerebral Hemisphere

In cases of damage to the right side of the cerebrum (**Fig. 1.3**) or the cerebral cortex, the following symptoms often appear:
* Damage to visual field
* Memory impairment
* Neglect of one side of the body

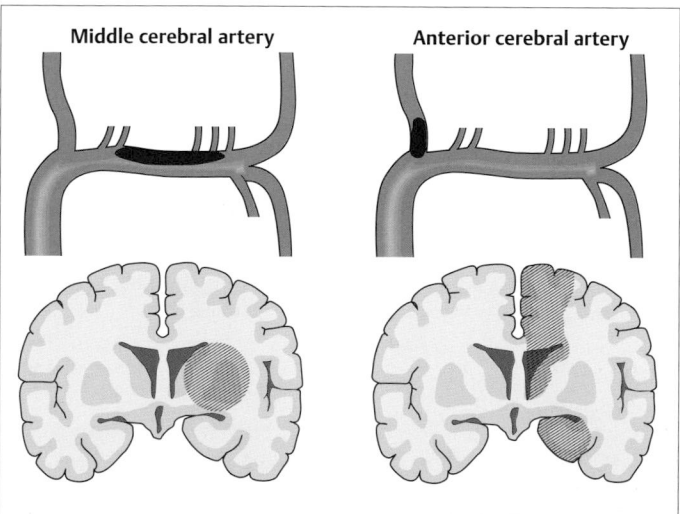

Middle cerebral artery   Anterior cerebral artery

Fig. 1.3 Infarctions in the areas supplied by the middle and anterior cerebral arteries.

Cerebellar Lesions

Strokes in the posterior cranial fossa affect the ipsilateral side of the body when a one-sided lesion is present, and the whole body when the lesion is on both sides. In this case, central damage to the cerebellum tends more often to give rise to disturbances in trunk coordination, whereas damage to the cerebellar hemispheres causes coordination disturbances in the ipsilateral extremities. Typical symptoms of cerebellar strokes include:
- Difficulty walking (due to ataxia)
- Decreased movement coordination (ataxia)
- Dizziness and problems maintaining balance

Brainstem Lesions

A stroke which affects the brainstem can cause functional disorders involving the cranial nerves (I–XII), for example:
- Altered sense of taste
- Hearing or visual impairment (partial or total)
- Drooping eyelids (ptosis) and paralysis of the ocular muscles
- Attenuation of defense reflexes (gagging and swallowing reflexes, pupil reflexes in response to light)
- Numbness in the face and weakening of the facial muscles (one side of the mouth droops)
- Difficulty maintaining balance
- Nystagmus
- Altered breathing and heart frequency
- Paralysis of the sternocleidomastoid muscle, which affects the proper turning of the head, and of the tongue muscles

■ Motor Convalescence and Rehabilitation Following Stroke

Motor deficits are among the most common symptoms found in stroke patients. The treatment of such impairments is among the special areas of expertise practiced by physical therapists.

Motor deficits such as paralysis (paresis) can affect patients' activities of daily living so drastically that they can no longer properly maintain their social roles. Only one-fourth of stroke survivors are able to attain the level of participation in nor-

mal daily life they had before the stroke. The most critical and essential improvements made in stroke patients are to be expected within the first 3 months after the stroke (Jørgensen et al. 1995, Kwakkel et al. 2004). However, around 35% of all survivors no longer have the skills necessary for functioning in normal everyday life, and a further 20%–25% are no longer able to walk (Kwakkel et al. 2002). Stroke is thus one of the most common causes of physical handicap; it generates considerable cost burdens for the health care and social care systems (Lierse et al. 2005).

Acute therapy should be performed as quickly, effectively, and efficiently as possible, but that is only the beginning: treatment must not then be considered complete. All standard modern forms of therapy used in the acute treatment of stroke aim, on the one hand, to reduce damage to the affected area of the brain, where the blood circulation has been dramatically reduced during the stroke; and on the other hand, to prevent the repeated occurrence of stroke. However, *no* form of medical treatment has any impact on symptoms (e.g., hemiparesis) that have been present in a stroke patient for more than 24 hours.

In specialized rehabilitation centers, stroke patients, after undergoing acute therapy, receive subsequent treatment from multidisciplinary teams. The ultimate aims of rehabilitation following stroke include maximum independence for the patients; recovery of walking skills is also included in this category. In specialized treatment centers, a multidisciplinary team is available to stroke patients, with services consisting of physician and nursing care, physical therapy, occupational therapy, sports, speech therapy, neuropsychology, social services, and other occupational groups. The organized care of patients in multidisciplinary stroke units can offset the negative effects of the stroke on their state of health, compared with less organized care (Duncan et al. 2002).

Early supported discharge (ESD), a system which enables a transfer of care from hospital to the home environment and allows for the continuation of rehabilitation and support with input from a specialist stroke team, is practiced mainly in the Scandinavian countries (Indredavik et al. 2008). Many studies are currently being conducted in the United States, the United Kingdom, and other major industrialized countries to measure the effectiveness of ESD in individual medical centers and to evaluate the possibility of integrating

ESD as a standard feature of national stroke care systems (Langhorne et al. 2005, Larsen et al. 2006, Norrving and Adams 2006).

More than 20% of patients are still wheelchair-bound 3 months after their stroke, 70% are still so walking-impaired that they cannot safely cross streets at traffic lights, and more than half of all patients remain impaired in their ability to perform normal daily activities. It is thus apparent that further developments are necessary in the area of rehabilitation following stroke (Bonita et al. 1997, Jørgensen et al. 1995, O'Mahony et al. 1999). For patients, the restoration and improvement of walking skills is a top priority (Bohannon 1988).

Walking rehabilitation has been the physical therapists' domain for many years. No other occupational group specializes in this particular area to the extent that physical therapists do (Barbeau and Fung 2001, Mehrholz and Pohl 2005, Wade 1993). In recent times, scientific substantiation of physical therapy in stroke patients has become increasingly important (Kwakkel et al. 1999). Studies demonstrate that the therapeutic objectives as well as the physical therapeutic methods employed are crucial for the optimal recovery of these patients, whose condition often becomes chronic (Ada et al. 1998, Carr and Shepherd 2003, Hendricks et al. 2002, Van Peppen et al. 2004).

Until the beginning of the 1990s, traditional but outdated therapeutic methods for improving patients' ability to walk following stroke were based on contradictory concepts: the inhibition of reflexes, "paving the way for normal movement" (Bobath 1977) on the one hand, and the activation of reflexes to promote recuperation following stroke on the other (Brunnstrom 1965). The field of physical therapy has veered away from such ideas, which were highly impracticable from a pathophysiological point of view. Practicing impaired everyday functions in patients who have suffered stroke has now moved into the foreground (Mehrholz and Pohl 2005, Mehrholz 2007, van Vliet et al. 2001).

Ultimately, there is an urgent need for pragmatic, scientific, and efficient physical therapy which is aimed at the individual goals of patients and their families. In 1999, Kwakkel and coworkers proved the effectiveness of physical therapy in stroke patients for the first time (Kwakkel et al. 1999). In addition, Carr and Shepherd (1998,

2003) are also considered to be pioneers in modern physical therapy for walking rehabilitation.

A summary of the basic assumptions making up the framework of modern walking rehabilitation is as follows:

1. Our knowledge of the acquisition and learning of motor skills is also applicable to stroke patients.
2. Focused training based on biomechanical knowledge improves the patients' ability to move, measured, among other ways, in terms of joint movements, movement speed, and strength. Improvements are attained through specific tasks.
3. The musculoskeletal system is also of critical importance for optimal recovery of stroke patients and thus for therapeutic success (Carr and Shepherd 2003).

The principles of task specificity ("one learns only what one practices") and repetition (frequent repetition of tasks in succession), as well as sports and physical therapy, as presented by Zander and Foerster, were formulated in the early 20th century (Foerster 1916). These ideas now form the basis of various modern developments in neurological rehabilitation (Hesse et al. 2003).

■ Course of Illness Following Stroke

Prognosis

Patients and their families often express the wish for the affected individuals to be restored as quickly as possible to a level of functioning that enables them to care for themselves at home. But what is the realistic prognosis for stroke patients, and what is the actual course of the illness?

Based on experience and studies, it is well known that, in the long term, a great many limitations in independence can be expected (Patel et al. 2006). Ungern-Sternberg and coworkers discovered different patterns in patients' courses of rehabilitation following stroke (Ungern-Sternberg et al. 1991):

- Pattern 1 (ca. 30% of the patients examined): continual improvement of everyday competence in the first 12 months after the event.
- Pattern 2 (ca. 20%): after initial acquisition of everyday competence, the patients' condition deteriorates to the condition found shortly after the stroke occurred.
- Pattern 3 (ca. 50%): patients are quite, or nearly completely, independent even at the beginning of rehabilitation; in the long term there is almost no deterioration in their state of health.

In a retrospective study, Davidoff and colleagues showed that rehabilitation proved to be effective for a specific type of patient group following stroke in terms of functional recovery, and that these improvements remained, for most patients, for over a year (Davidoff et al. 1991).

One common problem in stroke patients is pain (e.g., shoulder pain), which complicates rehabilitation (Jönsson et al. 2006). However, this study shows that patients' pain issues decrease with time (Jönsson et al. 2006). Risk factors for pain symptoms which persist for longer periods of time are, according to Jönsson et al., younger age, female gender, and high rating on the National Institutes of Health Stroke Scale (NIHSS) (i.e., severe motor impairment) (Goldstein et al. 1989, Jönsson et al. 2006).

Counsell and coworkers calculated a clinical prediction model using six variables present immediately following acute stroke; this model is used to help predict survival as well as the extent of everyday competence of acute stroke patients (Counsell et al. 2004). The six variables are:

- Age (the higher the age, the greater the risk)
- Status: living alone (risk)
- Status: independent before the event (chance)
- Status: normal orientation (maximum score on the Glasgow Coma Scale, chance)
- Ability to lift both arms from the horizontal position
- Ability to walk alone following stroke (chance) (Counsell et al. 2004)

Smith and colleagues evaluated the database of one sponsoring company and found that the main factors influencing patients' discharge status (to a nursing home, or back home) were competence in everyday activities at the beginning of rehabilitation and the age of the patient (Smith et al. 2002).

The NEMESIS Project (North East MElbourne Stroke Incidence Study) examined 264 patients in a study which included all cases of stroke in the northeastern part of Melbourne, 3 and 12 months after the event (Sturm et al. 2002). A lack of independence and unsuccessful occupational assimilation were the main limitations in terms of participation in "public" life. The most important determinants for these limitations were age, functional deficits, and motor impairment; on the other hand, severity of the illness at the time of admission to hospital was found not to be of such significance in this context (Sturm et al. 2004b).

In 2003 Appelros and coworkers explored the following independent variables (age, sex, cohabitation status, cigarette smoking, dementia, hypertension, ischemic heart disease, heart failure, atrial fibrillation, diabetes mellitus, transitory ischemic attack, peripheral atherosclerosis, and stroke severity) for risk factors predicting death within the first year following stroke: age, dementia, severity of infarction, and atrial fibrillation. The risk for recurrence of infarction was increased by the factors of age and dementia (Appelros et al. 2003).

In the Perth Community Study, an evaluation of the city's total population in 1989–1990, 370 stroke patients were examined (Hankey et al. 2002). Of the patients who survived the first 30 days following the event, over half were still alive 5 years later, one-third were severely handicapped, and 14% were living in a nursing home (Hankey et al. 2002). Risk factors for unfavorable long-term results were low level of everyday activities even before the stroke, and later stroke recurrence (Hankey et al. 2002).

One German study demonstrated that, 5 years after stroke, 40% of 289 patients over 65 years of age had survived and that the score on the Barthel Index (BI; the possible score range is 0–100) had been reduced by an average of 5 (Vogel 1994). The general condition in men deteriorated more rapidly than average, when compared to that of women. Vogel described the risk factors determining survival as a BI score of less than 60, a nursing home as the place of discharge, presence of diabetes mellitus, depression, cardiac illnesses, and psycho-organic syndromes at the time of the patients' discharge from stationary rehabilitation (Vogel 1994). Five years after their discharge, 65% of the patients were living at home and 33% were in nursing care or nursing homes; the rest were living with relatives (Vogel 1994).

A study performed in southwest London showed that, in a 5-year period, one-third of survivors were moderately to severely limited in their everyday activities and one-third were mildly limited. In addition, one-third of patients displayed signs of depression (Wilkinson et al. 1997).

In one cohort study from Moscow, consisting of 1538 stroke patients evaluated between 1972 and 1974, the analysis was repeated 7 years later. The results indicated that nearly 50% of all patients with TIA and 16% with heart attacks were affected, but 81% of the survivors were completely independent 7 years later (Scmidt et al. 1988). Factors contributing to a favorable long-term prognosis were young age, good motor skills, and absence of concomitant illnesses (Scmidt et al. 1988).

A study based upon the evaluation of the Erlangen Stroke Registry demonstrated that 24% of patients suffer a second stroke within 5 years after the first event (Kolominsky-Rabas et al. 2006). A mean residual life expectancy figure following the first stroke was calculated to be 8.6 years for men and 6.3 years for women (7.3 for both together) (Kolominsky-Rabas et al. 2006).

In a follow-up examination taking place 10 years after the event of stroke, Indredavik et al. reported survival rates of 13%–25%. Five percent of patients were living in a nursing home, 14% had a moderate to high BI score (>60, implying partial independence in everyday life), and 9% had a score above 95 (independence in everyday life) (Stroke Unit Trialists' Collaboration 2007).

In instances of ischemic infarction in which permanent damage is only mild (score <3 on the Rankin scale, which has six grades, 0–5; van Swieten et al. 1988), the 10-year survival rate, according to the results presented by Prencipe and coworkers, was determined to be 68% and the recurrence rate only 14% (Prencipe et al. 1998).

Within the context of the Perth Community Stroke Study, Hardie and colleagues reported 10-year survival rates of 21% and a recurrence rate of 25% (Hardie et al. 2004). Of the surviving patients, nearly half (47%) displayed severe impairment in performing everyday functions (Hardie et al. 2004).

In the Dutch TIA Trial, including patients with TIAs and minor infarctions and with only mild impairment (score <3 on the Rankin scale; van Swieten et al. 1988), van Wijk and coworkers found a 10-year survival rate of 40% and a recurrence rate of 44% (van Wijk et al. 2005).

Tuomilehto and coworkers described the results of a Finnish partial evaluation of the WHO Stroke Study (Tuomilehto et al. 1995), a survey conducted by telephone and letter. Out of an initial group of 1241 recruited patients, 19% were still alive 14 years after the stroke. More than 80% of patients who participated in the follow-up examination were living with a partner or in their own homes. Between 10% and 15% of the participants complained of depression. Half of the younger patients (<65 years) considered their state of health to be "good," compared to only one-fourth of patients over 65 years of age (Tuomilehto et al. 1995). Thirty-two percent of all patients interviewed reported having suffered either a heart attack or a stroke in the 14 years following their original stroke. One-third of the participants complained of speech difficulties, 31% reported bladder problems, 14% depression, 47% hemiparesis, and 16% hemiplegia (Tuomilehto et al. 1995).

Possibly one of the best-known cohort studies, the Framingham Study (Gresham et al. 1975, 1998), demonstrated that patients who had survived stroke for more than 20 years had higher mortality rates than an age- and gender-adjusted control group (Gresham et al. 1975, 1998). Long-term survivors, 20 years after the event, were more likely to be female, were more often comorbid, took more medication, drank less alcohol, and were less depressed than the control group (Gresham et al. 1998). It should however also be mentioned here that the results are based on only 10 individuals out of an initial group of 147 evaluated patients (20-year survival rate: 7%).

In summary, it can be said that prognosis and long-term course of illness following stroke are unfavorable. However, data pertaining to the evaluation of the stroke population deal with older patients. The advanced age of stroke patients puts the seemingly unfavorable prognosis into perspective. But regardless of this fact, the event of stroke will *always*, statistically speaking, reduce the patients' life expectancy.

Everyday Competence and Ability to Walk Following Stroke

Up to now there have been very few long-term follow-up studies conducted in connection with randomized controlled trials (RCTs) of therapy from the rehabilitation phase.

Langhammer described the 4-year follow-up of an RCT (Langhammer and Stanghelle 2000, 2003). Although it was shown that patients who had suffered stroke profited from the early employment of modern therapeutic techniques (shorter hospital stays due to faster recovery) (Langhammer and Stanghelle 2000), no differences whatsoever between the groups studied could be found 4 years after the event (Langhammer and Stanghelle 2003).

Three studies dealing with modern therapeutic applications designed to improve walking skills following stroke demonstrated a minimal, but nevertheless constant, effect lasting over 4–6 weeks:

1. Eich and coworkers described longer walking distances and higher walking speeds in patients who are initially able to walk, through sports-oriented treadmill training; the effects of this training lasted up to 18 weeks after the training period had ended (Eich et al. 2004).
2. Visintin and colleagues reported longer walking distances for stroke-impaired patients not initially able to walk, with effects of the training lasting up to 3 months after ending the training period, the type of training being treadmill exercise which eased the strain of the patients' body weight (Visintin et al. 1998).
3. Pohl and coworkers, in the context of the multicenter German Walking Trainer Study (DEutsche GAngtrainer Studie, DEGAS) included 155 acute stroke patients from 4 different clinics who were unable to walk. These patients whose cardiocirculatory status was determined to be stable, and who were at least able to remain in a sitting position at the edge of the bed while holding on, received either 20 minutes (net) of locomotion training on the walking trainer plus 25 minutes of physical therapy (Group A) or 45 minutes (net) of physical therapy (Group B) every weekday for 4 weeks. After the therapy had ended, significantly more patients in Group A had become

able to walk alone: 41 out of 77 (53%) in Group A as compared with 17 out of 78 (22%) in Group B. Changes in walking speed in the interval from the end of the study until the follow-up, on the other hand, were not found to be different when comparing the two groups. The DEGAS project also explored the area of competence in such daily activities as washing, using the toilet, eating, getting dressed, general mobility, and continence. The BI (0–100) was used as a measure for these everyday skills. The target criterion, together with a backup guideline provided by the German Federal Occupational Society of Rehabilitation (Bundesarbeitsgemeinschaft für Rehabilitation, BAR) was a BI of at least 75, which serves as a determining factor for ensuring a safe return to the home environment. This level was attained by 44 patients (57%) in Group A and only 21 (27%) in Group B at the end of the intervention (Pohl et al. 2007).

Thus far, RCTs on repetitive locomotion training (performed on a treadmill) have showed no superiority in terms of walking functions in stroke patients initially unable to walk (Kosak and Reding 2000, Moseley et al. 2005, Nilsson et al. 2001). Because these therapeutic efforts proved to be too arduous for physical therapists (repeatedly having to place the stroke patient's paralyzed foot in an ergonomically unfavorable position on the treadmill), there is some critical discussion to the effect that, in terms of the previous studies performed, too few measures have been taken to demonstrate the superiority of treadmill training in severely affected stroke patients (Hesse et al. 2003). With training using a special walking trainer, on the other hand, more steps are possible in any therapeutic context, as the therapists' additional burden of moving the patients' paralyzed feet is rendered unnecessary (Werner et al. 2002).

Seen from a neurophysiological point of view, early repetitive walking training aims at the activation of spinal and supraspinal locomotion centers (locomotor pattern generators), as discussed in connection with paraplegic patients, on the basis of animal experiments and clinical trials (MacKay-Lyons 2002). Imaging techniques employed in stroke patients revealed displacement of a bilateral cortical activation pattern to a unilateral pattern in the undamaged cerebral hemisphere (Dobkin et al. 2004, Luft et al. 2004, 2005).

A further hypothesis concerning the effects of repetitive walking training deals with the increased demands of repetitions, which could result in improvements in the level of cardiovascular fitness in otherwise immobile patients (Macko et al. 2005a, 2005b, Meek et al. 2003, Mehrholz and Pohl 2005). In the end, the integration of the partially automatized walking training during early rehabilitation is an adequate stimulus in terms of training for the cardiorespiratory system without overexerting stroke patients, who are often multimorbid (Pohl et al. 2003, 2004).

In the past 30 years, more than 300 RCTs have been published on stroke rehabilitation (Foley et al. 2003). These studies show two key elements of neurological rehabilitation in particular:

1. More therapy results in more effective recovery for the patient (principle of intensity of treatment: "more is better").
2. Therapeutic effects are task-specific (following the principle of task specificity: "one learns only what one practices").

Following a stroke, some patients demonstrate spontaneous recovery over time (Kwakkel et al. 2004, Twitchell 1951). In this context, Kollen and coworkers reported that 62% of the patients who initially could not walk were able to walk 6 months after the stroke (Kollen et al. 2006).

It is true that the extent of recovery can be predicted on the basis of the size of the damaged brain area and certain comorbidity factors; however, further variables also influence the course of convalescence following stroke. After consulting two systematic reviews, Meijer and colleagues found insufficient scientific evidence for prognostic factors in the subacute phase following stroke and called for increased research to be done on this topic, in particular on prognostic factors (Meijer et al. 2003a, 2003b). Prognostic factors which Meijer and colleagues suggested as variables, according to the current evidence, were age, side of lesion, motor function, and Barthel Index (6 months after illness) (Meijer et al. 2003a, 2003b).

One long-term observation and its corresponding evaluation revealed that the social factor of whether or not the patient had a partner was decisive in determining their ability to walk 3 years after the study was concluded (Mehrholz 2007). So far, these results are not comparable to any other study focusing on walking ability following stroke.

Singh and coworkers examined 255 patients in a retrospective cohort study and came to the conclusion that it was primarily patients who wheeled themselves from place to place in their wheelchairs who also, 3 years later, were able to walk alone. Continence following stroke was likewise an important predictor of independent walking (Singh et al. 2006). Mobility by means of a wheelchair, together with the factor of continence, make up nearly one-third of the possible score attainable on the BI.

According to calculations by Kollen and coworkers, the age of the patient and the BI score (during the first 10 weeks following infarction) are the two "sturdiest" independent predictors of independent walking 6 months after stroke (Kollen et al. 2006).

One study has drawn attention to the connection between ability to walk, measured by means of the 6-minute walking test, and handicaps in a large population of older people (Newman et al. 2006).

Two studies indicate the importance of walking speed. Goldie et al. demonstrated that for stroke-afflicted patients with a walking speed of less than 0.5 km/h (attained after 8 weeks of rehabilitation), long-term care is probably required (Goldie et al. 1996). A walking speed of over 1.5 km/h (toward the end of rehabilitation) could, on the other hand, serve as a predictor for independent walking in the home environment 3 months after concluding of rehabilitation, according to Perry (Perry et al. 1995).

The ultimate goal for many stroke patients is to attain a certain degree of independence which allows them to return to their familiar home, relationships, and roles. In spite of intensive efforts in acute medicine, a large number of patients are left with extensive damage due to the stroke. Thus, modern approaches to rehabilitation following stroke, which incorporate scientifically well-founded physical therapeutic methods, are especially in demand and in need of further development. Essential for modern rehabilitation is the work of Kwakkel et al. (e.g., Kwakkel et al. 2004), which elucidates the following:

- There is a so-called nonlinear pattern of recovery (optimal time frame of rehabilitation). This means that effects of stroke rehabilitation are most pronounced during the first 6 months after the event.

- Compared with improvements over time, the specific effects of therapy are minimal (ca. 10% of recovery variance). Certain forms of therapy (e.g., physical therapy) can accelerate recovery of functions, at least in the short term.
- Improvements in everyday activities can be explained in large part by adaptation strategies and compensation. Other hypotheses pertaining to the recovery of functions are neuronal plasticity, restitution of noninfarcted penumbral areas, regression of the diaschisis ("loss" of neighboring, functionally connected brain regions), and regeneration of brain tissue (Kollen et al. 2005, Kwakkel et al. 2004).

Pettersen and coworkers examined the functional results of 142 patients who had suffered stroke, of whom 83% still lived at home 3 years later (Pettersen et al. 2002). The condition of one-fifth of patients had worsened after 3 years, due to further strokes and comorbidity. Comorbidity (defined as "handicapping accompanying illness") was one of the most significant risk factors for dependence on a day-to-day basis, as judged using the BI (Pettersen et al. 2002). According to Pettersen et al., the BI score, measured during the early phase following stroke (before and after rehabilitation), was the most important predicting factor for favorable functional results 3 years after the event (Pettersen et al. 2002).

Kuo and colleagues pointed to a connection between walking speed and leg strength as well as limitations in everyday activities (Kuo et al. 2006). As the walking speed and the strength of the hemiparetic leg increased, it was found that stroke-affected patients had fewer limitations in their everyday activities.

Schiemanck and colleagues discovered, by calculating logistic regression models, that clinical variables such as severity of stroke (NIHSS), disturbances in the patients' state of consciousness (Glasgow Coma Scale), incontinence, age, gender, level of education, the hospital responsible for patient admission, sitting balance (trunk control test), level of strength (motricity index), and BI during the second week following stroke, were good predictors of independence for the long-term course of the illness (Schiemanck et al. 2006). Imaging techniques, such as the time of MRI, lesion volume and location (cortical, subcortical), and side of lesion, did not provide any additional predictive information with respect to the statistical model (Schiemanck et al. 2006).

In the past few years, a certain paradigm shift has been taking place in the field of rehabilitation research. Instead of evaluating individual clinical variables, it has now become increasingly common to extend the focus of the research to include the level of participation in everyday life, according to the ICF classification (Desrosiers et al. 2005a).

Initial studies pertaining to the prediction of long-term participation following stroke have already led to a whole array of new discoveries (Desrosiers et al. 2005a, 2006). Thus, it was determined in a comparative study that a considerable degree of limitation in participation is due not solely to the "condition" of stroke itself, but also to normal aging processes (Desrosiers et al. 2005a). Stroke is an illness affecting the older population, which means that more and more limitations in daily life become apparent with increasing age. The links between stroke, aging, and participation are the focus of further research. Desrosiers and coworkers have thus expressed the need for future interventions with the purpose of increasing participation in daily activities in stroke patients to aim at illness-specific limitations (Desrosiers et al. 2005a). This in turn means that improving stroke-induced handicaps should represent the main goal of rehabilitation efforts.

Another study published by Desrosiers demonstrated that the best prediction for long-term participation 2–4 years after stroke is made possible mainly through observation of four variables: age, comorbidity (comorbidity index, Charlson et al. 1987), depression (Beck Depression Index, Beck et al. 1961), and motor coordination of the lower extremities (Desrosiers et al. 2005b, 2006). The patients' own perceptions of such limitations are, however, not realistic (Patel et al. 2006). Hochstenbach and coworkers interviewed 172 patients and their families 9 months after a stroke and found a low concurrence between patients and their families in their perceptions of everyday and functional problems and issues (Hochstenbach et al. 2005). As potential causes, cognitive limitations (among others, anosognosia, the pathological failure to acknowledge an obvious handicap) have been discussed (Hochstenbach et al. 2005). The highest level of agreement between the partners in the perception of everyday problems was for speech, comprehension and writing difficulties, strength deficits, and seizures (Hochstenbach et al. 2005).

Although many patients experience improvements in motor skills, even years after the event, 40% of all patients follow a declining course of illness due rather to advancing age and comorbidity than to the repeated onset of stroke (Lindmark and Hamrin 1995, Viitanen et al. 1988, Wilkinson et al. 1997).

One year after the stroke, half of all patients require assistance with everyday activities, and a corresponding number of patients are unable to complete tasks which they feel to be social, creative, or in any way a meaningful occupation (Thorngren et al. 1990). It is precisely *here* that future measures which go above and beyond stationary rehabilitation should be taken. Such measures should be designed to include social welfare and should be oriented to occupation and activities, at the same time activating motor skills and coordination. This is a role that could be performed by physical therapists. A survey conducted in the Berlin area revealed that physical therapists represent the most important nonfamilial psychosocial contact partners for chronically ill patients following stroke (Hesse et al. 2001).

Quality of Life Following Stroke

Although the need for an evaluation aimed at determining the health-related quality of life in follow-up examinations for stroke patients is certainly recognized (Patel et al. 2006), so far there have been very few studies of this particular topic.

Teasdale and Engberg made use of a Danish hospital register to determine the health-related quality of life of stroke patients after 5, 10, and 15 years (Teasdale and Engberg 2005). In addition to a markedly reduced point score in the Nottingham Health Profile (NHP), they found limitations in particular for two of the six dimensions of the NHP (physical mobility and emotional control/reactions). This is not surprising: a large number of points in the NHP represent mobility problems in everyday life, and in addition, the variables of health-related quality of life correlate highly with daily living skills and participation in "public" life (Patel et al. 2006). Impairment in everyday activities is in turn a typical consequence of stroke.

According to Sturm and colleagues, the most important risk factors for everyday limitations following stroke are age, physical handicap, depression, and anxiety disorders (Sturm et al. 2004a, 2004b). Risk factors for poor quality of life for stroke-affected patients, as presented by Paul and coworkers, are age, hemiparesis, physical impairment, and socioeconomic status (Paul et al. 2005). Thus, the most significant predictive factors for everyday limitations and quality of life following stroke (with the exception of socioeconomic status, depression, and anxiety disorders) appear to be basically the same for limitation in everyday activities and quality of life following stroke.

In the NEMESIS Project, the health-related quality of life of patients was considerably reduced 2 years after the event and correlated very highly with everyday competence (Sturm et al. 2004a). Independent risk factors of health-related quality of life were reduced participation, physical handicap, anxiety, depression, place of residence (nursing home, own home), dementia, and age (Sturm et al. 2004a). Demographic variables such as age and place of residence were, on the other hand, not viewed as risk factors in this study.

Other authors have, however, come to different conclusions within the context and scope of various other projects. One example is the studies conducted by Hackett and Anderson. Hackett and coworkers used the SF-36 to evaluate health-related quality of life in patients 6 years after the event. In spite of moderate limitation of everyday activities (61% of all patients examined), they reported only minimal reduction of quality of life (Hackett et al. 2000). The authors concluded that patients in the long-term course of illness following stroke had access to adequate adaptation strategies (Hackett et al. 2000).

In a population-based study in Auckland, New Zealand, the health-related quality of life of patients was assessed 21 years after they had suffered a stroke (Anderson et al. 2004). With the exception of the subcategory of SF-36 vitality (VT), the patients' quality of life of was comparable to that of the standardized population of New Zealand (Anderson et al. 2004).

According to Naess and colleagues, only the symptoms of depression and fatigue appear to be considered as risk factors for a low health-oriented quality of life (Naess et al. 2006). Some 30%–40% of all stroke patients suffer from depressive disorders and 10%–15% have severe depression (Kauhanen

et al. 1999). The assessment and early consideration of depression thus appear to represent an important and useful approach. A poor quality of life
is, moreover, very highly dependent on the extent
of physical handicap (Naess et al. 2006). Therefore,
Naess and colleagues require as early an evaluation as possible of at-risk patients, along with the
effective treatment of depression, fatigue, and physical handicap (Naess et al. 2006).

■ Summary

Stroke presents a major global health challenge
and is one of the main causes of long-term disability in the major industrialized nations.

In the past, various forms of medical intervention have resulted in an improved survival rate
after stroke. This, as well as the ever-changing demographic developments, is the reason that more
and more people have to live with problems and
complications typically associated with stroke.

Besides the burden placed on stroke patients
and their families due to limitations in their daily
lives, questions of associated costs will become the
focus of further attention in the near future.

In addition to the effective acute medical care
provided for stroke patients, physical therapy oc-
cupies an essential, powerful, and significant role.
Physical therapeutic measures taken as soon as
possible after stroke, and which aim at improving
motor skills and the patient's proficiency in performing everyday activities, are very likely not
only to lessen the burden of the illness itself, but
also to improve everyday competence and quality
of life. They can ultimately reduce the economic
burden in the health care system.

2 Emergency and Acute Preclinical Management of Stroke

Gert Grellmann

It pays to devote one's attention to the smallest detail, for it is possible to interpret everything.
(Hermann Hesse, The Glass Bead Game)

This chapter is dedicated to the preclinical care of the stroke patient and illustrates the link between emergency care and subsequent clinical treatment. As our general awareness of the emergency of stroke and its implications has grown in the past 20 years and we now realize that time plays as critical a role here as in acute myocardial infarction, preclinical intervention has taken on a key position in treatment.

■ Introduction

Acute stroke is defined as a syndrome characterized by a suddenly occurring focal deficit of the central nervous system (CNS). Combinations with acute, nonfocal neurological deficits are possible; for example, reduction or loss of consciousness. A stroke can be brought on by acute cerebral ischemia or acute intracerebral hemorrhage (ICH). Cerebral ischemia is by far the most common cause, representing 85% of all cases of stroke. According to the common classification in emergency medicine, transitory cerebral ischemia (TIA, transient ischemic attack), in which reversal of symptoms takes place within 24 hours, is to be distinguished from a complete stroke. Intracerebral bleeding is responsible for strokes in 15% of cases; 10% are due to ICH and 5% to subarachnoidal hemorrhages (SAHs).

As paramedics cannot distinguish between bleeding and ischemia as causes of stroke, preclinical care does not take this into consideration. The aims of preclinical treatment thus lie primarily in the recognition of emergency symptoms, the securing of vital signs, and the preparation of the patient for transfer to the hospital and adequate in-patient therapy (Koennecke et al. 2005).

Stroke is among the obligatory educational topics for paramedics as well as for emergency room physicians. However, the general population must be made more aware of the urgency of the stroke situation, just as it already has been educated on the subject of acute myocardial infarction. It is only through increased awareness throughout the population groups that more patients can be adequately treated in the early phases of stroke, to minimize or even prevent long-term negative effects. The phrase "time is brain" has become an established term which effectively expresses and emphasizes the time factor.

Case Study 1
9:45 am An ambulance team (consisting of an paramedic and an emergency medical technician [EMT] is notified of an emergency. They find the following information on the pager: "Patient L.M., 68 years old, can no longer speak coherently, reduction in/loss of muscle strength in the arm," followed by the patient's address. Within 1 minute the ambulance team confirms the receipt of this information and sets out for the site of the emergency.

9:50 am The ambulance arrives at the patient's address. The team have with them an emergency case, a three-lead ECG, and a mobile respirator.

9:51 am The ambulance team enter patient L.M.'s house and find a 68-year-old, slightly overweight patient sitting at the breakfast table. The patient's wife reports that, while eating breakfast, her husband was suddenly unable to hold the coffee cup with his right hand and that his coffee began to dribble out of the right side of his mouth. His speech was slurred, but he was fully oriented and responsive. Upon observing these changes in her husband, the wife called their GP, who immediately dialed the emergency number and requested an ambulance.

The paramedic and EMT first help the patient out of the small, somewhat cramped kitchen and lay him down on the sofa so that his upper body is slightly elevated. As they do this, they note that the patient is unable to use his right leg while attempting to walk.

The paramedic measures the patient's blood pressure, sets up a three-lead ECG, and determines oxygen saturation. The patient's blood pressure is found to be 170/100 and oxygen saturation 97%; his heart rate is 90 beats per minute. It is quite clear to the paramedic that this patient has suffered an acute stroke and that this is a pressing emergency.

The paramedic inserts an IV needle into the unaffected arm and takes blood samples for subsequent laboratory tests. After this he attaches a prepared infusion (Ringer solution) to the IV line. The patient's blood glucose is measured and found to be 8.5 mmol/L (153 mg/dL). The ECG printout shows signs of absolute arrhythmia with atrial fibrillation. Meanwhile, the EMT has already informed the emergency headquarters of the situation and requested that preliminary arrangements be made at a district general hospital, roughly 10 minutes away, which has a large neurological department complete with a stroke unit. The EMT has also prepared a stretcher in the ambulance and brought a transfer sheet into the patient's house. After the team have positioned the patient on the transfer sheet, to maneuver him down the very narrow stairway and out to the ambulance, the paramedic again questions the patient's wife and makes a note of the names of the patient's medications as well as his previous illnesses. Apart from diabetes mellitus, kept under control through diet alone, and hypertension, which up to now has been successfully treated by means of medication, there are no special problems. The team make a note of the telephone numbers of the patient's wife and his GP. The paramedic again requests an exact description of the clinical symptoms and can now trace the beginning of the symptoms back to 9:30 am. After the patient's blood pressure is measured for the second time, he is taken out to the ambulance. He is placed onto the stretcher with his upper body elevated 30°; the IV infusion continues to run slowly. At the same time, ECG and oxygen saturation are being continually recorded. As the latter has dropped slightly to 94%, the paramedic administers oxygen to be given to the patient via an oxygen mask, at 2 L/min. The patient's oxygen saturation immediately rises again. Blood pressure and heart rate remain stable at their previous values. Meanwhile, the emergency headquarters has confirmed arrangements at the district hospital by phone.

10:15 am The paramedic contacts the neurology department physicians at the hospital, explains the current situation, and informs them of the patient's expected arrival at the hospital's interdisciplinary emergency department, estimated at 10:20.

10:31 am The ambulance arrives at the hospital, where a team of neurologists awaits the patient. The paramedic hands over the patient to the doctors and informs them of his status, the emergency measures already taken, information about the previous findings, and important telephone numbers. At the same time, the patient is being examined by the team of neurologists and is then taken in for a CT scan.

The initial tentative diagnosis by the paramedic of media infarction in the left hemisphere of the brain has been confirmed.

Because of the optimal time frame in which the stroke was diagnosed, the ensuing therapy—lysis using rt-PA (see Chapter 3) followed by further treatment in the stroke unit—can be considered a success, as the patient had only a minimal focal neurological deficit at the time of his transfer to a nearby rehabilitation clinic.

Case Study 2

At 6:35 am, the emergency headquarters receives a call from a very agitated man who explains that he woke up beside his wife this morning to find her much less responsive than usual. Upon making this discovery, he had attempted to lift her out of bed. During this maneuver he noticed that her speech was slurred and her answers to his questions were "jibberish," as he phrases it. His wife was unable to stay sitting up on the edge of the bed, and repeatedly fell over onto the bed.

Emergency headquarters arranges for an ambulance team, which arrives at the site of the emergency about 10 minutes later. There the paramedics find a 75-year-old obese woman lying in bed.

The patient has lost bladder control and is unable to answer the emergency team's questions adequately. The paramedic makes the diagnosis of aphasia and impaired language comprehension. The patient is only able to utter unvarying repetitive sequences. The paramedic also finds that the patient has paralysis of the entire right side of her body. The patient's husband reports that he and his wife had gone to bed at around 9:30 pm the night before, and that he had slept through the night, until early that morning. The patient's known previous illnesses include insulin-dependent diabetes mellitus which has been difficult to treat, hypertension, disturbances in lipid metabolism, and obesity.

The husband explains that the patient has an aversion to doctors, so she only visited her GP sporadically, did not take her medications for high blood pressure regularly, and only grudgingly took dietary advice. Her husband reports her as saying the "diabetes doctor" had repeatedly warned her about her "long-term sugar levels." This brief interview, combined with the clinical examination of the patient, confirms the paramedic's initial suspicion of acute stroke.

Because both the patient and her husband were asleep from 9:30 pm until 6:30 am, no exact information as to the onset of symptoms can be given and the time frame remains unclear. The patient's vital signs are again monitored. Her blood pressure is found to be 200/100 mmHg, her heart rate is irregular, at 120 per minute, and oxygen saturation is 92%. The patient's blood glucose level, determined from blood drawn from the IV line which has been inserted in the meantime, is 11.5 mmol/L (207 mg/dL). The patient's husband now reports that, starting about 8 weeks ago, his wife had complained of unsteadiness while walking, accompanied by dizziness and a tendency to collapse. Two weeks ago she had had similar symptoms, but this time, in addition to the other symptoms, she "saw double." Her GP, when making a house call, urged her to go to the hospital but she flatly refused to comply.

The team prepare to transfer the patient to the ambulance and at the same time the paramedic prepares to administer oxygen by means of an oxygen mask. After the patient has been taken to the ambulance and the oxygen mask has been applied, her oxygen saturation rises to 97%. The patient's heart rate is still 120 per minute and arrhythmic. The paramedic makes the diagnosis of absolute arrhythmia with atrial fibrillation.

The patient's blood pressure is 250/130 mmHg, so the paramedic decides to administer medication which will safely lower her blood pressure (12.5 urapidil fractionated IV). He terminates the procedure when the blood pressure has dropped to 180/100 mmHg. During the trip to the nearest hospital with a stroke unit, the paramedic phones the team of neurologists at the emergency department and gives them further details concerning the patient's status. On arrival at the emergency room, the paramedic hands over the patient to the on-call neurologist, who has opted for an initial cranial MRI because of the unclear time frame. Images reveal extensive infarction in the area of the brainstem. Subsequent Doppler sonography of the intracranial vessels shows free flow in the basilar artery. Ten days later, the patient is transferred to a suitable rehabilitation facility; at this time she still exhibits an extreme neurological deficit. Lysis therapy was not an option, because the time of occurrence of the stroke was unclear and the area of infarction was already clearly demarcated.

■ Symptoms of Stroke: Differential Diagnostics

The most important task of the paramedic who is called to treat a patient with neurological symptoms—in addition to securing vital functions—is to recognize the symptoms of a possible stroke and to deduce from this the necessary therapeutic actions. For this reason, a basic understanding of neurological symptoms is among the essential tools of every paramedic.

Not every patient presenting with sudden onset of hemiparesis has suffered a stroke! In a clinical situation, cerebral ischemia cannot be distinguished from intracranial hemorrhage. All of the disturbances listed below can occur alone or in combination with others.

Clinical symptoms of cerebral ischemia (**Table 2.1**) can affect different brain structures. If the cerebrum is affected, the emergency team will usually observe the following symptoms:

1. Hemiparesis (often with an emphasis on the brachiofacial region). Here, mild cases of paralysis are not discovered until the arm- or leg-holding test is performed. Loss of general strength does not necessarily occur. Flaccid hemiparesis, on the other hand, is quite easy to diagnose.

Table 2.1 The most important symptoms of acute stroke according to clinical symptoms

Deficit	Symptoms
Motor function	Hemiparesis (e.g., arm, leg, face), often emphasis on brachiofacial region
Sensitivity	Hemihypesthesia (e.g., arm, leg, face)
Coordination	Hemiataxia, ataxia of the extremities, asymmetry
Aphasia (affecting language)	Language comprehension, language production, reproduction of speech
Dysarthria (affecting speech)	Slurred, in some cases also "babbling"
Vision impairment	Amaurosis fugax, hemianopsia

2. Further, higher cortical language functions (aphasia) or speech (dysarthria) may be impaired. In cerebral regions, disturbances in the field of vision (e.g., homonymous hemianopsia) can occur. The absence of the Babinsky sign or weakened muscle reflexes on the affected side are *never* adequate criteria for ruling out acute stroke.

3. More difficult for the paramedic to differentiate are disturbances in the region of the brainstem or the cerebellum. Here, symptoms may occur such as diplopia, rotary vertigo or staggering and dizziness, nausea and vomiting, strongly slurred speech or difficulty swallowing, ataxia, or changes in level of consciousness. The clinical symptoms of occlusion of the posterior vessel region (basilar thrombosis) are particularly critical. As these are often partial obstructions, alterations in the patient's level of consciousness are often observed. If this is found in combination with some of the symptoms described in **Table 2.1**, then it is considered to be a top-priority neurological emergency.

Not every symptom mentioned above is, however, the result of a stroke. The paramedic must therefore consider other conditions, which may also be emergencies in their own right.

Common differential diagnoses of acute stroke

1. Focal neurological deficit following epileptic seizure (Todd paresis).
2. Unmasking of an older, pre-existing neurological deficit, as a result of a febrile infection or state of dehydration, for example. These conditions are very common in older, multimorbid patients in nursing homes. In such instances, the diagnosis is ultimately made much later, in the hospital, after therapy appropriate to the situation has been administered and the clinical symptoms have abated.
3. Hypoglycemia.
4. Vestibular neuropathy.
5. Transient global aphasia.
6. Intracranial tumor.
7. Inflammation in the region of the meninges or the brain (meningitis or encephalitis caused by various pathogens).
8. Cerebral sinus thrombosis.
9. Chronic subdural hematoma.
10. Migraine with or without an aura.

As the paramedic is only able to describe the symptoms, it is difficult to make an exact diagnosis. Nevertheless, differential therapeutic consequences do not arise in these circumstances. It is the paramedic's task to recognize the neurological emergency, to secure the patient's vital functions, and to guarantee transfer to a suitable hospital. It is thus crucial for the emergency team to be very familiar with the care facilities available within its assigned region.

Important questions when considering a target hospital:
- Is there a stroke unit?
- Is there round-the-clock neurological monitoring?
- Does the hospital have access to telemedicine?

Especially in the case of suspected basilar thrombosis, the paramedic must decide if the patient is to be taken to a district hospital which has a large neurological department complete with a stroke unit and a 24-hour angiography service. Thus, the emergency team has a crucial role to play in making an initial diagnosis in order to decide where the patient is to receive further care.

■ Measures Taken at the Scene of the Emergency

Patient's Medical History

In addition to the clinical examination, taking the patient history represents the most important task for the paramedic. In this situation, it is important to question the patient (if responsive) or the patient's family members, or the person responsible for placing the emergency call, as to the nature of the observed symptoms that prompted the emergency call. It is equally important to determine the chronology of the appearance of the patient's symptoms. The more accurately the time of the neurological emergency can be pinpointed, the easier it is to make decisions concerning whether to employ more aggressive treatment methods (lysis) at the destination hospital. In this context, the question of the patient's medical history is also of extreme importance. The paramedic makes a note of any previous illnesses, as well as any residual disability stemming from the original conditions and any medications the patient is taking.

Here, the emergency team should pay special attention to medications that influence blood coagulation or thrombocyte activity (oral anticoagulants such as vitamin K antagonists, e.g., phenprocoumon [Marcumar or Falithrom], and thrombocyte aggregation inhibitors, e.g., aspirin or clopidogrel).

To optimize further treatment in the hospital, the patient's GP and any other specialists who are familiar with the patient's illnesses should be contacted and questioned as to the patient's specific medical history. Their telephone numbers should be noted, so that hospital staff can, if necessary, contact these physicians before important therapeutic decisions are taken.

There may often be other relevant documents or records as well, for example, if the patient has already received nursing care. These should be made available to the paramedic and the hospital responsible for admitting the patient. The patient may also have saved discharge letters from previous hospital in-patient treatment; these letters can be of help. Finally, it is important to have the telephone numbers of family members at hand, in case questions concerning the patient's status arise.

It is also the task of the paramedic to explain what is going on to the patient's family members, and to provide reassurance. For legal reasons it may not be possible (or only in very rare exceptional cases) for family members to accompany the patient in the ambulance. It makes infinitely more sense for family and friends to stay at home and remain in close contact by telephone, rather than rush frantically after the ambulance to arrive at the hospital with the patient, much as they may wish to do so.

Clinical Examination

After taking the patient's medical history, the paramedic concentrates on the patient's physical status during a standard clinical examination. Often, this can be done at the same time as the interview. This saves time and is possible when there are enough emergency staff at the scene. The paramedic performs what is known as the "basic neurological check," to determine the patient's state of consciousness, the status of the pupils, eye movements (nystagmus), and make an assessment of the patient's speech. After the basic neurological check, any paralysis present is given further attention. To determine the extent of paralysis in patients who have had more minor strokes and who display only mild symptoms, the arm- or leg-holding test is of great importance. Mild cases of paresis and impairment of sensitivity can be revealed in this way. A brief test of reflex status is also part of the basic neurological check. If clinical symptoms improve or deteriorate, this must be documented in the patient's notes; this information is an important starting point for possible therapeutic decisions that may be made by the admitting hospital or for differential diagnostic considerations.

Basic Measures to be Taken by Paramedic

One of the most important tasks, in addition to determining the diagnosis or differential diagnosis, is securing the patient's vital functions. In every patient who is suspected of suffering ischemic infarction, the first action is to take IV blood samples for analysis at the target hospital. Blood glucose is determined on the spot to rule out the diagnosis of hypoglycemia. If the patient's blood sugar is found to be below normal, a 40% glucose solution is administered intravenously, after which the patient is observed to determine whether the condition is improving: hypoglycemia alone can be responsible for neurological symptoms, or can occur in combination with other conditions. If the neurological symptoms accompanying hypoglycemia do not disappear within a few minutes, then the additional diagnosis of stroke must be considered. The condition of hyperglycemia can be treated preclinically only in the rarest of cases, as insulin is almost never available among the emergency medications in ambulances. If insulin is available, a blood glucose level of less than 8 mmol/L (144 mg/dl) is desirable.

While one member of the emergency team is setting up the IV, another can be measuring the patient's blood pressure and oxygen saturation. Often, reactive blood pressure values are measured at this time. Systolic values of up to 200–220 mmHg and diastolic values between 100 and 110 mmHg are left untreated, as they are the result of a necessary increase in blood pressure following stroke. If the patient's systolic blood pressure is over 220 mmHg and diastolic over

120 mmHg, it must be lowered very carefully. This can be done using urapidil, a preparation that is easily titrated. Close monitoring of the patient's blood pressure (approximately every 5 minutes) is then required during the ride in the ambulance. When blood pressure values of under 180/110 mmHg have been reached, administration of medication is terminated. In rare cases, low blood pressure is found (hypotension, blood pressure systolic <100 mmHg). If the patient's medical history indicates that no cardiac insufficiency is present, colloidal fluids (e.g., Voluven 6%) can be administered. If the patient's blood pressure still cannot be stabilized, it may be necessary to administer catecholamines (substances which raise blood pressure by means of peripheral vasoconstriction). In addition, a three-lead ECG is set up. The results of the ECG are particularly important for the admitting hospital, in order to determine whether or not cardiac arrhythmia is present, which can lead to stroke (absolute arrhythmia in the presence of atrial fibrillation). By measuring peripheral oxygen saturation (Spo_2), it is possible to detect a state of hypoxia. A patient suspected of having suffered a stroke should be given liberal doses of oxygen, administered by means of a nasal tube. The usual amount given is 2–4 L/min of oxygen. An oxygen saturation level of more than 95% should be the aim (Dressel and Kessler 2003). Special care is needed when dealing with patients who suffer from chronic obstructive pulmonary disease. In these patients, high dosages of oxygen can provoke the reactive condition of CO_2 narcosis. For this reason, a medical history concerning the patient's previous related illnesses and medications should be obtained.

Body temperature must also be measured. If the patient's temperature is over 38°C, acetaminophen (paracetamol), 1 g in suppository form, may be given to bring down the fever (if this medication is available in the ambulance).

In cases of stroke, the patient may experience seizures. These nearly always resolve spontaneously, but if this proves not to be the case, the seizures may be treated intravenously with benzodiazepines (e.g., clonazepam). In patients with severe swallowing difficulties or severely impaired state of consciousness, the paramedic must make a quick decision as to whether or not to initiate artificial respiration before arrival at the hospital in an attempt to stabilize the patient's vital signs. This is more commonly required with strokes resulting from major brain hemorrhages than from ischemic conditions.

Transferring the affected patient into the emergency vehicle sometimes proves to be quite difficult and the paramedic has to decide how best to do this. It is not always possible to carry a patient on a transfer sheet down a very narrow stairway to a waiting emergency vehicle under the therapeutic conditions introduced above. In these instances, the emergency team may have to call for additional emergency equipment.

Once the patient has been examined, appropriate therapeutic measures have been initiated, and transfer to the emergency vehicle has been accomplished, the patient's upper body should be elevated slightly (30°). Naturally, the patient is constantly monitored during the drive to the target hospital, and the various therapeutic measures already taken are continued and allowed to take effect. The ambulance team must always remember to handle the patient's paralyzed side with special care and attention. IV needles should therefore always be inserted on the unaffected side.

While diagnostic and therapeutic measures are being undertaken, the EMT contacts the emergency headquarters to advise the patient's arrival. This serves to support the emergency team in its search for an appropriate target clinic. If direct cellphone contact between the emergency team and the target institution is possible, the admitting hospital will often contact the paramedic directly to elicit information important for the patient's further treatment. The following key elements should thus be incorporated into the patient's preregistration procedure: age; gender; intubation or respirator status; working diagnosis; whether the patient is awake, partially or fully responsive; long-term medications (in particular, those affecting coagulation and antihypertensive medications); and information pertaining to the expected time of arrival at the hospital.

The patient is transported to the target institution as quickly and carefully as possible. The paramedic has to decide at the scene of the emergency what form of emergency transport suits the particular circumstances. If road transport will take too long, they may opt for an emergency helicopter, for example. The emergency headquarters will assist in coordinating this.

During the ride to the hospital, the patient's vital signs are monitored and therapeutic measures are continued. It is also of critical importance for the paramedic to observe whether any neurological symptoms that are present worsen or improve, as well as whether or not it is necessary to initiate further therapeutic measures (e.g., when the patient's state of consciousness has worsened, and aspiration and accompanying decrease in oxygen saturation are suspected, forcing the decision to put the patient on a respirator even in this out-of-hospital context).

During the drive or upon arrival at the hospital, the paramedic records all findings and therapeutic measures taken, using a standardized emergency protocol. On arrival at the target institution, the paramedic hands the patient over to the admitting neurologist on duty. When the paramedic has successfully completed the handover procedure and the necessary documentation, the ambulance team can report to emergency headquarters for further instructions.

The above description of emergency procedures, with regard to preclinical options as well as any relevant differential diagnoses, illustrates exactly why differentiated therapy, such as preclinical lysis therapy which would be possible in the case of acute myocardial infarction, is unfortunately impossible for stroke patients.

Case Study 3

An emergency team is alerted at 10:30 pm by emergency headquarters and receives an emergency call with the following message:

"Seventy-five-year-old patient, not fully responsive, can no longer move independently."

Eight minutes later, they reach the site of the emergency to find a male patient sitting in a recliner in front of the television. The television is on, and the team observes that the last few minutes of an important football match are being shown.

The patient is hunched over in his chair, can only answer questions irregularly, and opens his eyes only in response to painful stimuli. When examining motor coordination, the paramedic notes a decrease in the strength of all four extremities, especially the right arm and leg. When examining the patient's pupils he further observes focal movement of the eye to the left, as well as a slightly dilated left pupil, which shows a delayed reaction to light.

The patient's vital signs are recorded to reveal the following information:

- Oxygen saturation 95%
- Blood pressure 200/100 mmHg
- Heart rate 90/min, arrhythmic

First, the paramedic inserts an IV, determines the patient's blood sugar level, which is normal, and administers a crystalloid Ringer infusion. Signs of absolute arrhythmia can be detected in the three-lead ECG. The patient's wife is too upset to give details of any medications the patient is taking, or any information concerning his previous illnesses. The EMT searches for containers or packets of medicine, but can only find medications already prepared for the patient to take during the day. The ambulance team is thus unable to determine the types of medication the patient is taking. The paramedic expresses a suspicion of stroke.

The patient is now carried to the emergency vehicle with the help of a transfer sheet. Upon reaching the ambulance, the paramedic notices that the patient's neurological symptoms have worsened. His condition has gone down three points according to the Glasgow Coma Scale, his oxygen saturation has dropped to 80%, and the left pupil is more dilated than it was on initial examination. For this reason, the paramedic decides to put the patient on out-of-hospital mechanical respiration. He applies short-term IV narcosis and inserts an orotracheal tube to ensure the patient now receives sufficient oxygen.

The paramedic reports the following working diagnoses to emergency headquarters:

- Acute stroke
- ICH ruled out
- Target hospital with CT scanner and neurosurgeons required

The emergency headquarters gives the orders by phone for the team to drive the patient to the university hospital, which is 20 minutes away. The patient's vital signs are stable, and the remainder of the drive is uneventful.

The paramedic hands the patient over to the neurologist on duty in the emergency department, who immediately orders a cranial CT scan. In the CT scan, a large intracranial area of hemorrhage is visible in the region of the left brain hemisphere with bleeding into the ventricular system and considerable displacement of the midline.

This case description serves again to illustrate how the paramedic can only make a tentative diagnosis on the basis of the clinical symptoms displayed. He is not in a position to discern whether the origin of the stroke symptoms is an ischemic infarction or intracranial hemorrhage. For this reason, lysis therapy is not included in the context of modern therapeutic methods for treating patients suspected of having suffered stroke (as opposed to the acute therapy of myocardial infarction).

■ Summary

The preclinical treatment initiated by the ambulance team represents an important link connecting the scene of the emergency and the hospital where further treatment takes place. The task to be performed by the paramedic is limited to taking a detailed patient medical history, securing vital functions, initiating accompanying therapeutic measures, and arranging a speedy yet safe transfer to a facility appropriate to the patient's needs.

The case studies introduced above serve to illuminate the immense significance of the preclinical treatment of the stroke patient with regard to further, more specialized, therapy options and methods, with the aim of keeping the neurological deficit at a minimum.

Emergency care is exhaustive and comprehensive. There is, however, still room for improvement in terms of educating the general population to increase their awareness of the classic symptoms accompanying the condition known as "stroke." The progress made, over the past 20 years, in the preclinical treatment of patients suffering from myocardial infarction illustrates that this is indeed possible.

3 Acute Therapy of Stroke

Ralf Schlosser

*Time is of the essence. Do not wait for a later, more conveni-
ent opportunity.*

(St. Catherine of Siena)

■ Therapy of Ischemic Stroke

Stroke patients are emergency patients! Strongly supported by the apt expression "time is brain," the care of these patients during the acute phase has improved greatly, in particular through the increased awareness of the general population as to what "stroke" means, the optimization of treatment procedures, and the care and guidance of patients in specialized stroke units. Moreover, progress has been made specifically through the introduction and approval of recombinant tissue plasminogen activator (rt-PA) for purposes of thrombolysis in a therapeutic context. Interventional techniques open up many possibilities, not only in terms of diagnostic options, but also for local thrombolysis and stent placement, among other procedures. Operative techniques are available as well, such as decompressive craniectomy in the case of space-occupying medial cerebral infarction, also termed malignant medial cerebral infarction.

This chapter offers an overview of the acute care of patients who have suffered ischemic stroke. It refers primarily to the guidelines of the German Association of Neurology (Hacke et al. 2008a) and the recommendations of the European Stroke Organization 2009.

General Information

Patients in whom acute stroke is suspected should be monitored in special stroke units. These wards specialize in the treatment of stroke patients and are characterized by the daily availability of a neurologist with extensive experience in the therapy of stroke. Further, there is 24-hour availability of CT scans and diagnostic neurosonography (DSG 2010). The function of stroke units is to perform thrombolysis, and, if necessary, to determine the indication for invasive therapeutic procedures, clarifying the cause of stroke and monitoring the patient intensively during the acute phase to detect complications early and thus to treat them. Stroke units therefore have special monitoring beds which make possible the continuous monitoring of blood pressure, oxygen saturation, ECG, respiration, temperature, and heart rate. Furthermore, hospitals possessing a stroke unit must also have an intensive care unit equipped with ventilators. Patients with a reduced level of consciousness, or those receiving ventilation, must be admitted directly to a (neurological) intensive care unit. One further important characteristic of stroke units is the interdisciplinary cooperation among physicians, caregivers, occupational therapists and physical therapists, speech therapists or swallowing therapists, and social workers (DSG 2010). Mortality and nursing effort may be greatly reduced in stroke patients who have been treated in a stroke unit, compared with patients who have been treated in nonspecialized wards (Candelise et al. 2007, Langhorne 1997). The intensive monitoring in particular appears to be responsible for the more favorable results (Sulter et al. 2003).

Most stroke units are found in major metropolitan areas. The quality of care of stroke patients outside of these centers can be ensured and improved through the cooperation and networking of several hospitals, as demonstrated for example in Bavaria (Germany), with the help of the TEMPiS program (Telemedicine Pilot Project for integrated Stroke treatment). In this program, regional clinics are connected to a stroke center. In addition, these clinics receive support in constructing and designing their own special stroke wards. When questions arise, clinic staff can make contact with the stroke center via telemedicine. Physicians in the stroke center can assess the patient by means of a video conference, and results of CT and MRI imaging may also be interpreted at the same time. Further procedures are then discussed within the group. In this way, not only the thrombolysis rate, but also the quality of the care for stroke patients, has been improved, and this in turn has resulted in an improved prognosis (Audebert et al. 2006).

Case Study 1 (Part 1 of 4)

A 72-year-old woman is sitting on a bench in her garden, knitting. Suddenly she finds that she is no longer able to use her left hand, and knitting has become impossible. As the knitting needle falls from her hand, she calls out to her grandson, who is playing on the lawn, and asks him to send for help. He soon returns with the woman's daughter. At this point, the woman can no longer move her left arm and attempts to explain, very excitedly and with slurred speech, what has happened to her. Her daughter immediately calls an ambulance, which takes her to a neurological clinic.

Case Study 2 (Part 1 of 4)

A 59-year-old man suddenly drops his coffee cup from his right hand while sitting at the breakfast table. As his wife looks up, startled, he tries excitedly to tell her something. However, his speech is very unclear and consists only of single words; he attempts to gesticulate but in doing so uses only his left arm. His right arm hangs limply at his side. It becomes apparent to his wife that he is no longer sitting up straight in his chair, but is now slumped over to the right side. She massages her husband's right arm with a wet washcloth. While doing this, she tries to reassure her husband, as he is still gesticulating wildly with his left arm. During the further course of events, the man does calm down somewhat. When the paralysis has still persisted for 2.5 hours, the wife calls for an ambulance. The patient, who is awake and displays signs of restlessness when being moved, is transferred to a nearby clinic.

In the Emergency Department

After the hospital physician has been informed by telephone about the patient's background by the paramedic or emergency headquarters staff, the hospital physician decides whether the patient is a candidate for thrombolytic therapy. This decision is made according to how long it is since the symptoms first appeared and whether the patient displays loss of consciousness, as well as whether or not he or she is taking anticoagulants. To save precious time in the hospital, admission of patients who are potential candidates for lysis therapy should take place in the relevant imaging department. After the patient has been admitted, patient history is recorded, the patient is examined (and blood pressure measured) and the relevant laboratory parameters are determined. The score on the National Institute of Health Stroke Scale (NIHSS) is determined as well (see **Table 3.2**). Next, the inclusion and exclusion criteria for lysis therapy are reviewed. In the meantime, a cranial CT scan is performed; if readily available, a cranial MRI scan may be used instead. By means of the imaging procedures, intracranial hemorrhage should be ruled out as the cause of the patient's symptoms. It is recommended that the patient is seen by a physician within 10 minutes of arrival at the hospital. The cranial CT scan should be initiated within 25 minutes of the patient's arrival, and the "door to needle" interval, that is, the time from the patient's arrival until the beginning of a possible thrombolysis procedure, should be no longer than 60 minutes (Hacke et al. 2008a).

Case Study 1 (Part 2 of 4)

The 72-year-old patient arrives at the emergency department of the hospital 40 minutes after the onset of her symptoms. The neurologist on call questions her as to her neurological deficits; the blood samples already taken by the paramedic are taken to the hospital laboratory. During clinical examination, left-sided hemiparalysis with a brachiofacial emphasis including paralysis of the left arm is discovered; during the leg-holding test, the patient's left leg drops slowly after approximately 4 seconds. The patient has slurred speech but displays no aphasia. The point score on the NIHSS is 9. The patient's blood pressure is found to be 170/100 mmHg and her heart rate is 95/min. The ECG reading shows a sinus rhythm. When asked about previous illnesses, she reports that she has suffered from high blood pressure for over 30 years; besides this, she has had mild diabetes for 3 years, for which she receives medication. The paramedic has already determined her blood sugar to be 7.5 mmol/L. After the patient has answered all the questions, the neurologist accompanies the patient to the CT department for a cranial CT scan.

Special Diagnostics

Cranial CT remains by far the most important diagnostic procedure for suspected stroke patients. To begin with, it makes it possible to differentiate between an ischemic and a hemorrhagic stroke.

With ischemic stroke, the CT scan shows, among other things, hypodense areas and initial swelling of the brain. Individual changes, so-called early infarction signs, can appear even within the first hour after the onset of symptoms and allow an estimate of the size of the ischemic infarction that is to be expected (Tomura et al. 1988, von Kummer et al. 1997). In addition, the "hyperdense media sign" (von Kummer et al. 1994) is present in cases of occlusion of the medial cerebral artery, in which instance the vessel is already visible in the native view as a hyperdense area (**Fig. 3.1**). In addition, CT angiography, performed after the native view procedure, can show vessel occlusion in the arterial and venous vascular territories. As a CT scan is readily available in many hospitals, it is the diagnostic method of choice.

A cranial MRI scan should only be performed when there is no risk of taking too much time over the procedure. MRI is actually the superior method for imaging ischemic infarctions in the posterior fossa. The diffusion and perfusion-weighted sequences play a significant role in MRI procedures (Köhrmann et al. 2006). This method could possibly identify potential patients who may well profit from thrombolysis even after the 3-hour time window, as the infarction core can thus be identified through the use of diffusion-weighted sequences, while tissue regions with a decreased blood supply can be identified by means of perfusion sequences. The difference between the size of both regions (mismatch) corresponds to the penumbra; that is, the region surrounding the infarction which receives a barely sufficient blood supply but has not

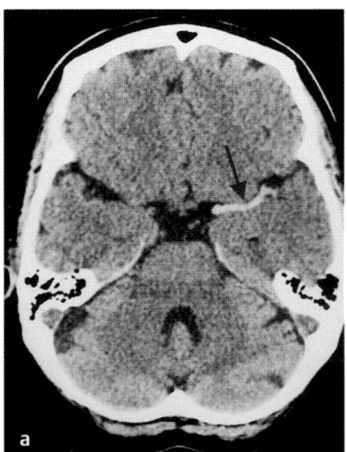

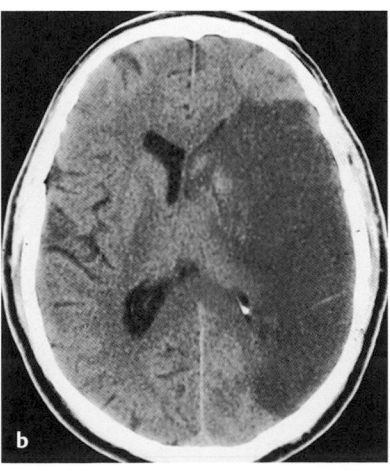

Fig. 3.1 a, b
a Occlusion of left middle cerebral artery. The thrombus appears as a hyperdense middle artery sign (arrow).
b Ischemic infarction in the region supplied by the left middle cerebral artery, with compression of the left ventricle and initial displacement of the midline to the right.

yet suffered irreversible damage. It is just this area that can be salvaged by means of thrombolysis. If a mismatch is no longer present, thrombolysis cannot be expected to bring about any further improvements. However, neither the use of perfusion MRI nor the "mismatch" concept can be generally recommended as a routine procedure with respect to therapeutic decisions to be made on this front (Hacke et al. 2008a).

Additional diagnostic techniques that can be employed are Doppler and duplex sonography, which make it possible to assess the major extracranial and intracranial vessels. During such procedures, signs of vessel occlusion and stenosis may be revealed; on occasion, these alterations can even be imaged directly. Special sonography contrast medium can be used to intensify the signal. It is advised that the procedure be performed as soon as possible (within the first 24 hours) (Hacke et al. 2008a). An EEG should be performed in cases of suspected status epilepticus, for example. An ECG is also done to rule out cardiac arrhythmia and myocardial ischemia as a possible cause of the cerebral infarction. Echocardiography can reveal intracardial thrombi. In the hospital laboratory, the patient's blood count, coagulation, blood sugar, renal values, and electrolytes are determined.

Of course, performing the complete diagnostic procedure (**Table 3.1**) requires a considerable amount of time. Since the management of these patients initially involves the question of whether or not thrombolysis is possible, there is an urgent need to work under extreme time pressure, as this therapy is only possible when initiated within the first 4.5 hours after the onset of symptoms. Before beginning thrombolysis, it is absolutely essential to rule out intracerebral hemorrhage by means of a CT or MRI scan. Further vessel diagnostics are not necessary before initiating lysis therapy (Szabo et al. 2005).

Case Study 1 (Part 3 of 4)

Apart from slight cerebral atrophy, the cranial CT scan of the 72-year-old patient does not reveal any early signs of infarction or bleeding. CT angiography shows no sign of vessel occlusion.

Table 3.1   Diagnostics and monitoring following admission to the stroke unit

Diagnostics	
Clinical findings, including NIHSS, blood pressure, heart rate	
Laboratory	Blood count, coagulation, blood glucose and renal function, electrolytes, CK, CK-Mb, in the further course of treatment, if necessary, special coagulation and vasculitis diagnostics
ECG at rest	
Cranial CT scan	Native image; if necessary, CT angiography, CT perfusion
Cranial MRI	Currently no routine application, only when readily available or time window > 3 hours
Doppler/duplex sonography (extra- and intracranial)	To be performed during further course of treatment, not necessary prior to thrombolysis
Chest radiograph	
Echocardiography, if necessary TEE	
Long-term ECG	
Long-term blood pressure	
Monitoring	
ECG, heart rate, blood pressure, respiration	If systemic thrombolysis is planned: RR systolic < 180 mmHg
Oxygen saturation	95%– 100%
Body temperature	< 37.5°C
Neurological findings	Regular NIHSS assessment
Laboratory (blood glucose, electrolytes)	Blood glucose < 8.3 mmol/L

Case Study 2 (Part 3 of 4)
In the cranial CT scan performed on the 59-year-old male patient, a hyperdense media sign on the left side is depicted about 3.5 hours after the onset of symptoms, as well as a hypodense area in the vascular territory supplied by the entire left medial cerebral artery and brain edema on the left side with compression of the left lateral ventricle already beginning to occur, as well as initial displacement of the midline to the right (**Fig. 3.1**). The ECG shows signs of absolute arrhythmia in the presence of atrial fibrillation.

2009). The aim is the early detection of life-threatening complications (pulmonary or cardiac) as well as any signs of deterioration in the patient's neurological status. Standardized neurological scales (e.g., NIHSS [**Table 3.2**], Scandinavian Stroke Scale, Glasgow Coma Scale) are most suitable for the assessment of neurological status.

Therapy

General Treatment Measures

After admission, the patient's neurological status and vital signs are monitored either regularly or continuously (European Stroke Organization

Respiratory Function

Stroke patients should undergo continuous pulse oximetry. An oxygen saturation value of 95%–100% is desirable (Nelles and Busse 2005) to guarantee sufficient blood supply to the penumbra. Oxygen can be administered via nasal tube (2–4 L/min; caution must be exercised with patients who suffer from chronic obstructive pulmonary disease). In cases of insufficient oxygenation, increase in CO_2, pneumonia, or increased risk of aspiration (e.g., when patients are unconscious or have suffered infarction of the brainstem), early intubation

Table 3.2   NIH Stroke Scale (1998, revised)

1a. State of con-sciousness	Awake: responding immediately	0
	Somnolent: drowsy, but awakens in response to mild stimulus	1
	Sopor: repeated or painful stimuli required to get patient's attention	2
	Coma: motor or vegetative reflex responses or none at all	3
1b. Orientation (questions concerning the date and age of patient)	Answers both questions correctly	0
	Answers one question correctly	1
	Answers neither question correctly	2
1c. Following instructions (opening and closing eyes and nonparetic hand)	Performs both tasks correctly	0
	Performs one task correctly	1
	Performs neither task correctly	2
2. Oculomotor coordination (following the examiner's finger, in the horizontal plane only)	Normal	0
	Partial visual paralysis	1
	Forced visual deviation or complete paralysis of eye muscles, which cannot be overcome by performing oculocephalic reflex	2
3. Field of vision (finger perimetric test)	No impairment of field of vision	0
	Partial hemianopsia	1
	Total hemianopsia	2
	Bilateral hemianopsia (blindness, including cortical blindness)	3
4. Facial paresis	No paralysis	0
	Slight paralysis (flattened nasolabial fold, asymmetry apparent when smiling	1
	Partial paralysis (complete or nearly complete paralysis of lower portion of face)	2
	Total paralysis on one or both sides (lower and upper portions of face)	3

Continued ▶

Table 3.2 Continued

5. Motor coordination of arms	Arms brought up to 90° position:	Left	Right
	• no lowering of arms in 10 seconds	0	0
	• lowering of arms over the course of 10 seconds, without touching the underlying surface	1	1
	• arm can be lifted against gravity, 90% position cannot be reached or maintained, arm is lowered to the underlying surface	2	2
	• no (active) lifting of arm to overcome gravity, arm falls	3	3
	• no movement	4	4
	In cases of amputation or joint stiffness	0	0
6. Motor coordination of legs	Legs brought to 45° position:	Left	Right
	• no lowering of leg in 5 seconds	0	0
	• lowering over 5 seconds without touching underlying surface	1	1
	• leg can be raised to overcome gravity, falls to the underlying surface within 5 seconds	2	2
	• leg cannot be lifted to overcome gravity, leg falls immediately	3	3
	• no movement	4	4
	In cases of amputation or joint stiffness	0	0
7. Extremity ataxia (finger to nose or knee to heel test)	Absent	0	
	Present in one extremity	1	
	Present in two extremities	2	
	In cases of paralysis or coma	0	
8. Sensitivity (needle, pain stimuli on arms, legs, body, face)	Normal, no loss of sensitivity	0	
	Mild to moderate loss of sensitivity	1	
	Severe to total loss of sensitivity	2	
	Coma	2	
9. Language (naming objects, describing pictures, reading series of sentences)	No aphasia, normal language	0	
	Mild to moderate aphasia (considerable limitation of word flow or language comprehension)	1	
	Severe aphasia (communication takes place by way of fragmented expressions)	2	
	Muteness, global aphasia, no meaningful speech production, no language comprehension	3	
	Coma	3	
10. Dysarthria (reading word lists)	Normal	0	
	Mild to moderate. Slurred articulation of at least a few words and can be understood with only great difficulty	1	
	Severe. Patient's slurred speech is incomprehensible and is not due to aphasia, or patient is anarthric	2	
	Coma	2	
	Intubation	0	
11. Neglect	No abnormal behavior observed	0	
	Visual, tactile, auditory or personal neglect observed when performing bilateral stimulation in one of the sensory qualities	1	
	Severe hemineglect or hemineglect in more than one quality. Patient does not recognize own hand, or orients him/herself only with respect to one side of the room	2	

is the best choice, taking into consideration the prognosis and the patient's own wishes (European Stroke Organization 2009).

Cardiac Function

Immediately following the stroke patient's admission, a 12-lead ECG must be recorded at rest. Subsequently the ECG should be monitored continuously; the reason for this is the more frequent occurrence of arrhythmia and changes in ECG findings during the first few days following the patient's stroke. For instance, a patient may develop atrial fibrillation (Vingerhoets et al. 1993) or supraventricular tachycardia (Lane et al. 1992), or demonstrate an increase in cardiac muscle enzymes (James et al. 2000). If there are no spontaneous blood pressure readings that are higher than normal, the cardiac output may be supported and increased by means of positive inotropes.

Blood Pressure

In the brain, cerebral blood flow is generally kept constant and is independent of systemic blood pressure. This adaptation takes place through what is known as autoregulation. By means of this process, dilation occurs in the arterioles when systemic blood pressure is low, and constriction when blood pressure is high. In the area that surrounds the infarction core, called the penumbra, this autoregulation becomes disturbed (Ringleb et al. 1998). The blood supply to this region is thus directly dependent on the systemic blood pressure or on the mean arterial pressure (Eames et al. 2002, Schwarz et al. 2002). In the first days following ischemic stroke, most patients display elevated blood pressure (Leonardi-Bee et al. 2002). These elevated values should not be treated in all cases, as sufficient circulation to the penumbra must be guaranteed during the acute phase of ischemic stroke, otherwise there is danger of the infarction zone becoming more extensive. Blood pressure should be treated with medication when values exceed 220 mmHg systolic and 120 mmHg diastolic. Sudden, extreme lowering of the blood pressure should, however, be avoided; for this reason, sublingual application of nifedipine, for example, cannot be recommended (European Stroke Organization 2009). In patients who are candidates for lysis or anticoagulation therapy, the systolic blood pressure should not exceed 180 mmHg because of the increased risk of bleeding when values are too high. Reduction of the blood pressure to normal values, based on the cause of infarction, can usually take place after 3 days. Most patients even experience a spontaneous decrease in the values within one week (Harper et al. 1994, Jansen et al. 1987). Hypotensive blood pressure values occur only very rarely in infarction patients (ca. 5%) but, as with like greatly elevated values, these also lead to less favorable results (Leonardi-Bee et al. 2002). Following a quick cardiologic diagnostic check, these patients should be given infusions of crystalloid or colloidal solutions. If elevation of blood pressure to the values mentioned above cannot be achieved, it is necessary to supplement therapy with catecholamines for these patients (Hacke et al. 2008a).

Glucose Metabolism

Over 50% of stroke patients present with elevated blood sugar levels; this is observed especially in those who have experienced extensive infarctions (Scott et al. 1999). Diabetics in particular may display drastic worsening of their glucose metabolism during the acute phase. During the course of their illness, patients with hyperglycemia have, in addition to poorer functional results, a two to three times higher mortality (Bruno et al. 1999, Capes et al. 2001, Williams et al. 2002). Therefore, blood glucose should be lowered consistently by means of insulin. As the further development during the course of the illness has been observed to be poorer in association with blood glucose levels of more than 150 mg/dL (8.3 mmol/L), therapy is recommended when these values are exceeded (Nelles and Busse 2005, Leigh et al. 2004). Here, intensive blood glucose monitoring is necessary to be able to detect hypoglycemia in time. Likewise, patients exhibiting hypoglycemia must be treated by the oral or intravenous administration of glucose (Hacke et al. 2008a).

Body Temperature

During the acute phase stroke patients often develop fever, which is quite frequently caused by a urinary or respiratory infection. (Georgilis et al. 1999), although elevated temperatures also occur in the absence of infection. A so-called central fever is a possible cause. Temperature elevation leads to an increase in blood flow, with subsequent elevation of intracerebral pressure by way of intensification of cerebral metabolism. Infarction patients who display elevated temperatures have poorer outcomes during the course of the illness (Hajat et al. 2000): with an increase in body temperature of only 1°C, the risk of a poor outcome doubles (Reith et al. 1996). Thus, patients whose temperature exceeds 37.5°C should be treated with antipyretic agents during the acute phase (Hacke et al. 2008b).

Fluids and Electrolytes

Well-balanced fluid and electrolyte metabolism is the aim in stroke patients. In most cases, intravenous fluids must be administered, as many patients exhibit exsiccosis (European Stroke Organization 2009). Any limitations due to pulmonary or cardiac illnesses must be carefully considered. Electrolytes should be checked daily and replaced, if necessary.

Nutrition

Stroke patients should receive enteral nutrition, if at all possible. During the acute phase, however, 50% of patients experience swallowing disturbances. Because of the associated risk of aspiration, oral nutrition should take place only after assessment of the patients' swallowing function by a speech therapist or an ear, nose, and throat specialist. If the patient is not able to swallow properly, nutrition can only be given by means of a gastric tube. If the patient's state of vigilance continues to deteriorate and intubation is imminent, temporary parenteral nutrition becomes necessary.

Pneumonia, Thrombosis, and Pressure Ulcer Prophylaxis

The development of pneumonia represents one of the main dangers for stroke patients. In most cases the patients suffer from aspiration pneumonia, since they quite often suffer from swallowing difficulties. This is caused by a reduction in the patient's state of vigilance, or is due to the actual location of the infarction. Oral nutrition should therefore be used only when the patient's swallowing function is sufficient. Furthermore, early mobilization and intensive breathing therapy (physical therapy, nursing, physical measures, and medication options) are practiced within the context of pneumonia prophylaxis.

With early mobilization, deep leg vein thrombosis does not develop as frequently. If mobilization is not possible, active or passive exercises can be performed as part of the physical therapy program. In addition, antithrombosis stockings and subcutaneous low molecular weight heparin (or in some cases unfractionated heparin) represent supplemental measures.

Mobilization plays an essential role in the prevention of pressure ulcers (decubitus ulcers). Immobile patients must be repositioned regularly. An alternating pressure mattress must be used if necessary.

The most important therapeutic measures are summarized in **Table 3.3**.

Table 3.3   Therapy of ischemic stroke

General Therapy (see also Table 3.1: Monitoring)	
Inhibition of thrombocyte aggregation	Neither prior to, nor within 24 hours following thrombolysis
Early mobilization	Not with elevated ICP
Enteral nutrition	Assessment of swallowing function, when inadequate, nasal stomach tube or PEG tube
Pneumonia prophylaxis	Respiratory therapy, mobilization
Pressure sore prophylaxis	Regular repositioning Pressure-adjustable mattress Mobilization
Thrombosis prophylaxis	Compression stockings Low-dose heparin
Specific Therapy	
Thrombolysis	With rt-PA within 3 hours, systemic In exceptional cases, local (not approved)
Stenoses of internal carotid artery, middle carotid artery	TEA (only with stenosis of internal carotid artery), PTA and subsequent stent implantation Also possible as emergency procedure
Therapy of cerebral edema	30° upper body positioning Osmotherapy Intubation/analgosedation/ short-term hyperventilation Decompressive craniectomy Hypothermia Barbiturate sedation

Specific Therapy

Thrombolysis

Recombinant Tissue Plasminogen Activator (rt-PA)

To be able to dissolve a fibrin clot, plasminogen must be activated by conversion to plasmin. Of all the endogenous plasminogen activators, the tissue plasminogen activator (t-PA, alteplase) plays the most significant role. It is synthesized by endothelial cells and released in the presence of different irritants or conditions (e.g., endothelial lesions, stasis, hypoxia, fibrin buildup). After its release, t-PA is responsible for the conversion of plasminogen into plasmin. Plasmin then splits the fibrin in the clot into fibrin monomers, through which process the clot is dissolved. Recombinant tissue plasminogen activator (rt-PA, alteplase), used for therapeutic purposes, is the product of genetic engineering. It is the only form of causal therapy approved for the treatment of acute ischemic stroke within the first 3 hours after the onset of symptoms. In addition, rt-PA has also been approved for the treatment of myocardial infarction and pulmonary embolism. In the case of acute ischemic stroke, the aim of lysis is to attempt to salvage nerve cells suffering reversible damage. Such cells are found surrounding the infarction core, in which the neurons are already irreversibly damaged a matter of minutes after vessel occlusion, as a result of oxygen deficiency. The cells in the peripheral area, called the penumbra, receive just enough of a residual oxygen supply to survive. The cell structure can thus be preserved, but neuronal activity is no longer present. Depending on the extent of residual circulation, the cells in the area of the penumbra die within a few hours. Thrombolysis may still allow reperfusion, but improvements in the patient's clinical status can no longer be achieved.

Scientific Background

In 1995, the NINDS study was published, in the context of which 624 patients received either rt-PA or a placebo (National Institute of Neurological Disorders and Stroke rt-PA Stroke Study Group 1995) within 3 hours following the onset of stroke symptoms. The study was able to demonstrate that the number of patients exhibiting a favorable outcome after 3 months was markedly higher in the group of patients receiving rt-PA (0.9 mg/kg body weight) than in the placebo group. These results were reached in all the scales used in the study (NIHSS 31% versus 20%, Barthel Index 50% versus 38%, Modified Ranking Scale 39% versus 26%, Glasgow Outcome Scale 44% versus 32%). In the group treated with rt-PA, however, significantly more cases of symptomatic bleeding occurred (6.4% versus 0.6%). In particular, patients with pronounced symptoms tended to develop bleeding, but no significant differences could be detected between the two groups with respect to mortality, nor did the number of patients with severe disabilities increase. After this study was published, rt-PA was approved in the United States in 1996 for the treatment of acute ischemic stroke in the 3-hour time window; in 2000, it was also approved in Europe.

Further studies followed in which therapy using rt-PA was investigated (among others, ECASS I in 1996, ECASS II in 1998, and ATLANTIS in 1999). In addition, meta-analyses were published which included previously performed individual studies of rt-PA. There it was confirmed that therapy using rt-PA leads to marked improvement of functional results (evaluated on the basis of the Modified Ranking Scale) (Hacke et al. 1999, Wardlaw et al. 2003). In an analysis of the four rt-PA studies it was demonstrated that the time factor plays an enormously important role in terms of outcome (Hacke et al. 2004): if the thrombolysis took place within the first 90 minutes following the onset of symptoms, the probability of favorable neurological results after 3 months was approximately 2.8 times higher than in the placebo group. When therapy was initiated after 4.5–6 hours, this probability was only 1.15 times higher. In 2008, the ECASS3 study was able to demonstrate that thrombolysis using rt-PA, administered 3–4.5 hours after the onset of symptoms, produced a significantly improved outcome compared with a placebo, in spite of the more frequent occurrence of symptomatic cerebral hemorrhage (2.4% versus 0.2%) (Hacke et al. 2008b). On the basis of these results, the European Stroke Organization 2009 and the guidelines presented by the German Society for Neurology recommend thrombolysis with rt-PA in the case of ischemic stroke, within a time window of up to 4.5 hours following the onset of symptoms (Hacke et al. 2008a). However, the treatment during the time frame between 3 and

4.5 hours has not been evaluated for the European approval of alteplase.

Indication

The administration of alteplase in patients suffering acute ischemic stroke is conditional on several factors (according to the technical information provided for Actilyse):
1. Onset of stroke symptoms not more than 3 hours previously.
2. Intracranial hemorrhage has been ruled out by means of appropriate imaging techniques.
3. The treatment must be administered by an experienced physician specially trained in the field of neurological intensive medicine.

Limiting the application of systemic (i.e., IV) lysis to the first 3 hours following the onset of symptoms means that there is considerable time pressure after the patient has been admitted to the hospital. The relevant data on patient history, images, and laboratory findings, including at least the coagulation parameters, must therefore be collected as quickly as possible, but with great care. Even when the patient arrives at the hospital promptly, allowing enough time to meet the 3-hour limit, this should not be a reason to take more time for the necessary procedures, because, as already mentioned, the earlier lysis therapy takes place, the higher the probability of favorable results (Hacke et al. 2004), even during the 3-hour time window. Ischemic stroke is after all a dynamic process; it is believed that the time interval associated with the development of infarction due to occlusion of a major vessel is around 10 hours from start to finish (Saver 2006). Any delay in therapy results in an increase in the number of neurons lost. Humans possess approximately 130 billion neurons. In every minute during which a supratentorial ischemic stroke remains untreated, the patient loses an average of 1.9 million neurons. In every hour during which no therapy takes place, the brain therefore loses as many neurons as it would in approximately 3.6 years of normal aging—around 120 million (Saver 2006). These figures serve to emphasize why the motto "time is brain" is so extraordinarily important in the context of acute therapy. It is therefore regrettable that, according to study analyses, only about 25% of all stroke patients reach the hospital within 3 hours and, despite the excellent results of this form of therapy, only 3%–8.5% of all stroke patients receive lysis (Reeves et al. 2005). Of patients with ischemic stroke in the California Acute Stroke Pilot Registry, 23.5% arrived at the emergency department within 3 hours of symptom onset, and 4.3% received thrombolysis (California Acute Stroke Pilot Registry [CASPR] Investigators 2005).

Contraindications

Besides the requirements for thrombolysis, there is also an range of contraindications (**Table 3.4**) to consider. The time window plays an important part in this context: thrombolysis has been approved for use within the time frame of up to 3 hours following the onset of symptoms. According to the most recent studies therapy is recommended during the time interval of 3–4.5 hours following the onset of symptoms (European Stroke Organization 2009, Hacke et al. 2008a), but the use of rt-PA has not yet been approved for this purpose.

Patients in whom the exact time of the appearance of their stroke symptoms is unknown, who have for example been found lying for unknown periods of time or who wake up in the morning displaying symptoms of stroke, are generally not considered candidates for lysis. In these cases, the patient history is crucial: for instance, a patient who goes to sleep one night at 23:00 and does not get up again until 6:00 the next morning, displaying no abnormalities when he gets up to use the toilet, then goes back to bed and wakes up again at 7:00, this time with symptoms of stroke, is in principle a patient who would profit from thrombolytic therapy because his symptoms have only been present for an hour (depending of course on the other inclusion and exclusion criteria as well). If the patient went to sleep at 23:00 and does not wake up until 7:00 the next morning, at which time he displays symptoms, then there is a possible time window of up to 8 hours during which the infarction could have occurred. Lysis is no longer possible, according to the inclusion conditions; it could, however, be performed in the context of an individual attempt at healing the condition. This also applies to patients in whom symptoms have persisted for up to 4.5 hours.

With regard to the severity of stroke and lysis therapy, there are currently differing points of view. A NIHSS score of 25 points or more indicates a severe stroke, clinically speaking. These patients

Table 3.4 Contraindications for thrombolysis using rt-PA (according to information provided for Actilyse)

Clinical	• Onset of stroke symptoms 3 hours or more previously, or unknown time of onset of symptoms • Minimal neurological deficits or symptoms which quickly become better before infusion is initiated • Severe stroke, confirmed either clinically (e. g., NIHSS ≥ 25) or through the use of imaging procedures • Seizures at the beginning of the stroke • Systolic blood pressure > 185 mmHg or diastolic blood pressure > 110 mmHg • Patient's age < 18 years or > 80 years
Imaging	• Confirmation of intracranial hemorrhage in the CT scan • Symptoms which indicate that subarachnoidal hemorrhage has occurred, even when CT scan is normal
Medical history	• Stroke within the past 3 months • History of stroke and accompanying diabetes mellitus • History of damage to central nervous system (e. g., neoplasm, aneurysm, intracranial or spinal surgery) • Known clotting disorders • Oral anticoagulation therapy (e. g., falithrom) • Current or recent severe or life-threatening bleeding • Major surgery or severe trauma in the past 3 months • Childbirth • Confirmed ulcerative illness in the gastrointestinal tract within the last 3 months • Severe liver disease • Neoplasia with increased risk of bleeding • Bacterial endocarditis
Labora-tory find-ings	• Thrombocytes < 100 000/mm^3 • Application of heparin in the past 48 hours and thromboplastin time above the normal value • Blood glucose level < 50 mg/100 mL or > 400 mg/100 mL
Risk-bene-fit relation in cases of	Recent minor traumas such as biopsies, punctures of major vessels, intramuscular injections, cardiac massage in connection with resuscitation

too can benefit from lysis within 3 hours (Hacke et al. 2004), but are still excluded from lysis therapy. Lysis should not be performed in patients whose symptoms are only mild or improving rapidly, according to the specialized information provided for Actilyse. Study results show, however, that approximately one-quarter to one-third of these patients not receiving this type of therapy were later disabled or even died (Barber et al. 2001, Nedeltchev et al. 2007). The criteria mentioned should therefore be considered very carefully (Grond 2005). Likewise, the risks and benefits should be weighed carefully following minor trauma or heart massage.

If the cause of the stroke symptoms is primary intracranial hemorrhage, there is no indication for systemic lysis. Neither is systemic thrombolysis used for intracerebral hemorrhage that develops later as secondary bleeding in the region of ischemic infarct (hemorrhagic transformation).

Complications

Bleeding is the main side effect to be expected; in particular, bleeding at the site of injection, hematomas, nosebleeds, bleeding from the gums, and, internally, gastrointestinal bleeding and bleeding in parenchymatous organs. Allergic reactions also occur occasionally.

Hemorrhagic transformation of the stroke region or major intracerebral hemorrhage can be problematic. Because of their short half-life, therapy with thrombocyte concentrate or coagulation factors is necessary only in very rare cases (Actilyse technical information).

Procedure

After the indications and contraindications have been considered and the decision to perform thrombolysis has been made, the patient receives an rt-PA dosage of 0.9 mg/kg body weight (but not more than 90 mg). Ten percent of the dosage is given initially as an intravenous bolus injection, and the remaining 90% as an infusion lasting an hour. The patients should be monitored during this time and up to 24 hours following therapy. Regular measuring of blood pressure, especially while the medication is being administered, is required. Likewise, neurological status must also be assessed regularly so that any worsening of the patient's condition (most likely in connection with intracranial hemorrhage) can be detected immediately. A control cranial CT scan is performed on the following day. During the first 24 hours after lysis, the patient may not receive aspirin (acetylsalicylic acid) or intravenous heparin.

Case Study 1 (Part 4 of 4)

The cranial CT scan performed on the 72-year-old patient has not revealed any early signs of infarction or bleeding. Eighty minutes have passed since the onset of her symptoms. After ruling out contraindications and reviewing the laboratory findings, the neurologist makes the decision to perform thrombolysis with rt-PA. The patient weighs approximately 80 kg, making the necessary dosage 72 mg. While still in the emergency room, she receives 7.2 mg of the medication as an intravenous bolus injection, the infusion is subsequently started and the patient is taken to the stroke unit, where she is hooked up to a monitor. Her blood pressure is now 160/95 mmHg and her heart rate is 90/min. She is receiving oxygen at a rate of 2 L/min and her oxygen saturation is 97%.

The patient is awake and still speaking indistinctly. Approximately 30 minutes after initiation of thrombolysis, she notices that she can now move her left upper arm; after 1 hour, she can lift her arm up off the mattress, and she has regained the ability to move her hands and fingers, if only with difficulty. The left-sided facial paralysis has disappeared almost completely, with the result that her dysarthria has also vanished. The patient is closely monitored over the next 2 days. On the third day, attempts are begun to optimize the medication for her hypertension. Due to drastically elevated blood glucose levels, it becomes necessary to switch to insulin. In addition, the patient receives a combination of aspirin and dipyridamol, as well as a lipid-lowering agent, as secondary prevention measures. On the sixth day, she is discharged to a rehabilitation unit.

Case Study 2 (Part 4 of 4)

The cranial CT scan performed on the 59-year-old man shows the start of a complete infarction of the medial cerebral artery. Because the time window has been exceeded, the infarction zone is already very large and well demarcated, and the clinical findings are extremely poor, thrombolysis is no longer possible. The patient is first transferred to the hospital's neurological intensive care unit. Because the patient is relatively young and the CT scan images showed cerebral edema and compression of the lateral ventricles already beginning to form after 3.5 hours, the decision is made to perform decompressive craniectomy. Postoperatively, deep analgosedation and, after insertion of an intravasal cooling catheter, hypothermia treatment (33°C) are per-

---

formed. In addition, osmotherapeutic agents are applied to combat the increase in cerebral pressure. After 5 days, no elevated cerebral pressure values are registered, and the patient is gradually warmed up again. In the meantime, a tracheotomy has been performed. After gradual reduction of the analgosedation, the patient can be weaned from the respirator, a process which is completed on the 16th day. At this point in time, he is alert and focused. He is able to move his left arm and left leg spontaneously and with force. Right-sided hemiplegia is still present. In addition, the patient suffers from global aphasia: he cannot follow instructions or form his own words (phonation is not possible because of the blocked tracheal cannula). On the 20th day he is moved to a rehabilitation unit for early rehabilitation.

The case studies demonstrate a very positive course of events for the 72-year-old woman, and quite a difficult one for the 59-year-old man. Not all patients receiving lysis therapy demonstrate such a favorable course of events as our first patient, although the probability of a positive outcome increases when the patient is taken to the hospital as early as possible.

The initial differences between the two cases are particularly worthy of note: in the first case the emergency services were contacted immediately, while in the second example precious time is lost. As a rule, ischemic stroke does not cause any pain, so patients and those around them apparently often do not consider it to be a threatening condition and just hope the paralysis will "go away by itself." It is therefore necessary to continue to raise awareness of this problematic situation in the general population.

Local Lysis

So far we have considered the IV application of rt-PA. In special cases, the local, intra-arterial application of rt-PA in the context of angiography may be an option. As yet there is no regulatory approval for this, so it should be attempted only at specialized centers. For one reason, these cases involve the posterior vascular territory, that is, occlusion of the vertebral artery and/or the basilar artery. Basilar thrombosis is associated with an extremely poor prognosis. In this case, local intra-arterial lysis has led to an increased rate of recanalization; however, the clinical results did not show any major differences (Lindsberg and Mattle 2006). The loss of time until local lysis can be initiated presents a problem (preparation of angiography, time needed to reach the vessel occlusion with the angiography catheter). Here the combination of initial IV lysis and subsequent local lysis could represent a possible solution, bridging the time until local lysis is initiated. In the anterior vascular territory, when the medial cerebral artery is occluded, the effectiveness of intra-arterial lysis has been confirmed (del Zoppo et al. 1998, Furlan et al. 1999). Here too the bridging concept appears to be a promising option (IMS Study Investigators 2004). In the case of occlusion of the medial cerebral artery, the German Association of Neurology recommends intra-arterial therapy using a plasminogen activating agent within a time window of 6 hours, due to greatly improved results in the context of individual curative attempts (Hacke et al. 2008a).

Secondary Prophylaxis

Early secondary prophylaxis for prevention of recurrence of ischemic stroke after a first event can take place using aspirin (100–300 mg/d)—however, not prior to lysis therapy or within the first 24 hours thereafter. In patients who have undergone decompressive craniectomy as part of cerebral edema treatment, this should also be decided on an individual basis. Aspirin appears to be effective especially in patients with a low risk of recurrence. If the risk is elevated, for example in cases of hypertension, diabetes mellitus, following myocardial infarction and other vascular events, and in smokers, then secondary prophylaxis should take place using either a combination of aspirin and dipyridamol, or clopidogrel (Diener et al. 2008). It is quite probable in such cases that patients will have to take thrombocyte aggregation inhibitors for the rest of their lives.

The use of low-dose heparin also plays a role in the prevention of thrombosis. In addition, upon weighing the risks and benefits, early heparinization may be found to be indicated in certain patients in whom a source of embolus is present, and who also have an elevated risk of recurrence (Hacke et al. 2008a). This category includes patients in whom cardiac or aortic thrombi have been detected, as well as those who have artificial heart valves (Diener et al. 2008). Patients with mechanical heart valves may continue oral anticoagulation, depending on the size of the infarc-

tion. In addition to this, oral anticoagulation is indicated in patients with chronic atrial fibrillation; depending on the size of infarction, this can be adjusted after 3–5 days. Patients in whom echocardiography has revealed a persisting foramen ovale (PFO) as the sole condition are given aspirin after the first ischemic event. If relapse occurs while the patient is taking the medication, or if an atrial septum aneurysm has been found in addition to the PFO, then the patient must begin oral anticoagulation. In cases of repeated ischemic events, or when oral anticoagulation is contraindicated, interventional occlusion of the PFO may be considered (Diener et al. 2008).

If, after an ischemic stroke, stenosis of the internal carotid artery of over 70% is diagnosed and is assumed to be responsible for the infarction, then it is referred to as a symptomatic stenosis. These stenoses should be treated surgically (endarterectomy), depending on the clinical findings, and in this case, within 2 weeks of the first event (Rothwell et al. 2004); after this time, surgery is no longer effective as a preventive measure. The time until surgery should be bridged by administering thrombocyte aggregation inhibitors. Operative therapy for a high-degree stenosis of the internal carotid artery has been shown to produce superior results to interventional treatment by stent-protected angioplasty (Kern et al. 2007), and is recommended as the therapy of choice (Diener et al 2008); however, long-term results are not yet available. The stenosis is occasionally also treated surgically or interventionally under emergency conditions when symptoms appear.

In the case of intracranial stenosis, the patient should be given aspirin. Sometimes it is necessary to insert a stent. Oral anticoagulation results in an increase in intracerebral hemorrhage (Chimowitz et al. 2005). In addition, the treatment of risk factors plays an important role in the context of secondary prevention. If hypertension, diabetes mellitus, or hyperlipidemia is present, it must also be adequately treated.

Therapy of Complications

Cerebral Edema

After ischemic infarction has occurred, brain edema develops. This is initially cytotoxic, and subsequently vasogenic. With extensive infarctions in particular, this edema can reach enormous proportions. The size of the cerebral edema is of critical significance in terms of further prognosis. Between the second and fifth day, cerebral edema and intracranial pressure reach their maximum (Hacke et al. 1996); they recede again over the course of the following 2 weeks (Shaw et al. 1959). In association with the growing cerebral edema and intracranial pressure, the patient develops headache and nausea. Finally, the patient's level of consciousness deteriorates. Without appropriate therapy, there is a danger that brain tissue may become entrapped, which is fatal.

General Measures

Patients in whom ischemic cerebral edema has developed are positioned with their upper body elevated (~30°). Elevation of the head to over 45° is associated with the risk of a drop in cerebral perfusion (Moraine et al. 2000); the head should therefore be in an intermediate position, with flexion and torsion avoided to prevent backup of venous blood, which would otherwise lead to an increase in intracranial pressure. A stress reaction can be reduced by means of sedatives and analgesics (Mayer and Chong 2002), but the associated decrease in the patient's level of consciousness must be kept in mind. Any fever must be treated vigorously with the help of medication; the initial aim is normothermia. A further aim is a well-regulated fluid balance, which can be monitored effectively by measurement of the patient's central venous pressure. Only isotonic solutions should be used, as hypotonic solutions may give rise to an increase in the volume of the edema and thus, in turn, a rise in intracerebral pressure (Mayer and Chong 2002). If measurement of the intracerebral pressure (ICP) is possible, the therapy may be oriented toward the cerebral perfusion pressure (CPP = mean arterial pressure [MAP] – intracerebral pressure [ICP]), in which case the target is a CPP of 70–110 mmHg (Mayer and Chong 2002). Particularly in patients with large infarctions, develop-

ing cerebral edema, and deteriorating consciousness level, the implantation of a parenchymatous cerebral pressure probe should be considered sooner rather than later. If epileptic seizures occur—which has been observed in 6% of patients during the first 72 hours (Vespa et al. 2003)—then they must be treated appropriately; prophylactic use of anticonvulsants is, however, not necessary. Depending on the further course of events, the option of intubation and respiration, with subsequent analgosedation of the patient, may also be considered. If the patient is receiving artificial respiration, the ICP can be reduced by means of hyperventilation. The background for this is the fact that CO_2 is an extremely potent vasodilator. The aim of hyperventilation is the reduction of pco_2, which in turn results in vasoconstriction. As a consequence, the intracranial blood volume decreases and the ICP falls. This procedure has been studied in detail, particularly in patients who have suffered cerebrocranial trauma. One crucial drawback is that, due to vasoconstriction, the cerebral blood flow in areas that are receiving a barely adequate blood supply continues to decrease, thus possibly leading to an increase in the size of the infarction. It therefore seems to be helpful to perform forced hyperventilation only for short periods of time when treating acute increases in cerebral pressure.

A further option for the therapy of elevated ICP is moderate hypothermia. Reducing the patient's body temperature to 32–33°C for 24–72 hours leads to a significant reduction in ICP (Schwab et al. 2001). The patient's temperature may be lowered by means of cooling blankets or intravasal catheter systems. However, complications may arise during hypothermia treatment, such as pneumonia, cardiac arrhythmia, and coagulation disturbances (Georgiadis et al. 2002). During the warming procedure in particular, the patient runs the risk of developing fatal cerebral pressure crises, which is why this process should be performed very slowly. Particular caution is required in the areas of nursing care and physical therapy during the phase of greatly increased cranial pressure, as even the most minimal changes in the patient's position may lead to massive increases in ICP.

Medication

Although this has not been confirmed by major controlled studies, the IV application of osmotherapeutic agents is of special importance in the therapy of elevated cerebral pressure. The agents in use include alcohols (mannitol, sorbitol, glycerol) or hypotonic saline solutions (including hydroxyethyl starch, e.g., HyperHAES). These substances function by creating an osmolarity gradient at the blood–brain barrier; they bond to water, thus leading, via a reduction in the intracranial tissue volume, to a corresponding decrease in cerebral pressure. Administration in bolus form is necessary each time, as it is otherwise impossible to build up a sufficient osmolarity gradient. This form of therapy requires careful monitoring of the patient's serum osmolarity and electrolytes, as conditions such as acute renal failure and considerable electrolyte imbalance can occur. In addition, there is a danger that a paradoxical increase in the intracerebral tissue may ensue, as a result of the substances permeating through the damaged blood–brain barrier into the brain tissue.

Barbiturates can lower the ICP, but there is at present no indication that would justify the routine use of high doses of barbiturates when cerebral pressure is elevated; in cases of ischemic stroke in particular, no convincing evidence has as yet been presented in the form of studies. Barbiturates also have significant side effects, and should therefore be used exclusively in the context of controlled studies and under continuous EEG and ICP monitoring.

Corticosteroids are not indicated for the therapy of cerebral edema associated with ischemia, due to the absence of any positive effects and the presence of side effects.

Operative Therapy

Decompressive craniectomy represents a surgical therapy option for cerebellar infarctions and in cases of major infarction in the vascular territory supplied by the medial cerebral artery, where as large a portion as possible of the skull is removed above the affected territory connected with the medial cerebral artery. During this procedure, an attempt is made to reduce the pressure-related effects of the cerebral edema on healthy brain tissue and also to prevent the entrapment of brain tissue. Particularly with the condition known as malignant medial cerebral artery infarction, Vahedi et al. (2007) demonstrated that decompressive craniectomy during the first 48 hours led not only to a significant increase in the survival rate compared with the patient group undergoing conser-

vative treatment (80% versus 28%), but also to considerable improvements in terms of functional results. It is especially notable that the number of patients who were most severely disabled did not increase. In association with the craniectomy procedure, a cerebral pressure probe is inserted which comes to lie in the brain parenchyma. In this way, the ICP may be monitored postoperatively, making it possible to monitor effectively the therapeutic measures intended to combat the elevated cerebral pressure. After the edema has receded, reimplantation of the portion of skull which has been removed can take place after approximately 3–5 months.

With cerebellar infarctions, as well as complications involving fluid drainage with ensuing hydrocephalus, there is also the associated risk of brainstem compression due to the edema. Thus, in addition to occipital decompressive craniectomy, external systems for drainage of ventricular fluids are often inserted in patients suffering from these complications.

Infections

As mentioned above, stroke patients have an elevated risk of developing aspiration pneumonia. In particular, patients experiencing decreased levels of consciousness may aspirate saliva and are often unable to cough up secretions in the respiratory tract, ultimately resulting in the accumulation of the secretions. If no improvements can be made in spite of antibiotic therapy as well as nursing care and physical therapy, these patients will require intubation and temporary artificial respiration. If the swallowing impairment does not improve over the further course of the illness, and the danger of aspiration persists, or if long-term respiration is necessary, a tracheotomy is performed. In addition, these patients should be supplied with a PEG tube to facilitate enteral nutrition.

Patients requiring intensive medical care, including stroke patients, are fitted with indwelling urinary catheters. These patients, in whom urine retention is often an issue, tend to develop urinary infections more often than other patients, thus requiring antibiotic therapy.

Pulmonary Embolism and Deep Venous Thrombosis

In stroke patients, who are often bedridden, the risk of thrombosis and thus the associated risk of developing pulmonary embolism can be reduced by adequate hydration and early mobilization. In addition, antithrombosis stockings and subcutaneous heparin can be used as supplementary therapy; however, the effectiveness of compression stockings in stroke patients has thus far not been proven (Hacke et al. 2008a). If pulmonary embolism occurs in spite of these measures, further treatment must be decided after considering the associated risks and benefits.

Pressure Sores (Decubital Ulcers)

The risk of developing pressure sores (decubital ulcers) can be reduced by the use of special padding, and when necessary, air mattresses, frequent changes in position, optimization of the patient's nutritional status, or application of cream to the skin (European Stroke Organization 2009). If the patient develops decubital ulcers in spite of prophylactic measures, these should be treated topically (e.g., using modern wound dressings). In some cases, antibiotics or surgical therapy may prove necessary.

Seizures

Approximately 6% of stroke patients develop focal or secondary generalized seizures during the acute phase (Vespa et al. 2003). These patients should be treated with anticonvulsants for 3–6 months. Prophylactic use of anticonvulsants is not necessary (European Stroke Organization 2009).

Special Cases

Dissection of Arteries Supplying Blood to the Brain

General Information

Especially in young patients, dissection of the vessels that supply blood to the brain often represents the cause of the stroke. Here, either the vessel wall becomes torn, which leads to bleeding within the wall, or primary bleeding occurs in the vessel wall. In both instances, the hematoma results in a narrowing of the vessel lumen, and in some cases even complete occlusion. In addition, a thrombus can form in the vessel lumen in this region, which can give rise to embolic brain infarctions when it becomes either completely or partially detached. Often a dissection develops as the consequence of trauma; even the most minor of traumas is sufficient to cause this damage. In some patients, fibromuscular dysplasia is observed, which causes the thinning out of certain layers of the vessel wall.

Diagnostics

The use of MRI is key in diagnostics. Not only wall hematomas but also alterations in the vessel lumen can be depicted using this technique (stenoses, "spikey" occlusions, tears in the intima). If the findings are unclear, arterial angiography can be done. Doppler and duplex sonography can also depict a dissection, but at the present time these are not sufficient as the sole diagnostic procedures.

Therapy

The option of recanalization therapy (either medical, with rt-PA, or interventional) is always available for cases of dissection. In addition, anticoagulation therapy should be initiated as soon as possible, depending on the size of infarction (as a rule, starting with full heparinization and later switching to oral anticoagulation) and should be continued for approximately 3–6 (maximum 24) months. The recommended therapy is 100 mg aspirin. In cases of recurring ischemic events in particular, or when pseudoaneurysms are present, an invasive procedure may also be considered (Ringelstein et al. 2008).

Sinus and Cerebral Vein Thrombosis

General Information

Up to now, only treatment pertaining to occlusion in those regions supplied by arteries has been mentioned, occlusions which lead to ischemic strokes due to disturbances in the blood supply. There are, however, also patients in whom occlusion develops in the cerebral venous vascular territory, referred to as sinus and cerebral vein thrombosis, which gives rise to disturbed cerebral blood drainage. As the arterial blood flow is not affected, blood therefore accumulates as a consequence. The intracranial blood volume is thus increased, ICP rises, and cerebral blood flow decreases. This ultimately results in hypoxia in the affected regions and also leads to the development of venous infarctions and congestion-related bleeding.

Diagnostics

Within the context of sinus and cerebral vein thrombosis diagnostics, the CT scan and MRI are the methods of choice. With the help of these imaging techniques, blood congestion bleeding can be visualized, and CT or MR venography make it possible to see occlusion in veins as well. Only very rarely (especially with cortical vein thromboses) is cerebral angiography necessary. The presence of elevated D-dimers helps to support the diagnosis. Special coagulation tests and other laboratory results are an essential part of the diagnostic procedure.

Therapy

The method of choice is the immediate PTT-controlled full heparinization of the patient for 10–14 days. As an alternative, low molecular weight heparin may also be given, although it appears to be less effective (Haberl et al. 2008). Complete heparinization must also be used when intracerebral hemorrhage has already occurred in connection with the illness. The patients must receive regular neurological monitoring, as any neurological symptoms present may worsen over the further course of events. Often insufficient anticoagulation is the reason for this. If the patient's condition worsens in spite of effective anticoagulation, local thrombolysis using rt-PA or urokinase represents a therapy option (Haberl et al. 2008). Peaks in cerebral pressure can be treated with osmotherapeutic agents, and decompressive craniectomy may be performed in cases of massive cerebral edema. If the patient has developed septic sinus thrombosis, additional antibiotic therapy is required to treat the original infection; it may also be necessary to clean the infectious wound surgically. Following the heparin therapy, oral coagulation is recommended for 3–6 months; if any coagulopathy is present, then anticoagulation therapy must be lifelong. If epileptic seizures occur, these must also be appropriately treated. Prophylactic anticonvulsive therapy may also be considered, since the risk of developing seizures is elevated in these patients (Ferro et al. 2003).

Outlook

New fibrinolytic agents with potentially longer time windows are currently being tested (e.g., desmoteplase, ancrod, tirofiban). Another hopeful prospect is that of ultrasound-assisted lysis using rt-PA; an increase in the effectiveness of the lysis appears to be achieved during this procedure, associated with higher rates of recanalization (Alexandrov et al. 2004). This would allow the dosage of the thrombolytic agent to be reduced. There is, however, the added risk that bleeding may occur during ultrasound-assisted lysis. The use of adult neuronal stem cells is also currently being studied as a treatment option for ischemic stroke. Substances that were hoped to display neuroprotective characteristics have, however, not yet been able to live up to researchers' expectations. It may well be the case that a combination of such substances with therapeutic hypothermia would produce more favorable results.

Summary

As already mentioned at the beginning of the chapter, stroke patients are emergency patients. Through improved care options in stroke units and therapy in the form of rt-PA, the prognosis for these patients has improved considerably over the past few years. During the acute phase, the main emphasis is on the decision as to whether or not the patient should receive systemic thrombolysis. In this particular phase there is enormous pressure to act very quickly, as there is only a period of 4.5 hours in which to perform therapy. If the contraindications for thrombolysis are taken into consideration, patients who receive this form of therapy have a much improved prognosis. Local lysis should only be performed at specialized centers. During the acute phase, stroke patients undergo intensive monitoring in the stroke unit, and the patient's vital signs and neurological status are recorded at regular intervals. In addition to the speedy clarification of the cause of the ischemic infarction with the aid of additional tests, the therapy of any risk factors as part of a secondary prevention program plays a critical role during the further course of the illness and treatment. While the patient is still in the stroke unit, early rehabilitative measures (occupational therapy, speech therapy, physical therapy) may be initiated following the acute therapy. If the patient's condition worsens, with an associated reduction in level of consciousness, repetition of cerebral diagnostic procedures (expansion of the infarction zone, development of cerebral edema) becomes necessary, with further care taking place on an neurological intensive care ward. Procedures such as intubation, artificial respiration, and analgosedation may also prove necessary. Decompressive craniectomy may be performed as part of the therapy plan in the case of cerebral edema.

■ Therapy of Hemorrhagic Stroke

Approximately 20% of all cases of stroke are caused by bleeding. This type of stroke usually involves bleeding in the brain parenchyma or into the subarachnoidal space. In a few cases, subdural or epidural hematomas occur directly beneath the skull. The therapy of cerebral hemorrhage has undergone major improvements during the past few years, in particular due to improved monitoring of these patients and the employment of interventional techniques. Patients suffering hemorrhagic stroke have a less favorable prognosis than those with ischemic stroke.

Intracerebral or Parenchymatous Hemorrhage

General Information

As with ischemic stroke, intracerebral hemorrhage gives rise to several different symptoms, depending on its location. The primary cause of intracerebral hemorrhage is hypertension, and in this case bleeding is typically located in the basal ganglia, the pons, and the cerebellum. In addition, coagulation disturbances (due to anticoagulation, illness, or a genetic trait) play a role in this context. Bleeding may also occur in connection with intracranial vessel anomalies, tumors or metastases, or following trauma. In older patients, the cause of bleeding is often the condition of amyloid angiopathy, in which the buildup of amyloid deposits in the vessel wall can cause the wall to rupture. Alcohol abuse, too, is associated with an increased risk of intracerebral hemorrhage. Lastly, patients who have undergone thrombolysis due to ischemic stroke may also develop intracerebral hemorrhage. If bleeding occurs, certain neurological symptoms and signs first become apparent due to direct damage to the parenchyma. As a result of the pressure exerted on the surrounding tissue, circulation and blood supply is reduced and ischemic damage ensues. A perifocal edema begins to form around the area where the bleeding has occurred. ICP increases, leading in turn to a further decrease in the cerebral perfusion pressure, thus reducing cerebral perfusion, which in turn intensifies the cerebral edema. In contrast to ischemic stroke, there is no penumbra present along the edge of the bleeding site, that is, an endangered area which is still theoretically salvageable (Schellinger et al. 2003). In some of these patients, the bleeding intensifies during the first 6 hours. This is relevant because the patient's prognosis worsens as the blood volume increases. The mortality associated with a blood volume loss of 30 cm^3 and a score of over 9 on the Glasgow Coma Scale after 30 days is 19%; this figure increases to 91% when the blood volume is to be over 60 cm^3 and the score on the Glasgow Coma Scale is less than 8 (Broderick et al. 1993). The size of the initial edema also plays an important prognostic role (Gebel et al. 2002). If the bleeding is not limited to the cerebral parenchyma, but also extends into the ventricle system, then the patient's prognosis also worsens. As a rule, intracerebral hemorrhage occurs as individual points of bleeding, but in some patients multiple bleeding sites are found when initial diagnostic procedures are performed. In these cases the cause is often associated with such conditions as amyloid angiopathy, sinus thrombosis, or vasculitis.

Diagnostics

It is not possible to distinguish intracerebral hemorrhage from ischemic stroke solely on the basis of clinical findings. Imaging diagnostics must therefore be performed immediately, in order to initiate specific therapeutic measures. The cranial CT scan is the method of choice when depicting recent intracerebral hemorrhage. In contrast to ischemic infarction, in which case a clear demarcation does not develop until later in the course of the illness, bleeding shows up even in the initial images as light, hyperdense areas with a dark border zone indicating the surrounding edema (**Fig. 3.2**). During the further course of events, the hematoma is reabsorbed; this is seen in the corresponding CT scan as a decrease in density. Cranial MRI scan is helpful to clarify atypically located areas of bleeding, that is, regions other than those typical of hypertensive bleeding. Tumor bleeding occasionally appears with a surrounding edema, which is quite pronounced even at an early stage. In some instances, however, a tumor as the cause of the bleeding cannot be clearly detected, in which case follow-up should take place after the blood mass has been reabsorbed. Blood vessel anomalies, among other findings, can also be detected with the help of MRI angiography. Digital subtraction angiography may also prove necessary to determine the cause of bleeding in some cases. This method should always be used when there is no previous history of hypertension, when the patient is young, and when the bleeding is in an atypical location and is considered to be hypertensive bleeding. While the initial imaging procedures are taking place, the patient's blood count, coagulation, liver and renal values are determined. In young patients, drug screening should also take place.

Therapy

Conservative Therapy

The basic therapy for patients suffering intracerebral hemorrhage does not differ greatly from that for patients with ischemic stroke. The European Stroke Initiative (Steiner et al. 2006) recommends that these patients be cared for in a stroke unit or, if necessary, in an intensive care unit. The patients' vital signs and neurological status must be monitored continuously. A standardized reporting scale

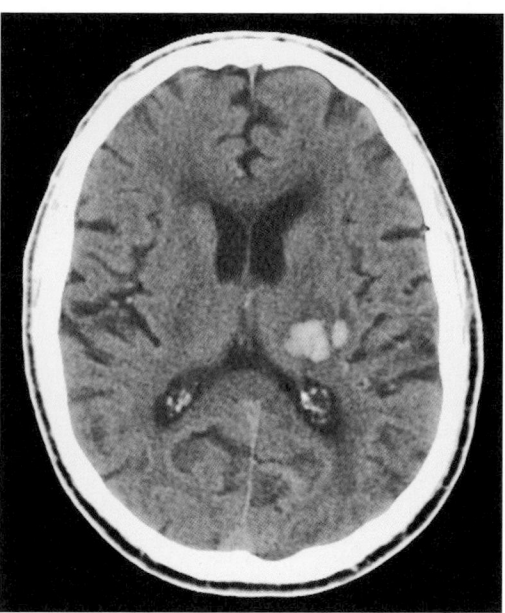

Fig. 3.2   Bleeding in the thalamus, left side.

(e.g., the NIHSS) should also be used to assess the status of these patients. The reason for this is the imminent risk of increased bleeding, even in patients who display only very mild neurological signs. Such an increase in the blood volume was observed in 38% of patients within 20 hours after the first cranial CT scan was performed (Brott et al. 1997). Sufficient oxygenation is crucial and, if values are too low, oxygen must be administered. To reduce the risk of aspiration and to improve the level of oxygenation, elective intubation should be considered at an early point. With respect to the management of the patient's blood pressure, it is generally recommended that systolic values of over 180 mmHg should be lowered (to reduce the risk of repeated bleeding); the CPP (= mean arterial pressure [MAP] – intracerebral pressure [ICP]) should not be allowed to drop to below 70 mmHg, to guarantee sufficient cerebral perfusion (Steiner et al. 2008). Invasive blood pressure measurement is a more effective form of monitoring the patient's blood pressure. For fluid balance, the aim is a state of euvolemia. Further measures include analgesia. Elevated body temperatures are to be treated appropriately. In addition, blood glucose levels must be determined at regular intervals and corrected if necessary. Early enteral nutrition should also be an aim. If the patient has difficulty in swallowing and/or a reduced level of consciousness, then nutrition must be given by way of a stomach tube or a PEG tube.

When the patient has suffered intracerebral hemorrhage, there is a high probability that symptomatic seizures will occur. This has been shown to be the case in 28% of patients during the first 72 hours, as recorded by continuous EEG measurements (Vespa et al. 2003). In connection with these findings, over half of the patients experienced nonconvulsive seizures, that is, there were no motor signs accompanying a loss of consciousness which would have indicated that a seizure was taking place—a condition that cannot be diagnosed without the aid of EEG readings. As patients who have had seizures tend to recover more slowly, anticonvulsive therapy must be given at an early stage, and prophylactic treatment may also be considered. In addition to the types of treatment already mentioned, measures pertaining to the prevention of pneumonia and pressure sores are also taken.

If any coagulation disturbances arise, they must be treated immediately. If the patient's coagulation disorder is drug-related, the medication must be promptly discontinued. If the bleeding is related to oral anticoagulation, the patient is given coagulation factors such as fresh frozen plasma (FFP) or prothrombin complex concentrate (PPSB) and vitamin K, whereby the latter displays delayed effects. In cases of bleeding associated with heparin treatment, the effects can be reversed by the use of the antagonist protamine sulfate. In instances of thrombocytopenia, thrombocyte concentrates are administered. As the patient's coagulation values begin to normalize, the risk of thrombosis and pulmonary embolism increases. In connection with thrombosis prophylaxis using heparin, the principal risk is that bleeding-associated complications may increase. At present, however, it is recommended that thrombosis prophylaxis using heparin should be initiated in stable patients starting on the second day (Albers et al. 2004). With regard to the risk of repeated bleeding, the practice of administering recombinant coagulation factor VIIa (rFVIIa) has been examined in the context of two studies. A reduction in the volume of bleeding was achieved, but this did not lead to an improvement in the clinical or functional results; in addition, the occurrence of thromboembolic events increased (Mayer et al 2005, Mayer et al. 2008). The use of rFVIIa therefore cannot be recommended at present.

A reduced level of consciousness, as well as headaches, nausea, and vomiting, indicate an increase in ICP. The cause of this may be the bleeding itself, the surrounding edema, and/or the accumulation of cerebrospinal fluid. In this case, the decision to insert a cerebral pressure probe or external ventricular drainage system should be made early, especially in patients who have a reduced level of consciousness, are on artificial respiration, or are sedated. For the treatment of edema, general and medicinal measures can be used which are described in the section on "Therapy of Complications" (p. 38), in particular the use of osmotherapeutic agents such as mannitol, temporary hyperventilation, and the use of barbiturates under EEG monitoring. As with ischemic stroke, the use of steroids is not recommended for the treatment of hemorrhagic stroke.

The decision as to whether, and when, any necessary anticoagulation therapy (e.g., following implantation of a mechanical heart valve) may be resumed after intracerebral hemorrhage has occurred, is a difficult one, which has to be made during the course of the illness and treatment (especially when the initial bleeding occurred during anticoagulation therapy). In each case, the individual risks and benefits must be carefully considered. Should the decision be made to initiate anticoagulation therapy, this may be started after 10–14 days in stable patients (European Stroke).

Operative Therapy

The question of which intercerebral hemorrhage patients should undergo surgery remains controversial. There is general agreement with regard to patients whose bleeding has extended into the ventricular system, or where the blood mass disturbs intracerebral fluid circulation, causing fluid to accumulate. In these patients an external ventricle drainage system (EVD) should be inserted to drain the fluid. This also makes it possible to monitor the patient's ICP by way of the drainage system. If the bleeding extends into the ventricular system, blood clots may sometimes block the tube, preventing drainage and requiring the insertion of a new drainage system. An EVD alone is, however, not sufficient to accelerate the reabsorption rate of the intraventricular blood. To achieve this, intraventricular application of a fibrinolytic agent (urokinase, rt-PA) is required. Whether or not this also yields improved functional results is still under investigation.

Patients who have suffered cerebellar hemorrhage should also undergo surgery, because in this case local pressure damages the brainstem, subsequently leading to accumulation of intracerebral fluid due to compression of the fluid drainage outlets. If the cause of bleeding is a blood vessel anomaly (e.g., angioma, aneurysms), then this should be treated neurosurgically and/or interventionally.

For all other patients, no such rules can be made as to who should receive surgical treatment. The problems presented by surgery, in addition to the injury inflicted on healthy parenchyma in addition to the already damaged tissue, include the increased risk of repeat bleeding, since the original tamponade effect caused by the bleeding is effectively cancelled out by the removal of the blood mass. The question of whether or not operative therapy improves the results in this case has been addressed by several studies. In the STICH (Surgical Trial in Intracerebral Haemorrhage) study, conservative and operative therapy options were compared for the treatment of patients with supratentorial bleeding (Mendelow et al. 2005). These author found that only patients with the most superficial bleeding sites profited from surgery. Results for the other patients were not significantly different. It should be mentioned, however, that the patients involved in this study were those for whom the treating physicians were not certain at the outset as to which form of therapy (conservative or operative) should be chosen. Surgery is currently recommended for superficial, minor cases of bleeding and for patients with progressive deterioration and loss of consciousness (Steiner et al. 2006). So far, studies have shown that patients with bleeding occurring at deeper levels do not benefit from surgery. If surgery is opted for, an open technique can be adopted. If an extensive hematoma has already developed, the cranial bone is not replaced after the procedure. There have also been attempts to drain the hematoma by means of endoscopic procedures. Another option for hematomas, even those located directly within the parenchymal tissue, is the local application of a fibrinolytic agent and regular aspiration of the blood mass as blood volume-reducing measures; however, further studies are necessary for this form of therapy.

Subarachnoid Hemorrhage

General Information

Bleeding into the subarachnoidal space usually occurs following the rupture of an aneurysm or a basal artery, or due to arteriovenous malformations. It may also occur in connection with coagulation disturbances or following cerebrocranial trauma. In the case of the latter, the question often arises as to whether the subarachnoid hemorrhage (SAH) occurred because of the trauma, or if it possibly represented the actual cause of the trauma. In around 20% of cases of SAH, intracerebral hemorrhage is detected as well. As a rule, the initial bleeding leads to dramatic symptoms; many patients become comatose immediately following the onset of bleeding. Blood collecting in the subarachnoidal space is subsequently reabsorbed, but does have the result, in some patients, of causing adhesions in the arachnoid granulations. Hydrocephalus may develop as a consequence of the decreased rate of fluid reabsorption. Another problem is the development of vasospasms, which generally occur after the third to the fifth day, and which nearly always last up to 3 weeks. Depending on their severity, these vasospasms may even lead to major ischemic strokes, due to the associated reduction in cerebral circulation. Patients suffering SAH often display cardiac arrhythmia as well.

Diagnostics

If SAH is suspected, a cranial CT scan (with CT angiography) is performed initially. As an alternative, MRI may also be used, especially for clarification of differential diagnoses. If no subarachnoidal blood can be seen using the available imaging techniques, but there is a strong suspicion of SAH on the basis of clinical findings, a lumbar puncture must be performed. If the cerebrospinal fluid is found to be normal, SAH can be safely ruled out. The best results in terms of detection of aneurysms are achieved by means of arterial angiography (depiction of four vessels) (**Fig. 3.3**). In addition, vasospasms can also be visualized using this method. In up to 20% of patients the source of the bleeding cannot be located in spite of extensive diagnostic efforts. If the initial angiographic find-

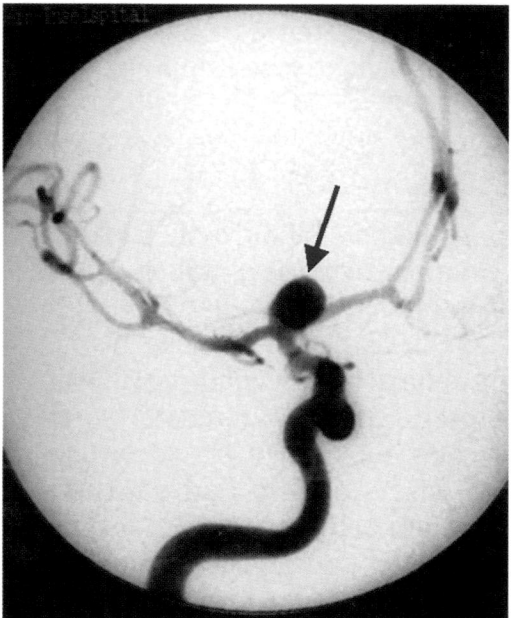

Fig. 3.3   Angiography: aneurysm located where the internal carotid artery divides.

ings do not show any signs of aneurysm, follow-up angiography is often performed during the later course of treatment in those patients who have suffered nonperimesencephalic SAH. The cause of perimesencephalic SAH, in which the blood fills only that part of the subarachnoid space surrounding the mesencephalon, is usually venous bleeding; follow-up angiography is therefore not recommended in this particular case. Accelerated blood flow, indicating the presence of vasospasms, can be detected by the use of transcranial Doppler/ duplex sonography. This method is also suitable for monitoring the patient's further progress and recovery.

Therapy

If an aneurysm has been detected and located, it must be treated immediately, because of the high risk of repeated bleeding. Two procedures are available for this:
1. Surgical clipping, performed by a neurosurgeon.
2. Insertion of platinum coils into the aneurysm by an experienced neuroradiologist.

Surgical clipping involves attaching a clip to the "neck" of the aneurysm, thus separating it from the main blood flow. In the coiling procedure, spiral platinum coils are placed in the aneurysm, guided by angiography. Blood then coagulates at this site, with the result that the blood stops flowing through the aneurysm. The choice of procedure should be made by an interdisciplinary team, drawing on the input of neurosurgeons, neuroradiologists, and neurologists. In the case of ruptured aneurysms whose location makes interventional therapy the most likely option, coiling is recommended (Steinmetz et al. 2008). When coils are used, it is sometimes necessary to insert a stent to protect the vessel lumen. In addition— and this is where the coiling procdure differs from clipping—heparin and/or thrombocyte aggregation inhibitors are administered during and after the placement of the coils. These measures are designed to prevent the formation of thrombi at those parts of the coils that have direct contact with the blood in the vessel lumen.

It is generally accepted that the patient must be on strict bed rest until the aneurysm can be treated. During this time, the patient's neurological status must be recorded regularly in order to detect any worsening of his or her condition (e.g., associated with repeated incidents of bleeding) as quickly as possible. Coagulation inhibitors must be discontinued; medications may be prescribed in the context of thrombosis prophylaxis after the aneurysm has been treated. In addition, the patient's vital signs should be monitored continuously, using invasive measures to determine blood pressure if necessary. Care should also be taken to maintain a sufficient level of oxygenation. Analgesics (including opiates) may be generously used. As a state of hypovolemia can favor the development of vasospasms, euvolemia, initially attained by the application of isotonic fluids, represents a further aim. Fluid balance can be regulated by the insertion of a central venous catheter and subsequent measurement of the patient's central venous pressure (>5 mmHg) (Grond 2005). The systolic blood pressure should not exceed 140 mmHg in patients with otherwise normal blood pressure. After the aneurysm has been treated (e.g., in connection with the treatment of vasospasms), considerably higher values are tolerated. Achieving and maintaining normoglycemia is also the aim in patients suffering SAH. Any occurrence of fever must be appropriately treated. Constipation should be strictly avoided at all times. If the patient experiences epileptic seizures, anticonvulsive therapy should be initiated.

Depending on the clinical findings (or in case of deterioration of the patient's clinical status), the patient must be intubated. It must also be determined whether the insertion of an EVD is necessary to treat or prevent accumulation of cerebrospinal fluid. With the help of this system, intracranial fluid, which is produced, but no longer adequatly reabsorbed, is deflected outward through a special drainage system. Because of the risk of infection, the fluid that has been drained off should undergo microbiological examination, as well as a cell count. If fluid reabsorption does not normalize during the further course of recovery, a permanent solution is necessary in the form of a ventriculo-peritoneal shunt (which drains the fluid from the intracerebral ventricular system into the abdomen) or a ventriculo-atrial shunt (drainage into the right atrium of the heart).

To prevent vasospasms from occurring, as already mentioned, hypovolemia must be avoided. Nimodipine (taken for 21 days, from the time of admission) has proven most effective in treating this condition, but attention must be paid to the blood pressure-lowering effects of the medication. Vasospasms can also be reduced by treatment with the statin simvastatin (Lynch et al. 2005). Intracranial blood flow velocity should be monitored daily, up until the tenth day, using transcranial Doppler/duplex sonography. If vasospasms do develop (detected by Doppler as an increase in the flow velocity) there is the associated risk of the patient's developing stroke symptoms. Restoration of sufficient circulation can be attempted by means of what is known as "triple H" therapy (hypertensive hypervolemic hemodilution); however, this can only take place after the aneurysm has been treated. With this method, hypertension is achieved by means of catecholamines and hydroxyethylstarch (HAES) and isotonic fluids produce the effects of hypervolemia and hemodilution.

Continuous intensive monitoring of the patient is required, as there is an associated risk of pulmonary and cardiac complications. If this form of therapy does not produce the desired effect, namely, improvement of the patient's neurological symptoms, an attempt to achieve dilation of the vessel by transluminal balloon angioplasty is still possible as a last resort, particularly in the case of proximal vasospasms. Another therapeutic option is the local intra-arterial application of calcium antagonists or papaverin (Steinmetz et al. 2008).

If cerebral edema develops, it must be treated immediately. The therapeutic measures are the same as those for edema occurring in the context of ischemic stroke.

Summary

In patients suffering hemorrhagic stroke, the initial diagnosis is made by imaging techniques (CT scan, CT angiography, MRI, MR angiography). In many cases, it is possible to determine the probable cause of the bleeding with the help of these procedures. Depending on the cause, decisions are made as to further treatment options: conservative, operative with the aim of removing the blood mass, insertion of an EVD system, craniectomy, placement of a tube for the measurement of cerebral pressure, or interventional with the purpose of inserting a coil in an aneurysm or embolization of vessels in the case of vascular malformations. Patients suffering hemorrhagic stroke, like those suffering ischemic stroke, must undergo continuous monitoring of their vital signs and neurological status. EEG monitoring is also helpful, especially in patients whose level of consciousness is reduced or who are sedated). In patients suffering SAH, transcranial Doppler/duplex sonography must be done on a daily basis to assess the flow velocity in the affected blood vessels.

4 Early Mobilization: Opportunity or Risk?

Jan Mehrholz

But men may construe things after their fashion,
Clean from the purpose of the things themselves.
(William Shakespeare, Julius Caesar)

It is now generally known that the chances of survival for stroke patients can be increased, and their independence in the home environment can be maximized, through early multidisciplinary rehabilitation in the proper setting—that is, in stroke units (Stroke Unit Trialists' Collaboration 2007). However, it is still not understood why specialized stroke units are so effective. Is their success due to individual factors such as fast, specific acute care, or early mobilization approaches? Is it the result of physical therapeutic measures, or is it the multidisciplinary concept of the stroke unit as a whole that is so effective?

One explanation of why care in stroke units increases survival rates and encourages independence possibly lies in the speedy acute diagnostic procedures and the rapid treatment of secondary complications following stroke (Stroke Unit Trialists Collaboration 1997). Analyses have shown that so-called secondary complications, such as deep vein thrombosis of the leg or respiratory infections, which can be attributed to immobilization, are responsible for more than half of the mortality rate after the event (Langhorne and Dennis 1998, Sinha and Warburton 2000). In other words, early mobilization more effectively prevents secondary complications due to immobilization of the patient. Having fewer secondary complications in turn increases the patient's chances of survival and possibly improves competency in day-to-day life. Studies have demonstrated indirectly that the complication rate can be reduced by means of early mobilization (Indredavik et al. 1991, 1999).

Critical voices, on the other hand, also make themselves heard. They suggest, on the basis of animal experimentation, that early mobilization may possibly have unfavorable effects. Although the results of such animal experiments are not unequivocal or uniform, their basic message is that the area surrounding the infarction region (penumbra) may be damaged if the patient is mobilized too early (Schädler and Beer 2007). Although animal experimental studies sometimes use outdated methods and are controversial with-

in the scientific community (Nudo 2003), the results of such experiments, among others, have led to a sort of "therapeutic nihilism." Thus, recommendations exist which advocate the use of conservative therapy during the first 4–7 days of the acute phase and further suggest the placement of stroke patients flat on their backs during the first 24 hours and the elevation of the patients, starting with the head end of the bed, beginning only after that (Schädler and Beer 2007). Is "mobilization in bed" (patient on back, upper body elevated) really to be considered mobilization? According to many therapists' definition, mobilization involves at least sitting or standing. At this point it must be added that it is not possible to mobilize all patients at a very early stage.

Should we discourage the application of intensive physical therapy during the first 24 hours following stroke, on the basis of the above-mentioned arguments? It can be generally stated that, when considering the individualized therapy of stroke patients, the net benefits to the individual patient, and thus the risk–benefit ratio, should be carefully weighed. It is equally clear that patients who have suffered stroke are much too inactive in the first few weeks following the stroke, and spend too little time learning the motor skills conducive to active and further training.

There are, to date, no definitive randomized controlled studies extending beyond the scope and status of already existing animal experiments which suggest that early and/or intensive mobilization may be harmful to stroke patients. On the contrary: Julie Bernhardt, a physical therapist and scientist from Melbourne, Australia, is currently conducting what is possibly the most important study on early mobilization and movement therapy during the acute phase following stroke. The AVERT study (A Very Early Rehabilitation Trial) was presented at the World Confederation for Physical Therapy (WCPT) congress in 2007 and subsequently published in the highly acclaimed journal *Stroke* (Bernhardt et al. 2008). Bernhardt and colleagues conducted a multicenter randomized controlled double-blinded pilot study in Melbourne (Bernhardt et al. 2008). The patients included in the study had suffered stroke up to 24 hours previously, had blood pressure values between 120 and 220 mmHg, oxygen saturation greater than 92%, resting heart rate between 40 and 100 beats per minute, and no signs of fever (body temperature <38.5°C). Patients who were experiencing a recurrence of stroke, or with progressive deterioration of their general state of health, or with leg fractures, and those undergoing palliative treatment, were excluded from the study. All patients received individualized rehabilitation, including physical therapy, for the duration of their stay. During the first 14 days, these patients were all mobilized out of bed—either very early, within the first 24 hours following stroke (VEM, very early mobilization), or according to standard procedure (SC, standard care), that is, without early mobilization. The primary dependent variable of the study was survival after 3 months. The most important target criterion for determining feasibility was the attainment of a higher level of early mobilization.

At the onset, after 7 and 14 days, and after 3, 6, and 12 months, a blinded investigator recorded results according to the Modified Rankin Scale (MRS) (Lees 2003). The MRS was, as recommended, subdivided into just two outcomes: clinically significant, or favorable, results (score 0–2), and unfavorable results (score 3–5) (de Haan et al. 1995).

Secondary parameters were severe and mild side effects, falls, and other injuries. Likewise, deterioration in the patient's condition according to the European Progression Stroke Definition (Barber et al. 2004) using the Scandinavian Stroke Scale, patient exhaustion (Borg Scale) (Borg 1970), and fall in blood pressure, were recorded. In addition, the investigators also examined whether the therapy scheme of the control group underwent any changes due to the installation of the study group ("contamination").

A total of 71 patients were included in phase II of the study (practicability study): 38 patients in the VEM group and 22 in the SC group. The patients included had an average age of 75 years and represented a relatively wide spectrum, as patients with both severe and mild cases of stroke were included in the study. At the beginning of the study, the two groups did not display differences with regard to important prognostic factors (Bernhardt et al. 2008). After 3 months, comparable numbers of patients had survived in both groups. Patients who had died tended to have been much more severely affected immediately following the stroke, compared to those who survived. According to the original plan, the patients in the VEM group were mobilized twice as long (167 minutes versus 69 minutes, $p = 0003$) and earlier (on average, 18 hours versus 31 hours following stroke). The groups did not show differences with regard to more severe side effects or complications. However, significantly fewer mild complications were found after 3 months: 61 in the VEM group versus 76 in the SC group ($p = 0.04$).

When the severity of the stroke was also included in the calculations, the proportion of patients in the VEM group with clinically favorable results was in some cases significantly higher than in the control group. The likelihood of obtaining favorable rehabilitation results after 3 and 6 months and after 1 year is, according to this study, markedly higher for patients undergoing early mobilization than for nonmobilized patients. The initial results produced by the AVERT study clearly demonstrate the following:

- There is no increased risk for stroke patients undergoing intensified early mobilization during the first 24 hours following the event.
- Early mobilization out of bed, that is, early physical therapy, is practicable.
- Early mobilization in a vertical position may produce even more favorable results, compared with a "wait and see" strategy.

Although these are only initial results of phase II of the AVERT study, plans exist for expanding it to include a total of 2104 patients. At present, there are only a few high-quality studies pertaining to this subject (with the exception of AVERT); a comprehensive and systematic Cochrane review appeared in 2008, available in the Cochrane Library (Bernhardt et al. 2009).

While further results of AVERT are awaited with interest, it is unlikely that the overall evaluation will produce drastically different results. We may conclude that the general suspicion of causing damage to stroke patients by practicing procedures too early can be maintained only under certain conditions. A new paradigm during the acute phase following stroke therefore appears to be required. We now know that very early mobilization during the first 24 hours following stroke is not harmful and, moreover, is both feasible and practicable. Yet—what is it that characterizes physical therapy practices during the acute phase following stroke? What are the most important "ingredients," and how is early mobilization to be practiced?

Although the acute medical treatment of stroke patients has been described extensively and in great detail, it is nevertheless remarkable how little we still know about early mobilization practices, and specifically, early mobilization following stroke. Initial results describing early mobilization of stroke patients are available, and these are sobering (Bernhardt et al. 2004, 2007a, 2007b). More than 50% of all patients are not only left alone most of the day (>60%), but are also inadequately treated for the remainder of the time, as their treatment does not involve any mobilization (>50% lying in bed, 28% sitting in a wheelchair). Results show that stroke patients may spend a mere 13% of the day practicing and performing potential activities that are useful in terms of the specific course of their illness and which support the rehabilitative process. In short, adequate therapy concepts, integrated into a rehabilitative program that is individually designed to suit each stroke patient, are badly needed (Carr and Shepherd 2003, 2010; see also Chapter 5).

5 Optimizing Functional Motor Recovery after Stroke

Janet H. Carr and Roberta B. Shepherd

A man who loves practice without theory is like the sailor who boards ship without a rudder and compass and never knows where he may cast.

(Leonardo da Vinci)

In this chapter we describe a scientific framework that forms the basis of clinical practice. Optimal functional recovery is the ultimate goal of neurorehabilitation after a brain lesion. The contribution of physical therapy to this process is the training of motor control with a particular focus on the optimization of motor performance in everyday actions. Methods used are designed to provide a stimulus to learning and to the acquisition of skill, and to increase muscle strength, endurance, aerobic fitness, and general wellbeing. Training is based on scientific research on impairments, and the secondary adaptations associated with physical inactivity; biomechanics, motor learning and cognitive science; exercise science; and the recognition of factors that may influence brain reorganization after injury (Carr and Shepherd 2003, 2010). It is the obligation of all health professionals to use current scientific evidence to improve the care of patients and to change clinical methods as knowledge changes.

■ Introduction

Experimental work indicates that physical activity in a stimulating environment is likely to facilitate neural reorganization and functional recovery. There is evidence that rehabilitation centers do not provide sufficient opportunity for physical activity and training to generate optimal recovery. Changes are needed in the delivery of rehabilitation to provide more active and intensive training, in an environment that promotes physical and mental activity and the acquisition of skill in functional actions. An environment is needed in which, early after stroke, the patient can be an active learner with opportunities for intensive exercise and training and not a passive recipient of therapy.

The goals of rehabilitation cannot be achieved if emphasis remains on one-to-one therapy for a short period each day. Good planning can ensure that each patient is physically and mentally engaged on learning how to regain former skills. Provision of small-group training and semi-supervised practice (one or two therapist/aides) can extend the time spent in meaningful and intensive rehabilitation.

■ Acute Stage after Stroke

The impact of a stroke on the individual, the family, and the workforce is substantial. Several systematic reviews have found that care on a stroke unit significantly reduces death and disability after stroke compared to conventional care in general wards (Indredavik et al. 1997, National Stroke Foundation 2010, Stroke Trialists' Collaboration 2001). A specialized stroke unit provides support, encouragement, and educational programs for patients and their families, with staff who have a special interest in the management of stroke, who are trained to provide coordinated multidisciplinary rehabilitation, and who have access to current scientific knowledge and continuing professional education programs.

Immediately after stroke it is difficult to predict the extent of eventual recovery. There are patients who improve unexpectedly and others who do poorly despite having a good prognosis. In Australia, of those who have had a stroke, approximately one-third of patients make a complete recovery, one-third are left with a disability that causes some reliance on others for assistance with everyday activities, and one-third die within the first 12 months (Clinical Guidelines for Stroke Rehabilitation and Recovery 2005). Many stroke survivors require ongoing support in the community and consideration should be given to planning and organizing ongoing postdischarge opportunities for training and exercise.

The central aspect of rehabilitation is the provision of a coordinated program by an interdisciplinary team of health professionals, doctors, nurses, physical therapists, occupational therapists, speech pathologists, and dietitians. The team may be expanded to include other disciplines, for example psychologists and/or neuropsychologists. The person with stroke and their family or friends should also be acknowledged as important members of the team. Working as a team enables occupational therapists and physical therapists with aides to work in the same environment, with agreed-upon goals and methods. Nurses and physicians have the opportunity to observe exercise and training sessions so they are aware of what individual patients can really achieve.

The impact of stroke on many body systems is particularly evident in the acute phase. Common complications include dysphagia or difficulty swallowing; urinary incontinence; communication deficits; injury to the paretic, unprotected shoulder; and excessive attentional focus toward the right side. It is necessary for all members of the team to be aware of and understand the effect of these on the patient and on their overall management, so that the most appropriate professional can be organized to give therapy. Rehabilitation is specific for each individual's needs, and includes not only a motor training program, but also programs designed to overcome visual, cognitive, perceptual, swallowing, communication, and continence difficulties, and depression.

Early and proactive physical therapy can reduce the likelihood of negative sequelae such as disuse weakness, soft tissue contracture, learned nonuse, physical deconditioning, and persistence and habituation of perceptual-cognitive impairments. Active training in sitting in the acute phase is critical to prevent complications associated with bed rest, and to stimulate the patient to reorient with gravity. Early mobilization can reduce secondary thromboembolic events, pneumonia, and mortality in stroke (Johansson 2000). Having the patient upright and active is also necessary to activate

their attentional state. It is possible that the longer the delay in starting active training of actions in sitting and standing, the more likely it is that the patient will become fearful and apprehensive at dealing with gravity. Active and frequent rehabilitation therefore starts as soon as vital signs are stable. Patients should be assisted to mobilize (i.e., sitting out of bed, standing up, and walking) as early and frequently as possible (Bernhardt et al. 2009), with monitoring of oxygen saturation, blood pressure, consciousness, and heart rate.

As soon as possible the focus changes from a sickness orientation to emphasize exercise and training planned around the patient's greatest need, which is to regain effective functioning in daily life. The general aims of physical therapy are to encourage patients to become physically and mentally active again, with a strong and flexible musculoskeletal system enabling them to regain the pleasures inherent in being physically and mentally active.

The rate and extent of mobilization depend on the patient's condition. However, even a weak person can be assisted to sit up with legs over the side of the bed, feet flat on the floor (**Fig. 5.1**). Active training is graded so the patient can experience early success—sitting with arms resting on a table enables even a very weak person to actively participate in controlling sitting balance. Since a firm surface is preferable to the compliant surface of a bed, a slide board and sheets can be used to move the patient on to a firm, height-adjustable surface. When necessary, a collar provides a more erect head position in sitting to encourage eye contact and spatial orientation. It is preferable that the patient is out of bed in sitting and standing (**Fig. 5.2a, b**), rather than spending time on bed mobility exercises in the supine position. Walking sideways around the bed builds confidence in shifting the weight in standing, loading the paretic limb, and regaining a sense of balance (**Fig. 5.3**).

The therapist records baseline motor performance, briefly estimates muscle strength and determines what actions the patient can attempt as improvements occur. The therapist's ability to establish contact with the patient through dialogue, positive feedback, and eye contact helps to generate a positive atmosphere and increase the patient's confidence (Talvitie 2000).

The typical stroke unit or rehabilitation environment is complex, unfamiliar, and unpredictable to individuals who suddenly find themselves there.

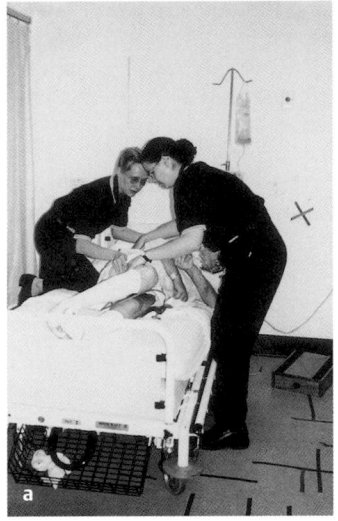
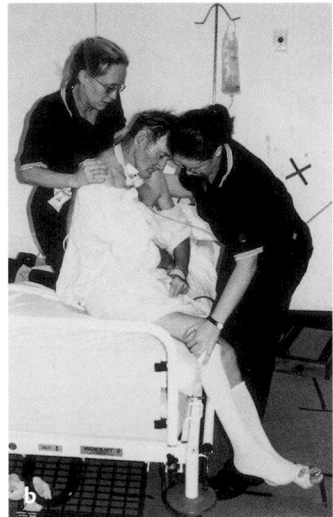
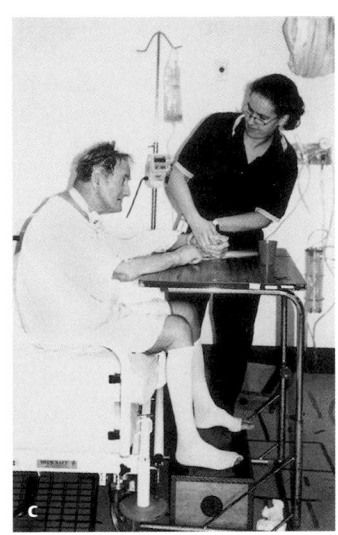

Fig. 5.1 a–c   Sitting over the side of the bed enables early physical activity in an erect position.
a, b The patient is assisted to turn on to his side and sit up.
c Feet are supported on a stool, arms on a table. The therapist encourages eye contact and vertical spatial orientation. The patient could only hold his head up momentarily—a soft collar would help provide a more erect sitting alignment. A firmer sitting surface would enable him to sit more upright.

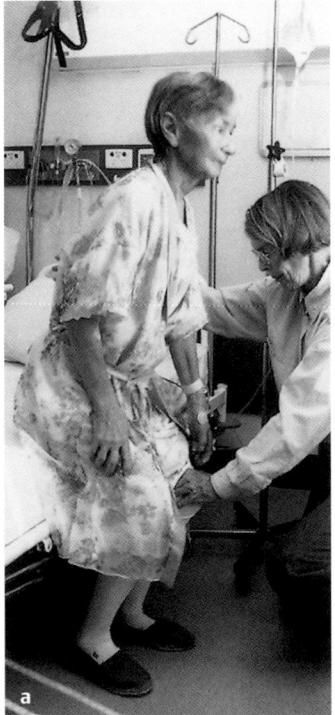
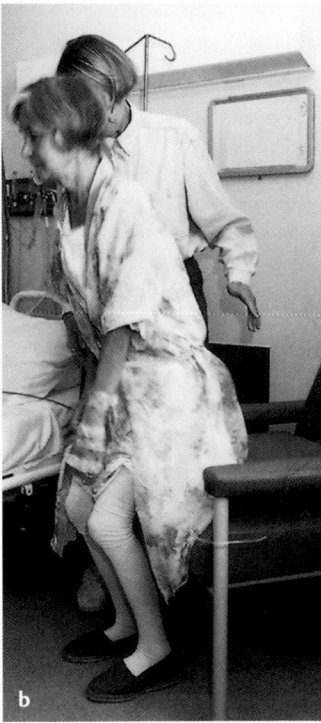
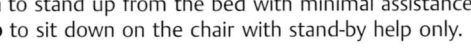
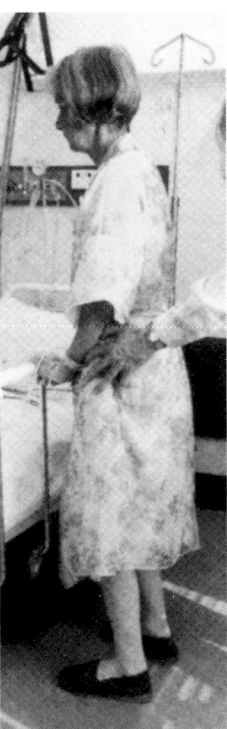

Fig. 5.2 a, b   The height of both the bed and chair are adjusted to enable the patient
a to stand up from the bed with minimal assistance,
b to sit down on the chair with stand-by help only.

Fig. 5.3   Walking sideways. The patient was able to practice walking around the bed semi-supervised and with the bed rail for support where necessary.

Patients have to get to know and interact with several different health professionals and other patients. This can be a stressful situation in itself, but after suffering a stroke, a patient is also coming to terms with a sense of loss and anxiety about the future. For a previously self-sufficient individual, adapting both to the disability and to the new environment may be difficult and can erode the feeling of competence.

Patient and family education is an integral part of rehabilitation. Education is introduced in the acute stage and reinforced during rehabilitation. It is adapted to the educational and cultural background of patient and family, the mental state of the patient, and to emotional factors that may interfere with learning. Discussions are held with the patient and family about their role in training and of the necessity for frequent, intensive, and vigorous physical activity. Families are encouraged to participate in training sessions. Since the patient and family are distressed and anxious in the acute phase, the opportunity to gain information needs to be ongoing. Members of stroke support groups who have themselves experienced a stroke can be helpful in talking to the patient.

The major focus in stroke rehabilitation research is typically on in-patient care. However, wider issues need to be addressed, especially as long-term disability and social and emotional sequelae of stroke affect the quality of life after discharge. Good discharge planning is crucial for reintegration into the community, for maximizing independence and participation, and for minimizing social isolation. The transfer of responsibility for management from in-patient facility to the community can be difficult; too little attention and resources may be provided. Many individuals are reported to suffer a loss of rehabilitation gains after they are discharged from rehabilitation (Paolucci et al. 2001) and to feel abandoned. A survey in the United Kingdom showed a paucity of follow-up services beyond the most basic level of community therapy or support. This was compounded by poor communication between professionals and between patients, carers, and professionals; high levels of patient dissatisfaction; and low expectations by professionals of patients' abilities (Tyson and Turner 2000).

Major oversights in postdischarge stroke management can include lack of community exercise facilities for the disabled, as well as lack of carer support and poor access to transport. There has been little emphasis on the obvious need for individuals with disability to continue with exercise and training postdischarge, not only to maintain progress but also to progress their functional abilities and levels of physical fitness. Participation in regular physical activity can have significant effects on increasing physical independence and quality of life, reducing the risk of falls, and preventing a recurrent stroke or a further cardiac event (Gordon et al. 2004).

Investigations of exercise programs provide evidence that many people, even several years after stroke, are able to make positive gains in strength, mobility, arm use fitness, endurance, and skill (Duncan et al. 2003, Eng et al. 2003, Harris et al. 2009, Pang et al. 2006a, Rimmer et al. 2000, Teixeira-Salmela et al. 2001). Furthermore, several of these programs had an impact upon activities such as getting on and off a bus or socializing with friends away from home—activities considered meaningful to the individuals concerned. Interviews with subjects and their families suggest that the gains in quality of life seemed to be critical factors in reintegrating stroke survivors into society (Eng et al. 2003, Rimmer et al. 2000, Teixeira-Salmela et al. 2001).

Friendships that develop among participants as members of a group can provide encouragement and support. A community-based stroke group can play an important role. For example, the Stroke Recovery Association of Australia is a social and self-help organization for stroke individuals and their families. Weekly group meetings organized by members at different locations provide emotional support and assistance in the transition back into the community, and in some cases these groups offer weekly exercise sessions and provide talking practice and encouragement for those with dysphasia.

■ Impairments and Adaptations

Effective motor performance in daily life requires sufficient coordination, balance, muscular strength, soft tissue extensibility, endurance, and cardiovascular fitness to fulfil the requirements of such actions as standing up and sitting down, walking, reaching, and bimanual grasping and manipulation. After a stroke affecting the motor sys-

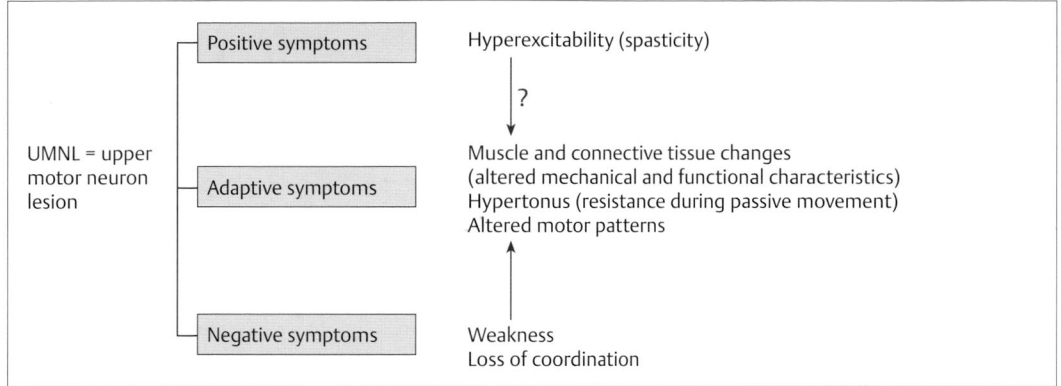

Fig. 5.4   Classification of positive and negative features of the UMN lesion and relationship to adaptive changes.

tem, the major impairments affecting function are muscle paralysis or weakness and loss of motor control. In addition, postlesion adaptive changes to muscle morphology, contractility and extensibility in response to paresis and disuse are major contributors to dysfunction.

Recent technological developments and scientific findings are enabling a clarification of the disordered mechanisms underlying impairments and of the extent and effect of postlesion adaptations to the neural and musculoskeletal systems that increase disability (**Fig. 5.4**). Contemporary scientific advances are driving a re-evaluation of the functional significance of different clinical signs.

Recent research findings are also driving a shift in the focus of rehabilitation. As part of this process, the current focus in neurological physical therapy has shifted from spasticity (reflex hyperactivity) as the major cause of disability to muscle weakness, lack of motor control, and secondary adaptive muscle changes. Rehabilitation professionals are developing methods of training to increase muscle strength, muscle contractility and motor control in functional actions, and to preserve soft tissue length and flexibility, minimizing the adaptive changes to muscle and spinal mechanisms that have negative effects. The focus in neurorehabilitation is now on a more active, intensive, and vigorous training program that begins early and requires the active mental and physical participation of the individual. The program focuses on optimizing task performance, specifically in terms of increasing muscle strength and energy efficiency for everyday actions. There are increas-

ing numbers of clinical studies reporting positive effects of intensive task-oriented training and exercise to improve muscle force generation, motor control, and performance.

Below is a summary of the mechanisms underlying impairments, the plastic changes occurring adaptively aftr stroke and their relationship to disability. An understanding of mechanisms underlying the physical disabilities provides a guide to poststroke physical therapy programs and gives a focus for training and exercise.

Weakness

Muscle force produced for an action is normally dependent on the number and type of motor units recruited; characteristics of the motor unit discharge, including the speed at which force is generated, called power (power = force × angular velocity); and the characteristics and size (cross-sectional area) of muscle. The tension output of a skeletal muscle results from its length, contraction velocity, and level of activity. We normally increase muscle force by increasing the number of active motor units and the firing rates and frequencies of those active units. Strength is therefore a neuromuscular phenomenon and, in terms of function, is activity-dependent. Muscles produce the appropriate amount of force for the particular action being performed, timing force production across joints as demanded both by the action and by the mechanical characteristics of the musculoskeletal linkage. The degree of muscle strength necessary for daily life is therefore not an absolute measure but is relative to the action being performed. For example, generation and control of quadriceps extensor force may be enough to straighten the knee in sitting but not for raising the body mass in standing up from a seat.

Paresis or paralysis after an upper motor neuron (UMN) lesion is defined as decreased motor unit recruitment with resultant inability or difficulty voluntarily recruiting skeletal muscle to generate movement (Gracies 2005a). Weakness is commonly the most disabling symptom after an UMN lesion. It arises from two sources: primarily from the lesion itself, as a result of a decrease in descending inputs converging on the final motoneuron population; secondarily from postlesion adaptations to disuse and decreased muscle activity. Weakness after stroke is characterized by impaired motor unit synchronization, slowness in generating peak force, and difficulty in generating the necessary force amplitude for an action and sustaining force output. Decreased central input results in a reduction in the number of motor units available for recruitment and a reduction in the firing rate of motor units (motor units normally fire at the rate necessary for fusion of twitches) (Frontera et al. 1997, Gemperline et al. 1995). These reduce the efficiency of muscle contractions, contribute to slowness of movement, perception of increased effort and fatigue and, with impaired motor unit synchronization, contribute to disorganized motor control. This failure of voluntary activation illustrates the direct effects on skeletal muscle of the neurological lesion (Newham 2005). Although decreased amplitude of force affects function, it is really the speed of force generation (power) that is the most critical parameter for effective motor performance. This is discussed below.

It is clear that deficits in the generation of force contribute significantly to functional disability (Farmer et al. 1993; see review by Ng and Shepherd 2000). However, since skeletal muscle adapts to the level of use imposed on it (Lieber 1988), secondary sources of weakness arise as a consequence of immobility (Farmer et al. 1993). In addition, secondary changes occur in the properties of motor units and in the morphological and mechanical properties of muscle itself.

Adaptive muscle length changes occurring after stroke can compound the effects of muscle weakness. The length of a muscle fiber is proportional to the speed at which a muscle can contract and relax. Any loss of muscle length with changes to sarcomeres will therefore result in reduced contractile speed. Changes in muscle stiffness (a mechanical response to a load on a noncontracting muscle; ratio of tension developed when a muscle is stretched) also affect contractile speed (Newham 2005). In a normally activated muscle, the muscle's length affects its ability to generate force. Muscle length affects actin and myosin overlap and the length of the moment arm (Winters and Kleweno 1993, Zajac 1989). Most torque is generated at mid-length and least torque at shortest length (Herzog et al. 1991); for example, plantar flexor muscles generate less torque as their length decreases.

Differential degrees of muscle weakness according to both joint angle and task have been reported in clinical studies. A person may be able to generate sufficient muscle force to bear weight in standing without leg collapse when the knee is flexed a few degrees, but not be able to hold the knee extended at 0° (Winter 1985). Ada and colleagues (2000) reported this differential effect of muscle length on strength in the upper limb, showing greater weakness of elbow flexors and extensors at shorter lengths.

Although the stroke lesion produces motor impairments on one side of the body, it has been shown that muscle activity on the other side of the body may also be affected. For example, bilateral muscle activation failure has been reported after stroke (Newham and Hsiao 2001), and significant weakness has been reported in muscles of the nonparetic lower limb (a 30% decrease in knee extensor strength) within the first week after stroke (Harris et al. 2001). The latter authors considered this to be a secondary weakness, attributing it to the effects of disuse, specifically lack of exercise and nutritional support. One advantage of task-oriented training programs is that the focus is on functional actions that naturally involve both right and left limbs, such as standing up, or walking on a treadmill. In these weightbearing exercises, both lower limbs are exercised and muscles throughout the body are trained to generate and control appropriate forces. Such a program can provide a means of minimizing secondary weakness, but must start early.

Contemporary research has found no evidence for several long-held therapy beliefs. Weakness is not primarily due to spasticity of antagonists (Newham and Hsiao 2001, Sahrmann and Norton 1977), and strength training has not been found to increase spasticity (Ada et al. 2006b, Sharp and Brouwer 1997). No pattern of muscle weakness has been found (Colebatch and Gandevia 1989), and no consistent difference between proximal and distal muscles, upper and lower limbs, flexors and extensors (Andrews and Bohannon 2000, Duncan et al. 1994). Rather, distribution of weakness may result from site and extent of lesion.

Loss of Motor Control

The mechanisms that underlie weakness of force generation also produce loss of motor control, that is, incoordination of limb segments during multi-segmental actions. There have been relatively few neurophysiological investigations of disordered motor control following stroke. However, kinematic and kinetic studies of reaching, walking, and standing up are providing insights into disordered control of limb segments during everyday actions. Training of motor control in the context of specific actions is a critical part of therapy that aims to train an individual toward optimal functional effectiveness. To implement this training the clinician needs an understanding of biomechanics and the mechanisms of dyscontrol.

Motor output is both reduced and disorganized and muscle activity may no longer be well enough coordinated to meet task and environmental demands, due to an impaired ability to fine-tune interactions between muscles (Kautz and Brown 1998). Coordination is not present in the motor act itself but rather in its interaction with the changing environment (Latash and Latash 1994).

After stroke it is typical for muscles to be slow to contract and relax. The time taken for a single quadriceps twitch to relax to half its peak force is significantly longer in the paretic than in the nonparetic limb (Newham et al. 1996). Slow angular velocities have been reported in knee flexion and extension (Davies et al. 1996). Several studies report that time taken to develop peak muscle force and to decrease it is impaired. In a study of individuals more than 1 year after stroke, McCrea and colleagues (2003) found that they took twice as long to reach peak torque with the paretic arm compared to their nonparetic arm and to able-bodied subjects. In other words, the ability to modulate force over time was impaired. Delayed contraction and relaxation times have been found to correlate significantly with physical disability (Chae et al. 2002) since the action being performed is disorganized and therefore ineffective. Canning and colleagues (1999) described a person who could generate peak elbow flexor torque of 9 N m, which was sufficient to lift her forearm and carry a small object. However, since it took her 7 seconds to reach peak torque, the strength of her elbow flexors was of limited functional use. There have been few studies specifically examining power output. One study of power output from quadriceps and hamstrings during leg cycling found abnormal timing of electromyelographic (EMG) activity in both muscles and less positive work (concentric) and more negative (eccentric) work than in able-bodied subjects (Kautz and Brown 1998). Olney (2005) investigated power output during gait and reported lower amplitudes and decreased speed of walking.

Cocontraction of muscles is commonly observed as the patient attempts to gain control over a limb. It is not itself abnormal. In able-bodied subjects, cocontraction is evident in active movement and increases when speed is increased. Cocontraction can illustrate lack of skill in able-bodied adults attempting a new or difficult task, decreasing as skill level increases (Enoka 1997). After acute brain lesion it can illustrate lack of skill in reorganizing action-specific muscle activation patterns in the presence of inadequate motor unit recruitment and muscle weakness. For example, a decrease in motor unit firing rate results in decreased muscle tension. Additional motor units may be recruited to enable greater force development. Hence stiffening the lower limb in stance can prevent limb collapse. Chae et al. (2002) reported a significant correlation between muscle weakness and the degree of cocontraction and motor disability.

However, cocontraction can also occur to an excessive degree, resulting from prolonged muscle activation; for example, carried over from agonist to antagonist phase in a reciprocal movement such as flexion-extension of the elbow (Kamper and Rymer 2001). Whether an abnormal degree of cocontraction illustrates motor control dysfunction or reflex hypersensitivity is not understood. Nevertheless, it is probable that the development of disabling cocontraction can be minimized or prevented by an exercise and motor training program designed to preserve the natural length of potentially short stiff muscles (Gracies 2005b).

Associated movements are unintended movements that accompany volitional movement but are not necessary for it. They may result from irradiation of neuronal excitation across the cortex or spinal cord during voluntary movement. They are seen in able-bodied individuals attempting complex tasks (Carey et al. 1983), under stress, and when generating maximum force levels, as well as illustrating lack of skill in attempts at a specific task. Using needle electrodes, experiments have shown that unnecessary muscle activation can be seen even when an associated movement is not present. Ada and O'Dwyer (2001) have reported no statistical relationship between associated movements and either stretch reflex activity or contracture.

Spasticity

A generally accepted definition of spasticity originating from a consensus conference and was reported by Lance (1980). Spasticity was defined as:

a motor disorder characterized by a velocity-dependent increase in tonic stretch reflexes (muscle tone) with exaggerated tendon jerks resulting from hyperexcitability of the stretch reflex as one component of the upper motor neuron syndrome.

This definition has the advantage of distinguishing spasticity from changes in passive muscle properties, which are commonly seen after stroke and do not appear to be related to spasticity.

The mechanisms producing spasticity are not understood. This is due to some extent to inadequate means of neurophysiological and clinical testing, difficulty interpreting results from individuals with different lesion sites and sizes, and difficulty in determining the effect of postlesion adaptations (Nielsen et al. 2007). Many theories have been put forward over the decades (see Table 2 in Gracies 2005a), but scientific support is lacking in humans. It used to be thought, for instance, that increased dynamic fusimotor drive

contributes to spasticity after stroke (e.g., Rushworth 1960). However, spindle behavior has been shown to be similar in both patients and controls (Wilson et al. 1999). More recent research has concluded that fusimotor dysfunction contributes little if anything to the deficit (Nielsen et al. 2007). Whatever its pathophysiological mechanisms, spasticity reflects a disorder of motor control, as suggested by the consensus definition above and acknowledged in an updated definition:

disordered sensorimotor control, resulting from an upper motor neuron lesion, presenting as intermittent or sustained involuntary activation of muscles (Pandyan et al. 2005).

Many reports indicate that stretch reflex hyperactivity can develop some time after the lesion, suggesting it may be an adaptive response to nonfunctional, stiff muscles. It can develop very early in the presence of muscle inactivity and/or muscle imbalance (Burke and Gandevia 1988, Gracies et al. 1997). Gracies (2005b) points out that progressive development of abnormal responses to muscle stretch probably occurs as a result of the gradual lesion- and activity-dependent adaptive changes in brain, spinal cord, and soft tissues, particularly muscles.

A major problem not only for the rehabilitation professional but also for research is that the term "spasticity" is typically used to cover a broad spectrum of diverse clinical signs, such as clonus, hypertonus, hyperreflexia, abnormal motor patterns, and even weakness (Paci 2003). However, it is clear that these clinical signs can exist independently from each other and result from different pathophysiological or mechanical mechanisms. An added complication is that the diagnosis of spasticity is typically arrived at by clinical tests such as the Modified Ashworth Scale that cannot distinguish the relative contributions of increased stiffness of muscles and reflex hyperactivity. This commonly used scale has poor inter-rater reliability and lacks validity (Pomeroy et al. 2000). It is a subjective measure of the resistance of a muscle to passive movement that does not take into account the velocity-dependent nature of hyperactive stretch reflex behavior. Singer and colleagues (2003) concluded from their study of resistance to passive stretching of calf muscles that an important component of resistance was mechanical and unrelated to stretch-induced reflex muscle contraction. The Tardieu Scale may be a more valid and reliable measure (see Appendix).

The term "hypertonus" originated more than a century ago as a way of describing an increase, after brain lesion, in what was termed "muscle or postural tone," perceived by the clinician as resistance to passive movement of a limb. The use of the word "tone" assumed that neural activity existed in a muscle even when at rest and that increased neural activity or hypertonus reflected spasticity due to the lesion. Normally, however, when a person relaxes completely, any resistance to passive movement is due to the elastic properties of soft tissues or failure to relax, and no electrical activity can be recorded in a resting muscle. Laboratory studies indicate that after stroke it is similar. Studies that have objectively measured stretch reflex activity at different velocities during passive movement in individuals after stroke have reported little or no electrical activity at rest (O'Dwyer et al. 1996, Salazar-Torres et al. 2004). In those subjects who demonstrate electrical activity there is no evidence that this is related to loss of function.

The results of tests of stretch reflexes at rest, that is, during passive movement, are unlikely to provide insights into the behavior of these reflexes during active movement. However, studies of stretch reflex response thresholds during active movement offer some insights. In a study of arm movement after stroke, Levin and colleagues (2000) reported limitations in regulating and coordinating stretch reflex response thresholds in flexor and extensor muscles. They suggested that reflex hyperactivity may not be the problem but rather the modulation of the stimulus-response as muscles are stretched during movement.

It is currently not clear from experimental findings to what extent stretch reflex hyperactivity (spasticity) is present in individuals after stroke during active movement, or whether and in what way it may contribute to functional disability. If spasticity has no functional significance and is not a problem for the patient, which appears to be the case in many individuals after stroke, then it need not be treated (Nielsen et al. 2007).

Some individuals after stroke develop excessive and persistent activity in paretic muscles called "dystonia." It is defined as a stretch-sensitive tonic muscle contraction that occurs in the absence of voluntary input (Gracies 2005b). Dystonia can contribute significantly to functional disability,

and may be due to continuous supraspinal drive to α motoneurons.

There is little to support the view that stretch reflex hypersensitivity is a significant contributor to movement dysfunction following stroke. Clinicians need to be aware that if they find increased resistance on passive movement of a limb in the first weeks after stroke, this may not indicate the presence of spasticity, and that mechanical and functional changes to muscle are more likely to be major contributors to the resistance. That is, in clinical practice, care must be taken not to misread a reduction in soft tissue compliance as emerging spasticity. If resistance to passive movement appears to be increasing, this might reflect a muscular rather than a neurological change (Sheean 2002).

Findings such as these require a change of focus in stroke rehabilitation. The clinical focus for many decades has been on spasticity as a major impairment interfering with motor function. As a consequence, many types of intervention directed at decreasing spasticity have been developed, including surgery, drug therapy, and physical inhibitory techniques. When spasticity is considered the primary cause of weakness of movement and functional disability, significant impairments such as impaired motor control, weakness of muscle, and a secondary increase in soft tissue stiffness may not be addressed at all in rehabilitation. Strengthening exercise or any activity that requires effort might be avoided in therapy sessions if it is assumed that the effort involved will increase spasticity. However, the evidence is that strength training does not cause an increase in spasticity. Stretch reflex amplitude may actually decrease after training (Bohannon 1988, Gregson et al 2000, Sharp and Brouwer 1997, Teixeira-Salmela et al. 1999, 2001). It is becoming recognized that much rehabilitation currently available may not be addressing the anatomical, biomechanical, and physiological mechanisms underlying the person's disability, and that, as a result, outcomes are poorer than they need be.

Adaptive Changes

The human system is highly adaptable and this underpins the natural flexibility of our behavior. Adaptations to lack of muscle activity and joint movement can occur at all levels of the neuromuscular system, from muscle fiber to motor cortex (McComas 1994). Changes in habitual levels of muscle activity and movement result in adaptive changes at any age and following any disruption to the system (Kleim et al. 2003). When the level of physical activity involving a limb declines, the ensuing reduction in physiological demands further decreases the capabilities of the limb (Duchateau and Enoka 2002). Paresis can result in inactivity of all muscles, not only those that are paretic since it leads to immobilization of a limb and absence of weightbearing. Prolonged periods without weightbearing are known to have a significant effect on skeletal muscle in able-bodied individuals, and bed rest can lead to decreased strength, poor balance, and increased fatigue, the extent depending on length of stay in bed. These conditions are reproduced after stroke and imposed immobility can be compounded by hospital procedures in the early stages after stroke (Gracies 2005a, b).

It is becoming increasingly clear that major anatomic, metabolic, mechanical, and functional changes within skeletal muscles occur after stroke in response to the lesion and to postlesion inactivity or disuse (for review, see Lieber et al. 2004). These peripheral changes can impact on the neural system itself and on functional motor performance. Adaptations occurring after stroke include increased muscle stiffness, changes in the characteristics of skeletal muscle (e.g., in the elastic properties of muscle cells), structural and functional reorganization of muscle and connective tissue (McComas 1994, Sinkjaer and Magnussen 1994), changed motor patterns during functional activities, and a process of learning not to use the paretic limb. Inactivity leads to a decline in muscular endurance, and changes in the cardiorespiratory system add to a decline in physical fitness and in the energy levels required for daily activities.

Adaptive physiological changes to muscle after brain lesion and associated with muscular inactivity and disuse include:

- Loss of functional motor units (McComas 1994)
- Changes in muscle fiber type and size; for example, severe atrophy of type II fibers with a predominance of slow-twitch (type I) fibers (Toffola et al. 2001)
- Cellular atrophy that may be load-dependent (Lieber et al. 2004)
- Changes in muscle metabolism such as reduced oxidative capacity (Potempa et al. 1996)

- Reduced capillary density compatible with endurance detraining or inactivity (Sunnerhagen et al. 1999)
- Changes in muscle mechanical properties including increased muscle stiffness (Mirbagheri et al. 2000)
- Reduction in muscle fascicle length
- Proliferation of extracellular connective tissue (Booth et al. 2001), with increased amount of collagen associated with resistance to passive stretch, muscle stiffness, and contracture

As a result of these changes, muscles become weaker, slower, and stiffer; the individual loses cardiovascular fitness and is easily fatigued. Changes may occur quite quickly, both in able-bodied people and after brain lesion. Quadriceps atrophy has been reported as early as 3 days after immobilization in able-bodied individuals (Lindboe and Platou 1984), with 30% reduction in cross-sectional area reported as occurring within a month (Halkjaer-Kristensen and Ingemann-Hansen 1985). After stroke, changes in muscle length can occur as early as 2 months after stroke (Malouin et al. 1997), and probably earlier.

Increased passive muscle stiffness, evident clinically when a muscle is passively stretched, appears to result from adaptive mechanical and morphological changes in muscle fibers and tendon and buildup of connective tissue related to lack of contractile activity. Increased stiffness is well documented after brain lesions (Given et al. 1995, Lamontagne et al. 2000, Sinkjaer and Magnussen 1994, Thilmann et al. 1991), with increases of 43% reported in plantar flexor muscles on the paretic compared to the nonparetic side (Malouin et al. 1997).

Stiffness has an active component, caused by muscle contraction, and a passive component. Several studies help us to understand something of the functional impact of increased passive stiffness. Passive stiffness reflects the viscoelastic properties of the muscle. One component of the resistance felt when a noncontracting muscle is passively lengthened is the inherent elasticity of the cross-bridges formed between actin and myosin filaments. Cross-bridge failure has also been suggested as a possible factor in the increased muscle stiffness found after a brain lesion (Carey and Burghardt 1993). In normal human muscle, stiffness due to cross-bridge attachment is partly dependent on the recent movement history of the muscle.

Muscle represents a classic biological example of the relationship between structure and function (Lieber et al. 1986). A muscle's length reflects the range of lengths it is subjected to throughout our daily lives and is therefore subject to change. Range of motion is reduced by shortening of muscle fiber length and by loss of muscle compliance. Muscle contracture can involve a shortening of muscle length as a result of changes to sarcomeres and an increase in resistance to passive stretch. It should be noted that contracture of one muscle group, for example the hip flexors, can have a similar effect on another group, in this case the hip adductors. A shorter than normal muscle is less extensible and a muscle that develops contracture at a shortened length fatigues more rapidly (Arendt-Nielsen et al. 1992). Adaptive changes also occur in joints and include proliferation of fatty tissue in joint space, cartilage atrophy, weakening of ligament insertion sites, osteoporosis (Akeson et al. 1987), and joint malalignment.

Adaptive neural changes, including impaired motor (supraspinal) drive and secondary changes related to morphological plasticity (e.g., collateral sprouting) at spinal cord level (Nielsen et al 2007), can result both from the lesion and from postlesion disuse (McComas 1994). Studies of the effects of immobilization in able-bodied individuals have shown decreased maximum firing rate of muscles and increases in recruitment threshold after a period of immobilization (Duchateau and Hainaut 1990). A larger number of motor units must be recruited to develop a submaximal contraction, since all motor units have lost part of their contractile tension.

Increased muscle stiffness, changes in muscle length, and accumulation of connective tissue occurring postlesion can also affect stretch receptor sensitivity (O'Dwyer et al. 1996, Salazar-Torres et al. 2004). Increased spindle sensitivity due to intrafusal shortening may cause the stretch reflex to be elicited earlier in joint range because a given change of joint angle stretches the spindles more than normal.

Adaptive motor patterns seen during attempts at functional actions early after stroke can result from muscle weakness or paralysis, the muscle imbalance observed being due to greater weakness in some muscles relative to others (**Fig. 5.5**). Later, lack of muscle extensibility occurring as a result of stiffness and muscle contracture can contribute to adaptive patterns. Both muscle weakness and contracture affect the dynamics of the segmental linkage, and the movement patterns that occur illustrate adaptive changes in the synergic relationships between muscles due to muscle imbalance, with stronger muscles acting relatively unopposed. These movements appear to be the individual's best attempt at an action given the state of the neural and musculoskeletal systems together with the dynamic possibilities inherent in the musculoskeletal linkage (Carr and Shepherd 2010). Lance (1990), in a letter to the *Lancet*, reminded us that impaired voluntary movement and abnormal posture do not reflect spasticity but that these signs reflect adaptations to muscle weakness, changes in motoneuron firing patterns, soft tissue stiffness, and contracture.

A behavioral adaptation with negative consequences after a unilateral lesion such as stroke is the phenomenon of *"learned nonuse"* of the paretic arm (Taub 1980). The person responds to difficulty in moving the limb by not using it. A similar phenomenon is observable in the lower limbs, when an individual relies on loading the nonparetic limb to stand up.

In summary, enforced inactivity due to weakness can lead to adaptive anatomic, mechanical, and functional changes in soft tissues and motor behavior. Progressive muscle hypoextensibility, stiffness, and contracture can be major causes of disability and have a major effect on attempts to regain function. Adaptive motor performance reflects muscle paresis, imbalance, stiffness, and muscle length. However, neither scientific investigation nor clinical practice places sufficient emphasis on investigating the adaptive phenomena as causative agents, the effects of which may be minimized by a vigorous program of task-oriented exercise and training.

Evidence from research findings related to impairments and adaptation strongly supports a change in focus for rehabilitation therapists to a training model that includes active practice of tasks that must be relearned as quickly as possible, and exercises aimed at increasing muscle strength, motor control, and physical endurance. In planning clinical practice, certain clinical implications can be derived from our current understanding of impairments and adaptive sequelae and these provide three principal goals:

- Optimize functional motor performance by task-oriented training of motor control.

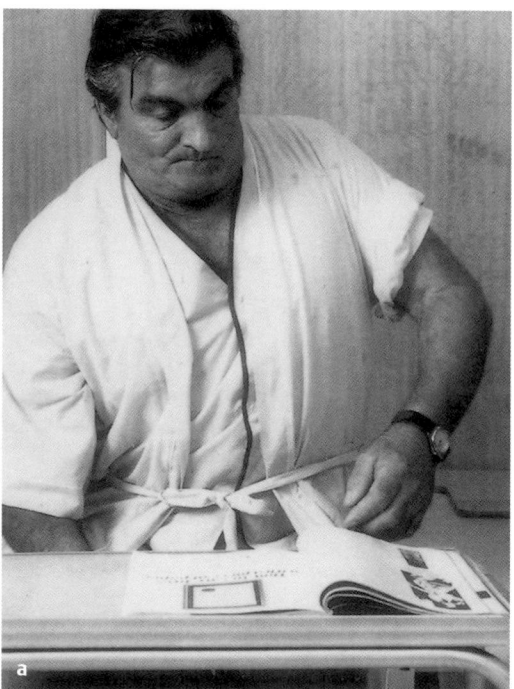

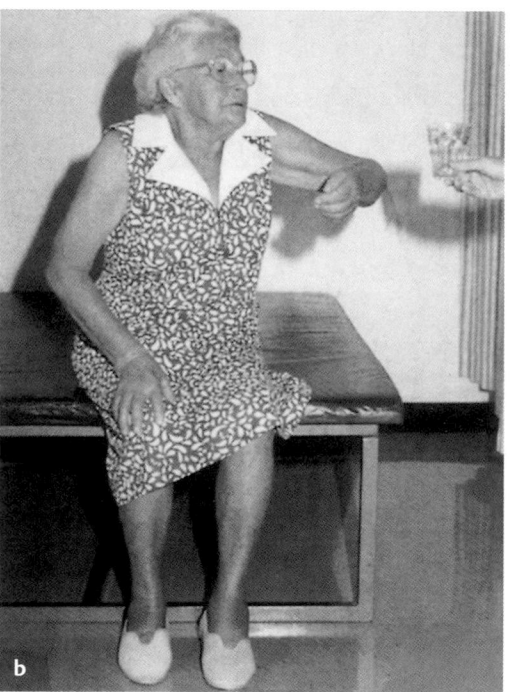

Fig. 5.5 a, b   Common adaptations to muscle weakness and paralysis of shoulder muscles.
a Attempting to point to a picture, the patient elevates the shoulder girdle, laterally flexes, and rotates at the spine to swing his arm forward.

b Two-joint biceps brachii flexes the elbow as well as the shoulder when triceps brachii is weak and limb control is poor.

- At the same time, prevent or minimize adaptive disuse changes to the structure, mechanics, and contractile function of muscles.
- Minimize adaptive physical and mental deconditioning that occurs in response to inactivity.

To achieve these goals, therapists depend on their knowledge of how people learn to be skilled in motor performance, and on an understanding of the relationship between learning and the environment in which rehabilitation is performed. Understanding the possibilities inherent in the brain's capacity to reorganize after a neural lesion in response to what the individual experiences can provide important insights for the therapist into the development of effective methods of rehabilitation.

■ Interrelationships between Motor Learning, Brain Plasticity, and Environments

Motor Learning

Skill is defined as any activity that has become better organized and more effective as a result of practice (Annett 1971) and also as the ability to consistently attain a goal with some economy of effort (Gentile 2000). Everyday actions constitute motor skills—they are complex actions made up of segmental movements linked together in the appropriate spatial and temporal sequence.

Skill development takes place in overlapping stages described as first getting the idea of the movement (the cognitive stage), then developing the ability to adapt the movement pattern to the demands of the environment (Gentile 2000). We make the assumption that the acquisition of skill, involving practice and exercise, is a manifestation of internal processes making up what is called "motor learning." Motor learning itself cannot be directly observed but can only be inferred from our observations of a relatively consistent improvement in performance of an action. That is, we note a relatively stable change in motor behavior as a result of a set of processes involving exercise and practice (Magill 2001, Schmidt 1988). This is why we measure certain characteristics of motor performance at the start of training and at various stages throughout and after training (Magill 2001). However, although improved performance is of course a positive finding, it is not in itself evidence of learning. This is obtained by follow-up testing of retention a few weeks later.

The major aim of intervention is ultimately the optimization of motor performance, that is, the regaining of effective performance in the motor actions of daily living. Physical therapists are increasingly aware of patients as active participants and learners rather than as passive recipients of therapy. It is due to some extent to our increasing knowledge of how people learn and relearn motor skills that we now understand that rehabilitation is principally a learning process. Patients have to learn again how to perform the functional motor actions in which they were previously skilled.

The process of acquiring skill is typically investigated by biomechanical studies of able-bodied adults as they learn a novel task or train to improve a specific skill, and increasingly in the re-learning of everyday skills by people with motor disability. The obvious clinical implications of motor learning research have been demonstrated over several decades (Carr and Shepherd 2010, Magill 2001, Shumway-Cook and Woollacott 2007). Considering the patient as a learner requires rehabilitation therapists to set up conditions under which skill learning can take place. Awareness of the characteristics of each stage of learning enables the therapist to provide appropriate practice conditions to optimize performance (Carr and Shepherd 2003, 2010).

Skilled performance is characterized by the ability to perform complex movements, with the flexibility to vary movement to meet ongoing environmental demands. This applies as much to everyday actions such as walking and standing up from a seat as it does to recreational, sporting, or work-related actions. Skill is task-specific. Although such actions as level walking and stair walking may

share similar biomechanical characteristics, the demands placed on the individual by each action are different. The individual learns to reshape and adapt the basic movement pattern according to different contexts; for example, crossing the street at pedestrian lights may require an increase in walking speed, negotiating obstacles in the house requires other changes in the walking pattern.

To improve the efficacy of a particular action requires many hours of practice if the goal is to be achieved. For some individuals, speeding up the action and improving power generation may be major performance goals. However, for those whose muscle strength and motor control is below a certain threshold, exercises to increase strength and control are necessary, together with practice of the action under modified conditions. For example, reaching to grasp an object can be practiced with the arm resting on a table at 90° shoulder flexion; this reduces the complexity of the action and the muscle force to be generated from shoulder muscles such as deltoid.

Several factors are known to be important in motor learning and the acquisition of skill:

- Ability to focus attention
- Prioritizing and setting of goals
- Effects of contextual information on motor performance
- Perceived locus of control—therapist or patient?
- Effects of interactive practice with others who have similar difficulties
- Information in the form of instruction, demonstration, and feedback
- Frequent practice with many repetitions (for strength, control, and learning) and in different contexts (for flexibility of performance)
- Modification of task or environment to simplify practice or to make the task more challenging

Focusing Attention

The ability to focus attention on a task, to sustain concentration, to shift attention from one environmental feature to another, and to ignore irrelevant inputs, are critical to everyday functional ability. They are also critical when a patient is practicing to relearn once well-learned skills. This stage of task learning involves identifying what has to be learned, and understanding the ways by which the goal can be accomplished. Patients themselves re-

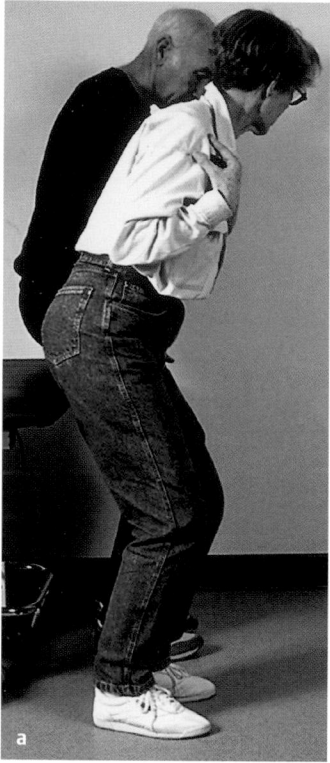

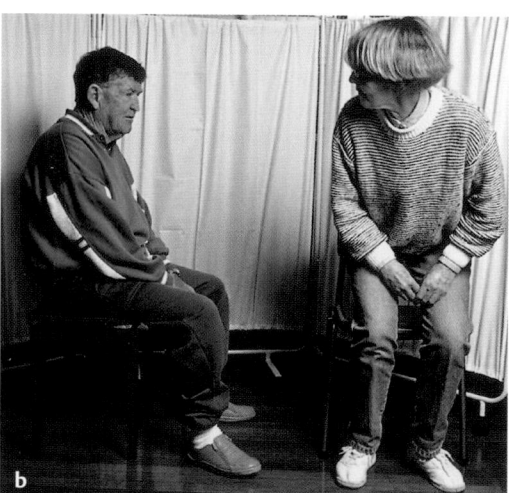

Fig. 5.6 a, b Demonstrating the extent of trunk flexion at the hips for standing up.
a Therapist beside the patient so he can align his shoulders with hers;
b Sagittal plane view shows him how far forward the shoulders are moved.

port that attempts to perform everyday activities poststroke require purposeful effort and increased attention to the task that are imposed on the individual by their reduced functional ability (Brodal 1973).

In clinical practice, the learner's focus of attention shifts as muscle strength, motor control, and skill increase. In walking, for example, the focus may shift from the feet to the surrounding environment; in sit-to-stand it may change from initial foot placement and increasing the speed of forward rotation of the upper body to steadying a glass of water while standing up. As part of the training process, the therapist directs the patient's attention away from an internal body-oriented focus (foot position, forward rotation of the upper body at the hips) to an external focus that is directly related to the goal of the action (steadying a glass of water while standing up, stepping over/avoiding obstacles on the floor while walking). Some recent findings with healthy subjects have shown what a difference it can make to performance and skill development if the learner directs attention toward the effect of the movement (an external focus) rather than to the movement itself (an internal focus). There is increasing evidence that directing learners to the effects of their movements, that is, whether or not the goal has been achieved, may be more effective than attending to the movement itself (Wulf et al. 1999a, 1999b). Wulf and colleagues suggest that paying attention to the outcome and not the movement helps the system to self-organize (Wulf et al. 1998).

A patient in the early stages after stroke, who is confused, depressed, and weak, may need frequent cues about where to focus attention; for example, looking at the object not at the hand, or looking at a target straight ahead when standing up, not at the floor. Commonly used methods include the therapist demonstrating (modelling) the action being practiced (**Fig. 5.6**) and giving clear, simple instructions. Written instructions of what to practice are useful for encouraging independent practice.

Demonstration, Modelling, Verbal Instructions

Instructions may degrade performance if they are inappropriate or too numerous. They may make the task so attention-demanding that the learner experiences information overload (Wulf and Wei-gelt 1997). In the early stages of learning, instructions from the therapist should be brief. They should cue the person to one or two critical features of the action. A figure drawing can reinforce these key elements (**Fig. 5.7**). As the person internalizes these details, they can start to think more of the goal of the action; for example, to stand up and shake hands, or to walk to another room. At this later stage instructing the person to focus on details of their performance can be detrimental.

A skilled model (the therapist) may command greater attention than an unskilled model (the patient herself). Demonstration of an action by the therapist assists the patient to get the idea of what the movement looks like—the "shape" of the movement (see Magill 2001). Research has shown that the visual system automatically detects invariant information in determining how to produce the observed action. A combination of observation and physical practice seems to permit unique opportunities for learning beyond those available from physical practice alone (Shea et al. 2000).

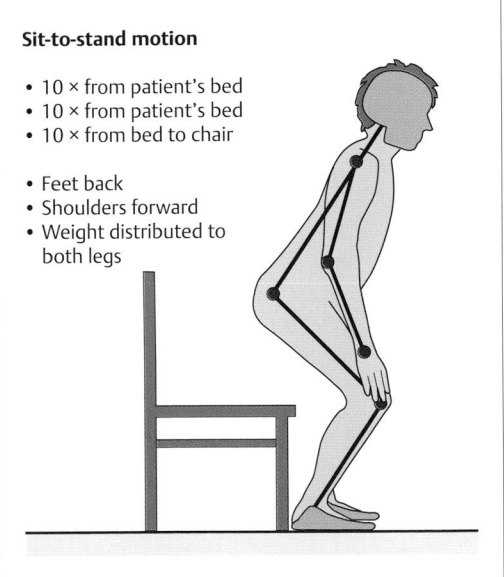

Sit-to-stand motion

- 10 × from patient's bed
- 10 × from patient's bed
- 10 × from bed to chair

- Feet back
- Shoulders forward
- Weight distributed to both legs

Fig. 5.7   A diagram illustrating critical features of STS and the number of repetitions to perform.

Goal Setting

The goal must be worthwhile to the patient and it must also be challenging. In training functional tasks, the therapist sets the goals in consultation with the individual and based on evaluation of the patient's capabilities. As teacher or trainer, the therapist may point out a key component of a task (e.g., move the paretic foot back before standing up); provide verbal instructions, feedback, or demonstration; direct the person's visual attention; or highlight regulatory cues in the environment (e.g., the height of an obstacle). However, it is the patient who must learn to organize a movement that matches the environment to achieve these goals.

In clinical practice, pragmatism can lead to a clash of goals that may have deleterious effects on learning. If a major goal of training is to improve walking, opportunities need to be provided for practice in meaningful contexts; for example, moving from physical therapy to speech therapy provides an opportunity to practice walking for at least part of the way rather than travelling in a wheelchair. If a major goal is to prevent the development of learned nonuse of paretic limbs, providing a one-arm propelled wheelchair with the goal of independence conflicts with the goal of encouraging use of the paretic limbs. More time each day will be spent propelling the chair with the nonparetic limb than in using the paretic limbs. Similarly, providing a sling that holds the upper limb in shoulder adduction/internal rotation with the aim of protecting the shoulder may cause collateral damage—avoidance of paretic limb use or "learned nonuse." Such dilemmas must be carefully considered. Consistency in working toward important goals is critical to optimizing functional performance. For example, practicing standing up with the foot of the stronger leg placed behind the paretic leg, a common adaptation, is inconsistent with the goal of loading of the paretic limb. The foot placed furthest back takes more of the load of raising the body mass to standing, that is, foot placement affects load distribution.

Meaningful goal setting involves organizing the environment to be functionally relevant; that is, by providing meaningful objects of different sizes, weight, and graspability, which allow for different tasks to be trained. Goals should be concrete rather than abstract: "Reach out and take the glass from the table" rather than "Raise your arm"; "Reach sideways to take the glass" rather than "Shift your weight over to the left."

Contextual Information Has Been Shown to Affect Performance

Concrete goals differ from abstract goals in the degree to which the required action is directed toward controlling a physical interaction with the environment as opposed to movement for its own sake. Recent research has illustrated the different outcomes when individuals after stroke work with concrete goals linked to real objects rather than with more abstract goals (van Vliet et al. 1995, Wu et al. 2000). Wu and colleagues examined a task in which subjects used one hand to scoop coins from a table into the other hand. Able-bodied and stroke subjects took part, sometimes with coins, sometimes mimicking the movement without coins. Both groups of subjects demonstrated faster movements that were smoother and straighter when they scooped the coins compared with when they mimicked the action.

Practice

Practice is the single most important factor responsible for permanent improvement in the ability to perform a motor skill, that is, for learning to occur (Magill 2001). As a general rule the action to be acquired should be practiced in its entirety since one component of the action depends on preceding components, and the required neuromotor and biomechanical mechanisms can only be activated by performance of the action itself. For example, contraction of plantar flexors at the end of stance phase produces power generation for push-off that is critical not only for forward progression but also for the upcoming swing phase. Power generation affects walking speed and ensures energy exchange (Olney et al. 1986). These complex neuromuscular mechanisms can only be optimized through the practice of walking, and therefore walking on a treadmill (with body weight support and assistance from the therapist) can help the system to reorganize early after stroke. However, strengthening exercises that are oriented to a major action component (e.g., ankle

plantarflexion) also need to be practiced if the muscles are too weak to perform the task itself effectively.

Transfer of learning lies at the heart of motor learning (Magill 2001). One of the goals of practicing a task such as walking is the ability to transfer what we have learned into different contexts. To function in the community, the patient practices walking in the rehabilitation department, but the limb control and balance achieved must also transfer into different contexts—walking to the next appointment or to a shop, walking up a hill, crossing the road, carrying a bag. After stroke, this capacity to transfer skill may also depend on practicing exercises that strengthen and improve endurance of leg muscles, and aerobic training to improve fitness.

Repetitions

Many repetitions of an action are required to increase muscle strength and limb control, and for the patient to develop an optimal way of performing the action (Bernstein in Latash and Latash 1994). Thousands of repetitions may be necessary to improve strength and control, and to embed the organization of the action in the system. Acquiring skill does not only mean to repeat and consolidate, but also to invent and progress (Whiting 1980), so-called "repetition without repetition" (Bernstein 1967). Skill acquisition involves the ability to solve motor problems posed by the environment. However, physical therapy may neglect the repetitive element of skill acquisition that is an essential prerequisite for motor rehabilitation (Bütefisch et al. 1995). Patients need the opportunity to practice motor actions repeatedly in different task and environmental conditions to develop this flexibility and to be encouraged to see themselves as problem-solvers.

Practice is a continuum from overt physical practice to covert or *mental practice*. For many decades (Deiber et al. 1998, Driskell et al. 1994) mental practice combined with physical practice has been effectively used to promote the learning of motor skills in athletes and to preserve skill when physical practice was not possible. Mental practice can involve motor imagery—the mental rehearsal of a physical action without overt movement. Several studies have found electrical activity evident in muscles when individuals were asked to imagine themselves performing an action; for example, bending the arm to lift a weight. These results suggest that appropriate motor connections may be activated during mental practice and support the proposal that the initial stage of learning a task involves a high degree of cognitive activity. Mental practice is likely to be most effective when the individual has developed a basic understanding of the action itself, and when combined with physical practice. Observing a demonstration of the action can help an individual develop a mental picture of the action to be performed.

Malouin and colleagues (2004a, 2004b) tested 12 subjects after stroke and 14 able-bodied subjects before and after a single session of mental practice using motor imagery. They were asked to reduce the loading through the nonparetic leg and increase the load on the paretic leg. Subjects were shown a vertical force signal indicating magnitude and timing of force under either the nonparetic or the paretic leg. The results showed that loading the paretic leg improved, and working memory scores (recall in visuospatial, verbal, kinaesthetic domains) at follow-up correlated significantly with the level of improvement.

How difficult a functional task is for a individual depends on how challenging the task is relative to the skill level of that person (Guadagnoli and Lee 2004). This is a useful concept for clinical practice, as even very simple tasks may be difficult for an individual with severe impairment early after a stroke. If this is the case, the task and/or the environment in which it is performed must be modified to enable practice to take place. A task can be modified so less force is required. This may increase the effectiveness of the prime mover muscles and avoid unnecessary adaptive behavior. A task can be made less difficult by decreasing the number of segments to be moved. The distance to be moved can be decreased so that the person has more control over the movement. Challenges to balance can be decreased to enable the person to gain some control over balance mechanisms while performing the task; wearing a harness, for example, gives the person confidence and allows practice of different tasks in standing without fear of falling (see **Fig. 5.31**, p. 95).

As the person improves, the task itself can be made more difficult and the action can be practiced under different and more difficult environmental conditions (**Fig. 5.8**, **Fig. 5.18**); for example, walking around and over obstacles, performing

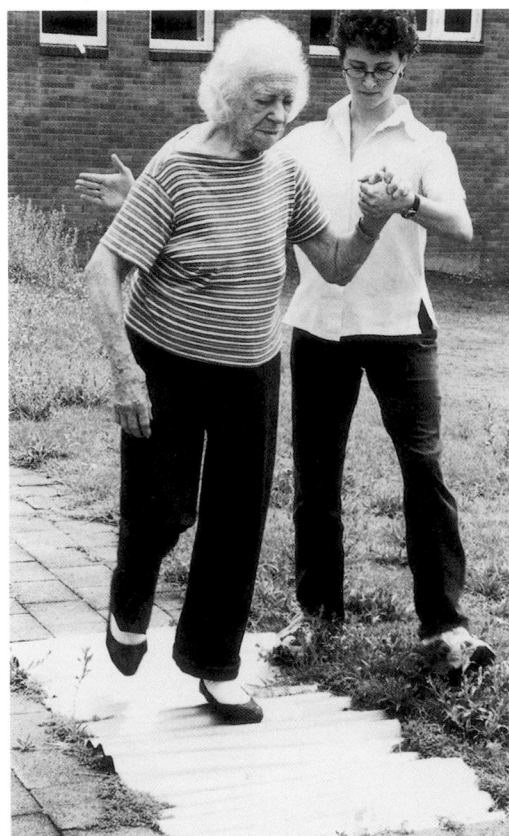

Fig. 5.8 Training flexibility and improving confidence —walking on an uneven surface (corrugated iron).

more repetitions, increasing resistance or load. Progressing training may also involve increasing the distance walked, or carrying out two tasks at once such as holding a glass full of water while standing up, or walking and talking.

Delivery of Physical Therapy—Providing Opportunities for Practice

Changes in physical therapy practice are required to make better use of the time allotted for rehabilitation, not only in methods used but also in delivery. It is clear from several studies of clinical practice that it is common for only a small part of the patient's day to be made available for practice and learning. To some extent this reflects typical work practices. However, we now have clear evidence that recovery of reasonable functional efficacy after stroke demands a great deal of practice and that rehabilitation methods in large part involve learning processes. It is therefore important that therapists move away from reliance of hands-on, one-to-one therapy to a model in which the person practices, not only in individualized training sessions with the therapist, but also in small groups with supervision and individual assistance, and training as necessary (**Fig. 5.9**). One or two therapists with the assistance of an aide can supervise several individuals in a group, with relatives helping if they are willing and able (**Fig. 5.11**). Patients can move from one work-station to another in a circuit training class (**Fig. 5.10**) where they practice specific motor activities with both simple and technological aids to promote strength and skill, such as photographs or videotapes of the action to be learned, and printed or

electronic exercise guidelines (e.g., www.rehab. ubc.ca/jeng/Our_Exercise_Manuals/GRASP.htm).

Providing semi-supervised practice can increase the time the patient spends training without substantially increasing the therapist's load. Patients can work together in pairs in group practice, one observing, one physically practicing. Alternating practice with a partner can be more effective than practice alone, and Shea and colleagues (1999) describe the effects of interactive practice between two people. Their results suggest that physical practice, observation, and dialogue (suggestions, motivating comments) between learners in an interactive way can produce an effective learning protocol. The introduction of group classes has been found to increase the level of social interaction during the day. In one study, patients spent 25% more time with their peers (De Weerdt et al. 2001). Barreca and colleagues found that participants assigned to the group developed

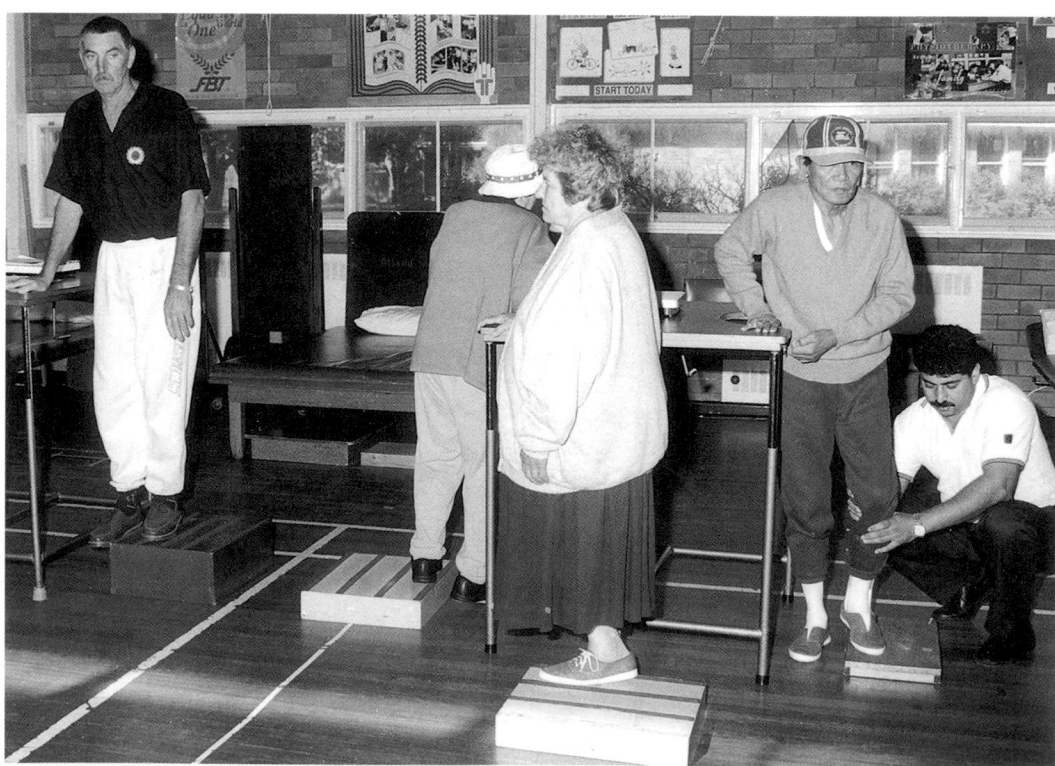

Fig. 5.9 Training in a group in an in-patient rehabilitation setting. Safe, semi-supervised practice of lateral step-ups for each individual is ensured by having a high table close by for support. (*Reprinted with kind permission from PRO-ED Inc, Austin Tx, USA.*)

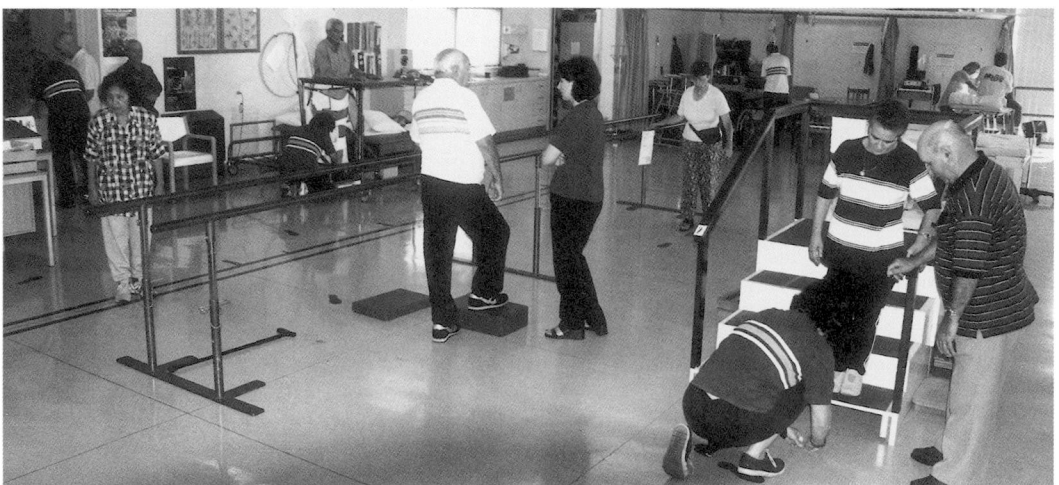

Fig. 5.10 Overview of a community lower limb circuit class. The aims of the class are
1. to improve the ability to stand up, balance and walk;
2. to improve the ability to walk up and down stairs; and
3. to improve fitness and ability to walk longer distances.
(Courtesy of F Mackey, and colleagues, Illawarra Area Health Service, Australia.)

a camaraderie, encouraging each other and celebrating successes (Barreca et al. 2004).

Practicing with another person in an interactive way increases the learners' motivation by adding competitive and cooperative components to the practice situation (McNevin et al. 2000). The presence of others with similar disabilities may motivate and encourage individuals to do better and increase their sense of wellbeing and their communication skills by engaging with others. There are also benefits to be gained from observing another person learning a task (Hebert and Landin 1994). Working with another person provides rest intervals when training is physically challenging, yet particpants have to remain focused to assist their partner. The delivery of physical therapy in circuit and exercise classes is shown to be effective and feasible (Ada et al. 2006a, Eng et al. 2003, Teixeira-Salmela et al. 1999, 2001). Semi-supervised practice can help bridge the gap between individualized training and unsupervised practice in rehabilitation and at home. If patients feel they have some control over practice conditions and are encouraged to see the therapist as a resource person, their problem-solving abilities can improve. These skills are essential to enable practice at home.

Many promising new technological aids to improve motor performance and increase practice time are currently being developed and investi-

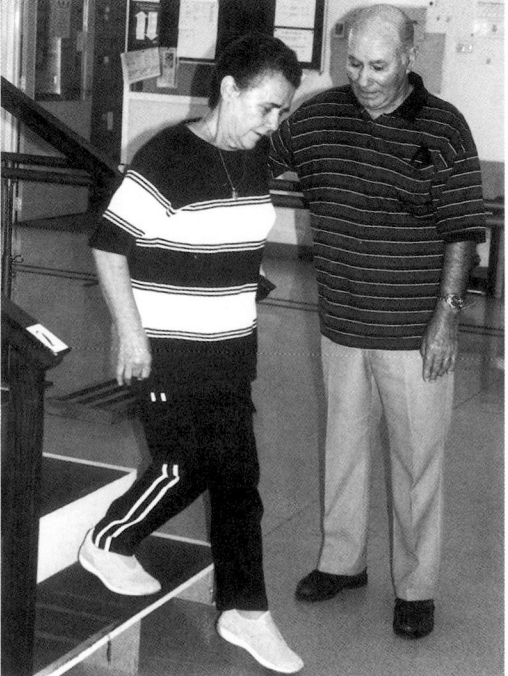

Fig. 5.11 A participant's husband supervises her at the stair walking station. *(Courtesy of F Mackey, and colleagues, Illawarra Area Health Service, Australia.)*

gated, and may increase time spent in physical and mental activity by enabling patients to practice independently. These developments include robot-aided training (Hidler et al. 2005) and computer games activated and controlled by manipulanda of different types. It is too early for substantial evidence of the positive effects of these methods. There are some early indications that virtual reality training can result in improvements in motor skills (Holden and Dyar 2002, Merians et al. 2002).

Many therapists already acknowledge that functional improvement can take place without the therapist's constant presence and that it is unrealistic to expect that any patient will reach their potential if they spend only a short period each day in physical activity with a therapist. It is possible that many hours of each patient's day spent in specialized stroke units and rehabilitation facilities are hours wasted. However, challenges to the customary delivery of therapy can be difficult for clinicians and may require a change in culture within a department.

Programs of exercise and training are described later in this chapter. They are designed to promote the relearning of skilled performance specifically in standing up and sitting down, walking, reaching, and manipulation. From early after stroke the opportunity exists to retrain the existing neural circuitry so that optimal function can be restored. The neurological goal is to stimulate brain organization and thereby optimize functional skill.

Effects of Skill Training and the Environment on Neuroplasticity

Training skill and organizing an active learning environment appear to affect brain plasticity. Positive effects seem to depend on practice of meaningful activities in task-oriented and intensive training. In general, findings support Lemon's suggestion that the mechanisms underlying development of skill are also the mechanisms of motor learning (Lemon 1993). The term "neuroplasticity" refers to the capacity of the central nervous system to adapt to functional demands and to reorganize. In contrast to an earlier view of the brain as functionally static, substantial evidence has emerged that the human brain is dynamic, flex-

ible, and engaged in problem-solving throughout our lives (Buonomano and Merzenich 1998, Johansson 2000, Nudo et al. 2001, Weiller 1998,). Results from both animal and human studies are converging to show that cortical plasticity also occurs after a lesion to the cortical system such as a stroke. Evidence suggests that, in both animals and humans, postinjury behavior and experience play a critical role in modifying the functional reorganization of undamaged cortical tissue and that such changes correlate with function (Nudo et al. 2001). Results currently available imply that treatment programs can be either adaptive or maladaptive depending on what patients do and the experiences they have (Walker-Batson et al. 2004).

While neuroscientists are exploring the influence of neural plasticity on functional recovery, clinicians need to identify the impact of this new scientific evidence on clinical practice in the rehabilitation of neurological patients. At present it appears that a patient's experiences in occupational and physical therapy and the environment in which rehabilitation is performed can drive neural changes and brain reorganization with positive or negative effects depending on those experiences.

Within the organization of the sensory cortical system there are multiple representations of the external world and these are topographically represented as maps. These maps change in ways that reflect use and experience. The size and organization of motor maps is examined by stimulating the cortex either directly with microelectrodes or transcranially using magnetic stimulation to induce movements, and by using functional imaging to map the area of activation when subjects are engaged in different behaviors.

Insights into mechanisms mediating motor recovery after injury to the sensorimotor cortex and its subcortical connections are emerging from both animal and human studies. Several lines of investigation provide evidence that supports a role for poststroke motor learning and task-specific training in the production of positive functional changes in the motor cortex. Studies in normal rats, monkeys, and humans have demonstrated that specific motor training can increase the size of different components of motor maps. Studies of brain maps in humans have shown that cortical representations of muscles of the fingers of the left but not the right hand were expanded in right-handed skilled violin players who perform regularly (Elbert et al. 1995). We know that many repetitions are required for an individual to become skilled at a complex motor task. Extensive stimulation of the reading finger experienced by proficient Braille readers is associated with an increase in that finger's representation compared with the nonreading hand and either hand of the controls (Pascual-Leone et al. 1993). In addition, the size of the representation fluctuated with the amount of reading activity.

The use of animal models permits tight control of factors that may confound the outcomes of human studies, given the complexities inherent in working with people who are active participants in the recovery process. It is in the patient's best interest for those working in rehabilitation to remain current with advances in this area.

To examine lesion-induced plasticity in the primary motor cortex of primates, Nudo and colleagues have used intracortical microstimulation techniques (ICMS) to map the hand representation in adult squirrel monkeys before and after focal ischemic lesions. Unilateral damage to the forelimb area of the sensorimotor cortex resulted in preferential use of the unimpaired limb. It was found that hand movement representations that were adjacent to the infarct but were spared from direct injury underwent a loss of cortical tissue (Nudo and Milliken 1996). Since the animals in this study did not have any specific training after injury, the losses in the representational area of the paretic hand may have been the direct result of diminished use (Nudo and Milliken 1996). Therefore, in a subsequent study, lesioned monkeys were trained on a small-object retrieval task. To obtain a food pellet, they were trained to insert one or two fingers into a small-diameter container to pick out a food pellet, a task that required fine control of the digits and hand. The unimpaired limb was restrained. For the first few days after the infarct, movements were slow and monkeys had difficulty placing the digits into the small holes. However, skill improved over time and the number of misses decreased rapidly. Comparison of ICMS maps before and after the infarct showed that the spared hand representation area adjacent to the infarct had expanded (Nudo et al. 1996). These results suggest that specific training to induce motor learning can shape subsequent reorganization in the undamaged motor cortex and that this may play an important part in functional recovery (Nudo et al. 1996). Interestingly, in a

further study, restraint of the unimpaired limb without additional training of the paretic limb resulted in a decrease of total hand representation. Specifically, the size of finger, wrist, and forearm representations of the paretic limb decreased. That is to say, it was the enforced practice of a desirable task with the paretic limb that brought about improved limb performance (Friel and Nudo 1998).

In a further study using identical neurophysiological techniques, monkeys were trained on the reach and retrieval task, this time with a large-diameter container. The lesioned monkeys were able to perform the retrieval task efficiently early in training, and performance remained stereotypic and unchanged over time. In addition, comparison of pre-and postinjury ICMS revealed no task-related representational changes. These results suggest that simple use of the limb was insufficient to produce plasticity in cortical maps. Apparently there was no particular driving force for the development of motor skill or new strategies (Plautz et al. 2000). Since motor skill learning can only be inferred when there is a stable and measurable change in motor performance over time, the results suggest that the task was too easy and further practice had no benefit and indeed had a negative effect (Plautz et al. 2000). This has particular significance for physical therapy practice, pointing out the importance of patients practicing actions that are difficult and challenging rather than those that are too easy and can already be attempted.

The mechanisms underlying recovery from brain damage in humans are known to be complex and multifactorial, including functional and anatomical reorganization, altered neurotransmission, and metabolism. Only recently have direct studies of brain function in humans become possible with the introduction of imaging techniques such as positron emission tomography (PET), functional magnetic resonance imaging (fMRI), and transcranial magnetic stimulation (TMS). The results of these investigations have demonstrated functional reorganization in intact cortical tissue both adjacent to the injury and in more remote cortical areas (e.g., Johansson 2000, Kolb 2003, Liepert et al. 2001, Nelles 2004, Nelles et al. 2001, Nudo 2003, Nudo et al. 2001). Reorganization may take several forms, including unmasking of existing circuits, growth of new synapses via axonal sprouting or dendritic proliferation, and the development of compensatory processes.

Of critical importance for rehabilitation is that experience, with the opportunity to acquire motor skill by active use of the paretic limbs, appears to modulate the adaptive reorganization that inevitably occurs. However, postinjury changes occurring over time may be either adaptive or maladaptive; that is, brain reorganization can have beneficial or negative effects driven by positive or negative events or experiences that the individual has following the stroke. Disuse can induce a negative effect. Liepert and colleagues (1995) found a significant shrinkage in the cortical representation of inactive muscles after 4–6 weeks of ankle immobilization in able-bodied subjects, and this increased with duration of immobilization. Following amputation, neighboring networks expand into the area previously devoted to activity of the amputated segment (Fuhr et al. 1992).

In the absence of appropriate experience and specific training of a paretic limb, an individual may learn not to use the limb. As in animal studies, focusing on tasks that are engaging, challenging, and meaningful to the individual seems to be effective in optimizing the neural plasticity associated with functional recovery. Evidence of brain changes related to task-specific training poststroke suggest that it is possible to entrain or "force" the brain toward a more efficient activation pattern (Calautti and Baron 2003). The results of a multi-centre study of constraint-induced movement therapy (CIMT) for improving upper-extremity function after stroke in humans (Wolf et al. 2006) show that constraining the nonparetic limb combined with task-oriented practice can improve upper limb function in subjects who have some active movement in the hand. The results indicate that both intensity and task-specificity are critical in overcoming learned nonuse after stroke. Associated with improved function after stroke, there is also evidence of significant enlargement in the representation of the paretic limb in the cortex (Liepert et al. 1998, 2000). These studies provide clear evidence of brain changes related to task training methods used in rehabilitation therapy.

It is reported that early mobilization can reduce secondary thromboembolic events, pneumonia, and mortality after stroke (Indredavik et al. 1997, Stroke Trialists' Collaboration 2001). There have been some limited data from studies of rats by Kozlowski and colleagues (1996), suggesting that training starting 24 hours after onset may increase cortical tissue loss. The authors suggested that there may be a period of vulnerability of neuronal tissue very early after stroke in humans. Nudo (2003), however, has commented that the risk of an exaggeration of the injury in humans is low. He pointed out that the rats in Kozlowski's study had large lesions and a body cast that included the unaffected forelimb that was fixed to the thorax within the first 24 hours after injury. Since rats are quadrupeds, the forced use of the paretic limb would have been extreme as the animal attempted to use it for support, locomotion, grooming, and feeding. Immediate poststroke use is self-limiting in humans with infarcts and other comorbid conditions, and it is therefore unlikely that patients will be involved in events that might lead to exaggeration of the injury. Since early mobilization is known to be important in the prevention of life-threatening medical complications, several authors have cautioned against changing the current policy of early mobilization after stroke (Bernhardt et al. 2009, Johansson 2000, Nudo 2003). Although evidence of the value of specific rehabilitation intervention after stroke is limited, clinical data so far strongly support early mobilization with task-oriented training.

Nudo (2003) summarizes the empirical evidence underpinning our understanding of the neuroplasticity that can modulate functional recovery with active rehabilitation strategies:

- Injury to the motor cortex as in stroke induces functional changes in cortical tissue that is spared by the injury.
- The acquisition of skilled movement induces predictable functional changes within the motor cortex.
- The two events interact so that, following cortical injury, the acquisition of motor skill influences the type and growth of functional plasticity that occurs in the undamaged cortex.

Clinicians are well positioned to use and test concepts in clinical practice, with the ultimate goal of maximizing the potential benefits of rehabilitation and eliminating interventions that may have no benefit or even have negative consequences for the patient. Guidelines for clinical practice can be gained from research findings on brain reorganization:

- Neural reorganization and motor skill learning are optimized when the focus is on tasks that are engaging, challenging, and meaningful.

- Repetition of simple movements or of a meaningless task are insufficient to produce long-term neural organization.

■ The Rehabilitation Environment

The formation of new and different networks and the regaining of skill in everyday actions with a damaged neural system requires training and exercise in an environment that encourages and facilitates mental and physical activity and the process of learning. The rehabilitation environment can be a direct facilitator of rehabilitation goals if it is an environment oriented toward health, fitness, mental and social stimulation, and learning.

There is extensive evidence in laboratory animals that the rehabilitation environment can influence outcome after brain damage. Rats housed in enriched environments after brain infarction performed significantly better on motor tasks such as narrow beam-walking, ladder-rung walking, or skilled forearm reaching than rats housed alone or in standard laboratory cages (Held et al. 1985, Ohlsson and Johansson 1995). The aspect of the enriched environment found to result in the best performance was the opportunity for physical activity combined with social interaction (Johansson and Ohlsson 1996, Biernaskie and Corbett 2001, Risedal et al. 2002). Complex environments with a variety of objects to stimulate limb use are thought to stimulate the animal to incorporate the use of the impaired side in meaningful behavior (Teasell et al. 2005).

The stroke patient's rehabilitation environment is made up of the physical or built environment, consisting of the objects within the environment, other patients, families, and staff. The physical structures in the rehabilitation area have meaning for the patient. It appears from research into both animal and human behavior that the nature of the environment—its physical structure, possibilities for social interaction, physical activity, and exercise—affect brain reorganization after a lesion. Behavioral and ecological studies of humans illustrate the close relationship between the environment and behavior, including the extent and type of physical activity the individual engages in.

Motor control research indicates that objects, their position and orientation in space, drive the action in terms of the pattern or shape of the movement. How the arm segments move when reaching to pick up an object is dependent on the characteristics of the object and where it is in the environment as well as what is to be done with it. The environmental features in this example are a potent facilitator of motor behavior.

Data from clinical studies suggest that providing an environment that encourages social and physical activity is a major challenge that is not being sufficiently met. Observational studies of how stroke patients spend their day in rehabilitation units show that a large part of a patient's day may be spent inactive and alone, watching others or looking out the window (Esmonde et al. 1997, Keith 1980, Lincoln et al. 1989, Mackey et al. 1996, Tinson 1989). Although any physical activity that occurred during the day was in the therapy area, in a study by van Vliet and colleagues (2005) it was found to occur for only a small part of the day, on average 23 minutes. Even less physical activity occurred on weekends and there was little evidence of independent exercise (Tinson 1989, Tyson and Selley 2006). A recent observation of physical activity within the first 14 days of acute stroke found that, although most patients (84.5%) were free to move out of bed, only 13% were engaged in activities that might have the potential to improve mobility and prevent secondary complications (Bernhardt et al. 2004). More than 50% of the patients' time was spent resting in bed. Given its known negative effects, the high levels of bed rest in this study should be of concern.

The most striking finding of these studies is the high proportion of physical and social inactivity. Whatever the relationship between intensity of physical activity and outcome poststroke, the time spent in physical activity in some neurological rehabilitation departments appears minimal compared with normal daily activity, even for healthy elderly people. As such, this minimal time spent in active rehabilitation may not be sufficient to prevent the known negative effects of disuse poststroke.

In recent years, there have been several attempts to investigate whether augmenting exercise training by physical therapists and occupational therapists results in improved outcomes. The results of these studies, in which an additional small increase of time is spent in physical therapy or occupational therapy, are inconclusive. They range from no measurable benefit (Lincoln et al.

1999, Partridge et al. 2000, Rodgers et al. 2003) to significant positive effects (Blennerhassett and Dite 2004, Foley et al. 2003, Kwakkel et al. 1999, 2004). There are many reasons for these discrepancies, including lack of detail of the protocols used in therapy (what the patient actually did, how much, and for how long), differences in outcome measures, insufficient contrast between experimental and control groups, and methodological quality. However, merely increasing the time spent in a therapy session is unlikely to result in improved outcomes—what the patient is actually doing in the session must itself be effective if increasing the time spent is to improve the outcome.

Stroke and coronary artery disease share common risk factors and pathophysiological processes. However, there is a distinct difference in the physical rehabilitation provided and in the environment in which it is performed. Cardiac surgery patients are likely to be rehabilitated in facilities where exercise equipment, including treadmills, exercise bicycles, and heart rate monitors, is in full view. Their purpose is unlikely to be misunderstood—the patients know they will have to work hard to recover strength, endurance, and fitness. Emphasis in stroke rehabilitation is commonly placed primarily on the neurological impairments, with little attention to cardiovascular adaptation to physical inactivity, whereas cardiac rehabilitation has consisted for many years of retraining the cardiorespiratory system through carefully monitored and progressed aerobic exercise. It is becoming clear that functional recovery after stroke with return to independence cannot be explained solely by the state of the neuromuscular system. Adaptation to physical inactivity threatens the individual's ability to meet the elevated energy demands of gait and activities of daily living.

■ Task-Oriented Training to Increase Skill and Motor Control

The physiological factors that affect muscle force generation are *structural* (cross-sectional area (i.e., size) of muscle, density of fibers, and efficiency of mechanical leverage across joints) and *functional* (number, type, and frequency of motor units recruited during a contraction, initial muscle length, and efficiency of cooperation between muscles in a synergy). The goal of physical therapy in neurological rehabilitation is the optimization of functional motor performance. After stroke, the major impairments limiting motor performance are muscle weakness or paralysis, adaptive changes to soft tissues, lack of endurance, and physical fitness.

It is common for patients to experience varying degrees of muscle weakness and the resultant immobility is likely to lead to further and more general adaptive decreases in strength. In addition, elderly individuals may have had muscle weakness due to declining physical activity pre-stroke. Weakness secondary to movement limitations imposed by the brain lesion may actually be more debilitating for the individual than the direct effects of brain injury, but these secondary changes may be preventable or reversible. A study by Hachisuka and colleagues (1997) reported that muscle weakness and atrophy due to disuse are essentially preventable by exercise that activates high threshold motor units such as sit-to-stand, stair walking, and eccentric knee extension training.

In able-bodied individuals, strength training has been shown to stimulate neuromuscular changes. Specifically, it leads to increases in muscle excitation, motor unit activation, recruitment of the motoneuron pool, inhibition of antagonist muscles, and improved synchronization of motor unit firing patterns. Strength training also stimulates metabolic, mechanical, and structural muscle fiber changes that lead to an increase in strength and muscle size as well as endurance. Exercises have the potential to alter passive viscoelastic properties of muscle and tendon. There may also be some advantageous effect of increase in muscle size after stroke (Häkkinen et al. 1998), since muscle atrophy can become a factor in disuse weakness. Even in very elderly individuals, an increase in muscle mass may have functional and metabolic benefits (Harridge et al. 1999).

It follows that strength training is necessary after stroke to increase the force-generating capacity and efficiency of weak muscles to improve functional motor performance. In general two types of exercise are included, weightbearing (closed kinetic chain) and nonweightbearing (open chain) exercises (**Fig. 5.12**). Functional weightbearing exercises to improve strength and control of the lower limb involve moving the body

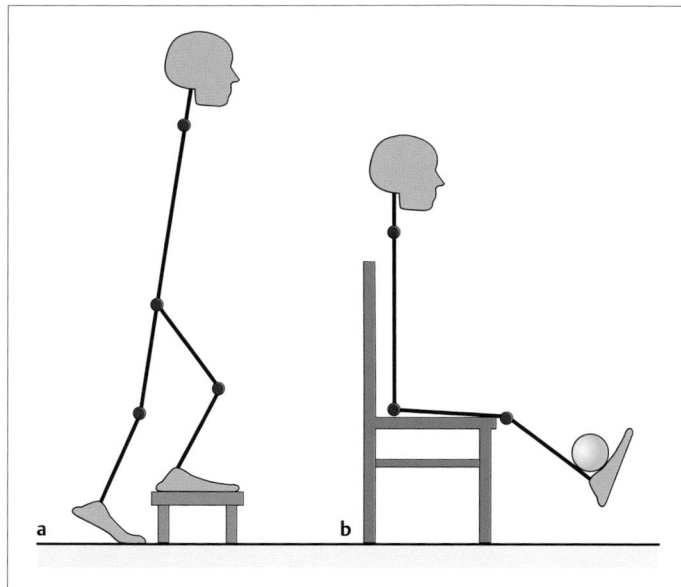

Fig. 5.12 a, b
a Hip, knee, and ankle muscles contract concentrically and eccentrically in kinetic chain body weight-resisted exercises such as step-ups.
b A single-joint, free weight-resisted exercise for quadriceps femoris.

mass over the feet as base of support, with body weight (and added weight where necessary) providing resistance. Open chain exercise includes single-joint exercises with resistance applied in various ways including free weights and dynamometry. There is increasing evidence that strengthening exercise increases strength and physical activity (Ada et al. 2006b).

The relationship between strength and functional performance is complex. The amount of strength required depends on a person's physical size, and on the task to be performed (e.g., walking on a flat surface compared with stair walking). That is, strength is relative. Sufficient muscle strength alone is not sufficient for skilled functional performance—it is factors such as timing of muscle forces and coordination of body segments that underlie motor control of a limb and enable effective and efficient movement. Biomechanical study of the coordination of the lower limbs provides insights into what needs to be regained after stroke.

■ The Lower Limbs in Support, Propulsion, and Balance

The principal functions of the lower limbs in activities performed with feet in contact with the ground are to support the body mass, balance it over the base of support, and propel it in the desired direction (Forssberg 1982).

Support of the large upper body requires the generation of sufficient lower limb extensor activity to maintain segmental alignment in the presence of gravitational and other forces working to collapse the limb. Many mono- and biarticular muscles that span hip, knee, and ankle joints contribute to support by working cooperatively across the three joints. This cooperation is illustrated by the "support moment of force," an algebraic summation of the moments of force acting over the three joints (Winter 1987), demonstrated in studies of walking and of sit-to-stand (Shepherd and Gentile 1994). Any reduction of force at one joint can be made up for by increased moments of force at the other two joints.

Balance of the body mass relative to the base of support enables us to perform everyday actions under a variety of different conditions. The mechanical problem of remaining balanced in the presence of the destabilizing forces that occur as we move around is a particular challenge to the central nervous system. Both anticipatory and ongoing postural adjustments ensure the body is aligned and balanced over the base of support, stabilizing parts of the body while others move (Ghez 1991). Even the simple action of raising the arm in standing requires initial and ongoing muscle activations. Muscle activation patterns and joint rotations that balance us as we move about are flexible and vary specifically according to task and context (Belen'kiĭ et al. 1967, Eng et al. 1992).

In weightbearing actions (e.g., walking, stair walking, standing up and sitting down, reaching for an object in standing, squatting), ground reaction forces occur at the support surface in response to body movement. *Propulsion* of the body mass requires the generation and timing of muscle forces to accelerate the body in the desired direction.

The basic pattern of intersegmental coordination in many actions significant to daily life consists of flexion and extension at hips, knees, and ankles over the feet (**Fig. 5.13**). The body mass is raised and lowered over the supporting feet, the three joints acting as a single functional unit. Foot, shank, and thigh make up a segmental linkage, movement at one joint necessarily producing movement of the other two joints.

The motor control system appears to use simplifying strategies to control the segmental linkage, with cooperation between muscle forces produced over the three joints varying according to the task and the conditions under which it is performed. Regaining skill in motor performance therefore requires not only the ability to generate muscle forces but also to time the forces produced by a large number of muscles. Control of complex intersegmental relationships is required to bring about an effective movement. Studies of human movement in neuroscience and biomechanics have led to the development of specifically targeted task-oriented exercises designed to increase muscle strength, preserve soft tissue flexibility, and train functional motor control.

Weightbearing actions can be trained and practiced concurrently within a few days after stroke. As a general rule the action to be learned should be practiced in its entirety, since one component of the action depends on preceding components. The required neuromotor and biomechanical mechanisms involved in any action can only be organized during performance of that action. Motor training (including strength training) research has shown that exercise effects tend to be specific to task and context (Morrissey et al. 1995, Rutherford 1988) with the greatest changes occurring in the training exercise itself (**Fig. 5.14**). However, there

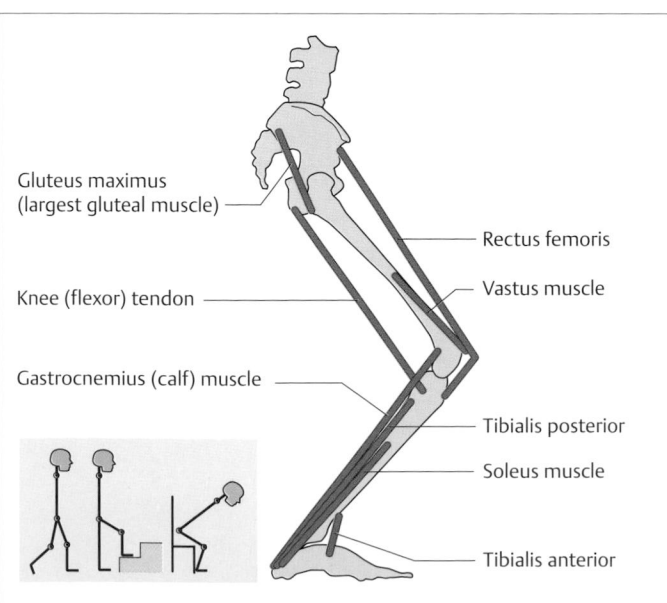

Gluteus maximus
(largest gluteal muscle)

Knee (flexor) tendon

Gastrocnemius (calf) muscle

Rectus femoris

Vastus muscle

Tibialis posterior

Soleus muscle

Tibialis anterior

Fig. 5.13 Diagram showing lower limb segments and eight major muscles involved in concentric and eccentric flexion and extension of the lower limbs over a fixed foot. G max, gluteus maximus; gastroc, gastrocnemius; hamstr, hamstrings; rect fem, rectus femoris; tib ant, tibialis anterior; tib post, tibilias posterior. *(Reprinted from Journal of Biomechanics, AD Kuo and FE Zajac, 1993, with permission from Elsevier Science.)*

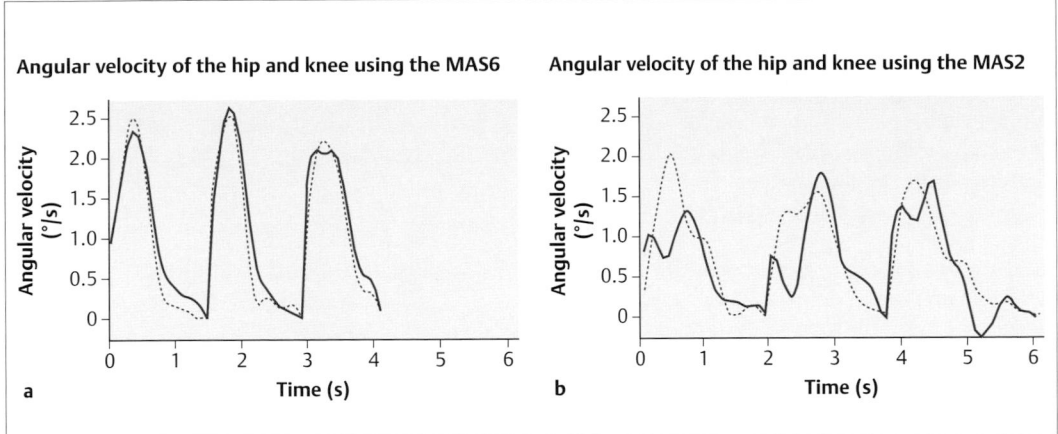

Angular velocity of the hip and knee using the MAS6

Angular velocity of the hip and knee using the MAS2

Fig. 5.14 a, b Improvement in kinematic characteristics and coordination following task training of standing up quantified by linear analysis.
a Hip (solid line) and knee (dashed line) joint velocities are almost perfectly coupled at MAS6, whereas **b** there was significant independent activity at MAS2. *(Reprinted from Human Movement Science, L Ada, NJ O'Dwyer, PD Neilsen, 1993, with permission from Elsevier Science.)*

is also evidence that transfer of the training effect can occur between actions that share similar biomechanical characteristics (Gottlieb et al. 1988). Exercises such as step-ups, heels raise and lower, standing up and sitting down, and modified squats strengthen weak muscles concentrically and eccentrically using body weight resistance and can improve segmental limb control. They take advantage of the specificity principle in that they provide similar functional stresses to the actions being trained. Muscles are therefore exercised in an action pattern that shares some of the dynamic characteristics of many weightbearing actions that are a major focus of the patient's rehabilitation. These exercises train the ability of extensor muscles to switch from shortening to lengthening contractions in muscles spanning several joints (e.g., biceps femoris, gastrocnemius). In addition, they require contraction of other muscles that also play a part in controlling the limb.

Transfer from practice of one action to improvement in another with similar dynamics was illustrated in a study of individuals more than 1 year after stroke (Dean and Shepherd 1997), in which seated subjects reached forward quickly to grasp an object placed on a table at the limit of reachability. The results showed that repetitive practice of the reaching action not only improved the distance reached and the speed of reaching but also the performance of an action not practiced, sit-to-

stand. Beyond-arm's-length reaching in sitting shares similar biomechanical characteristics with sit-to-stand. Both involve an initial major horizontal shift of body weight forward over the feet and the production of vertical ground reaction forces generated through the feet.

It is apparent from clinical observation that after stroke there can be difficulty switching between concentric and eccentric activity, especially when weightbearing. The force-producing capacity (tension regulation) of muscle differs according to whether the contraction is concentric or eccentric (Pinniger et al. 2000). Voluntary eccentric contractions produce greater force than concentric contractions yet involve lower rates of motor unit discharge (Tax et al. 1990). In able-bodied individuals, exercises involving concentric and eccentric contractions produce better gains in strength than exercises with concentric contractions alone. When the muscle is actively stretched in an eccentric contraction, tension in the series elasticity component increases and the stored elastic energy is used in the subsequent concentric contraction (Svantesson and Sunnerhagen 1997).

The effect of what is called the *stretch–shortening cycle* is seen when an eccentric contraction immediately precedes a concentric contraction, as in the brief flexion counter-movement seen in performance of the vertical jump. The concentric phase generates more force when it follows the flexion movement and the person jumps higher. A similar mechanism probably exists in walking (Komi 1986) and in standing up (Shepherd and Gentile 1994). The brief flexion at the knees in standing up, occurring at movement onset, provides a stretch to the knee extensor muscles, immediately prior to limb extension. In stroke patients, it is reported that a significantly larger concentric force occurred during limb loading in standing up after eccentric exercise on an isokinetic dynamometer (Engardt et al. 1995). From their research into changes in the mechanical properties of muscles in the affected limb after stroke, Svantesson and colleagues (2000) suggest that training activities in rehabilitation that emphasize eccentric–concentric exercise may result in more normal function and enhance recovery.

It follows that functional weightbearing exercises, practiced repetitively, can provide a focus for training control of the limb at the same time as providing an action-specific strength training stimulus. These exercises directly address the weakness and lack of motor control which are major neural impairments following stroke, compounded over time by the adaptive effects of disuse and immobility. Preparatory and ongoing balance adjustments are also made during practice of weightbearing exercises so the individual is also practicing the skill of balancing the body mass over the feet while moving.

If muscles are below a certain task-related functional threshold (Buchner et al. 1996), exercises oriented to a particular action component may need to be practiced. For example, contraction of plantar flexors at the end of stance phase of gait produces the power generation at push-off that is critical to the upcoming swing phase. Power generation affects walking speed and ensures energy exchange between segments (Olney et al. 1986). It is likely that these mechanisms can be optimized by exercises to strengthen the calf muscles at the joint angle at which the major burst is required, between about 10° dorsiflexion and 20° plantarflexion (Olney et al. 1988), e.g., by faster treadmill and level walking, and walking up a ramp.

In summary, training of an action such as walking or standing up involves practice of the action itself with task-oriented exercises that incorporate similar dynamic characteristics to the action. Research into movement dynamics indicates that the control system utilizes simplifying strategies as a means of controlling the many degrees of freedom

inherent in the body's segmental linkage. This information enables us to plan a program of training incorporating exercises that increase muscle force generation and are likely to transfer into improved performance of several similar actions, as well as specific training of the action to be learned.

■ Task-Oriented Training

Functional Weightbearing Exercises

Step Up and Step Down

Hip, knee, and ankle extensor muscles are trained to work cooperatively, concentrically and eccentrically, to raise and lower the body mass. Forces are distributed evenly over the three joints when stepping up and down in a forward direction (**Fig. 5.15**), and are more concentrated at the knee in lateral step-ups (Agahari et al. 1996). Resistance is supplied by the body mass, and can be increased by raising step height. These exercises can also be practiced in a safety harness if necessary (**Fig. 5.16**).

Heels Lower and Raise On a Step

Ankle plantar flexors are critical muscles, providing power for propulsion in the stance phase of walking, and enabling walking up a slope (**Fig. 5.17**). They contribute to ankle stability and control forward postural sway. This exercise actively stretches the eccentrically contracting calf muscles when the heel is lowered and is important for preserving the calf muscle length critical for push-off in gait and to performance of many weightbearing actions.

Squatting

Semi-squatting (**Fig. 5.18**) is practiced by reaching down to pick up (or touch) a target object. The depth of squat can be modified, with the target object placed on a stool or on the floor.

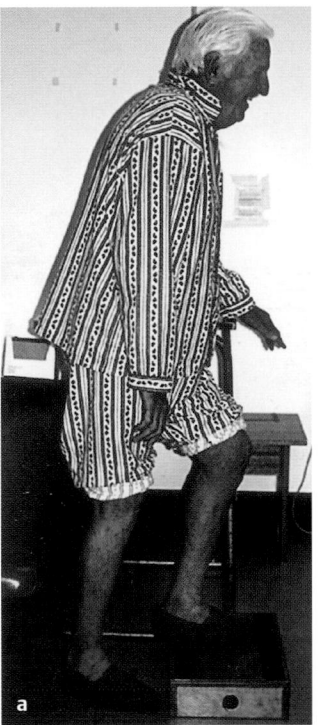
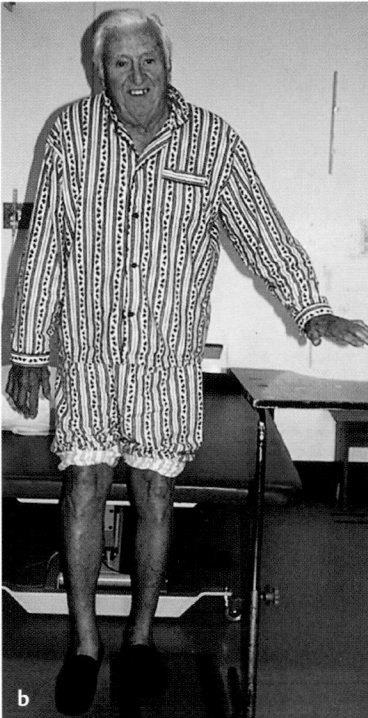
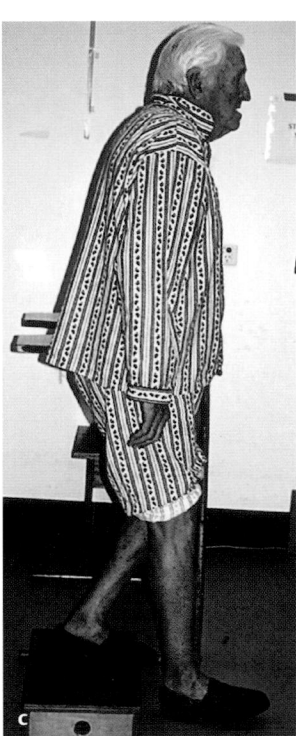

Fig. 5.15 a–c
a Step-up exercises forward,
b laterally and
c forward step-downs, to train hip and knee extensors and ankle plantar flexors to work together, both con-

centrically and eccentrically, to raise and lower the body mass against body weight resistance. These exercises also train ankle dorsiflexors and place an active stretch on the soleus muscle.

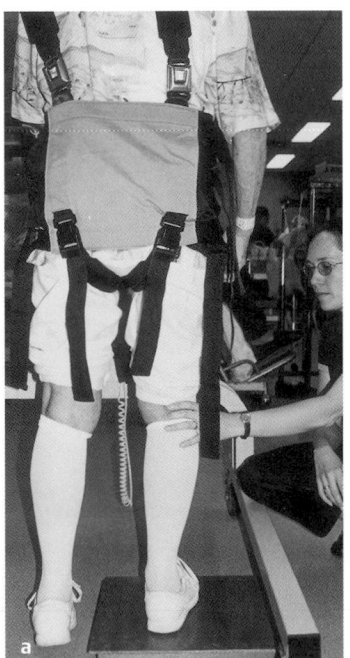
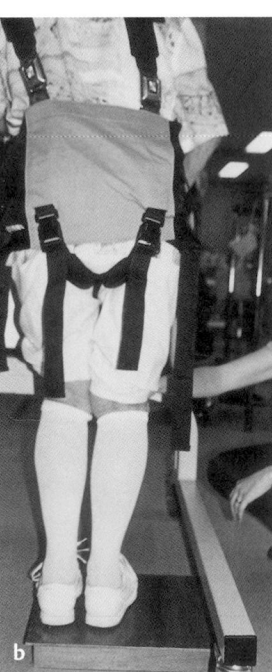

Fig. 5.16 Step-ups can be practiced in a harness. This provides confidence while strengthening the lower limb extensor muscles concentrically and eccentrically. The patient has her paretic foot on the step. She raises and lowers her body weight to place her nonparetic foot on to the step. This is less challenging than repetitive raising and lowering as demonstrated in **Fig 5.15 b**.

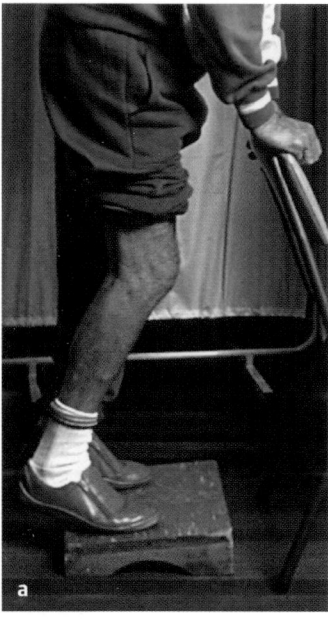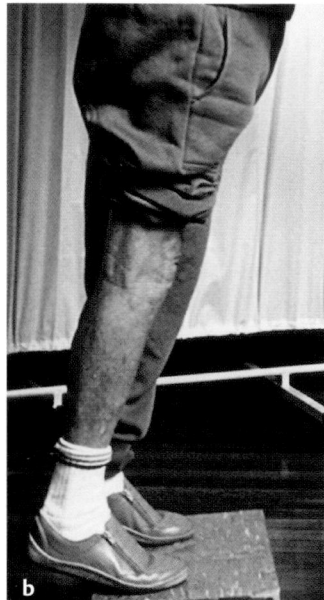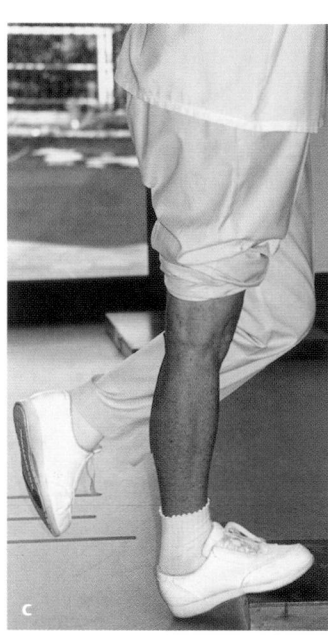

Fig. 5.17 a–c   Heels raised to plantigrade and lowered to strengthen and actively stretch the plantar flexors. This exercise trains the calf muscles specifically at the length required for push-off at the end of stance. The patient holds on to a stable object as he practices.
a When he attempts to raise his heels to plantigrade, his paretic knee flexes. It is difficult for him to control

the paretic knee in extension when the two-joint gas- trocnemius contracts.
b He has got the idea of controlling the muscles that cross the ankle and knee.
c This woman can control her quadriceps to keep her knee extended while soleus and gastrocnemius con- tract to plantarflex the ankle. Now she increases repe- titions and speed to improve control and endurance.

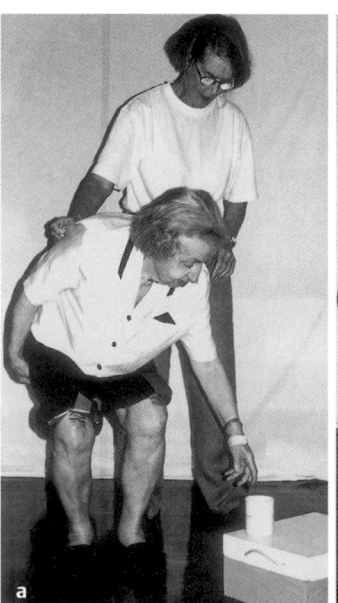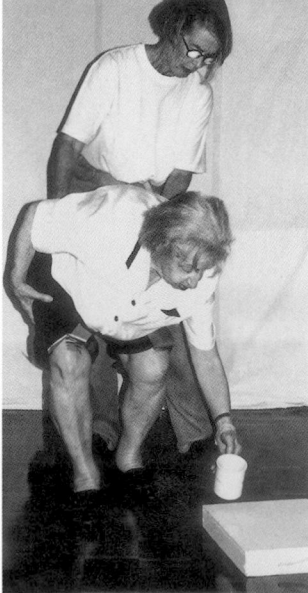

Fig. 5.18 a, b   Squatting exercise: adapting the task by modifying the environment to enable an individual to train.
a Practice with the object on a box develops confidence to reach even lower.

b This man practices loading his paretic limb in a more difficult position for balance. His right leg is also weak so he practices to both sides.

Repetitive Sit-to-Stand (Fig. 5.19)

Major force generation comes from quadriceps muscles with assistance of other lower limb extensors. If muscles are weak, seat height is increased so less muscle force is required. As muscles become stronger, seat height is lowered and a prescribed number of repetitions are increased to improve endurance. The paretic limb is forced to bear weight by placing the paretic foot behind the nonparetic foot before movement starts. The action is performed at close to normal speed, that is, not too slowly.

The above exercises are practiced repetitively, with maximum repetitions (up to 10 with no breaks) in sets of three, with a short break between sets. A counter is a useful aid for the patient to count repetitions.

Nonweightbearing Exercises

In these exercises, resistance is provided by free weights, weight machines (e.g., dynamometer), and elastic bands (**Fig. 5.20**). With the goal of increasing the ability of a muscle or group of muscles to generate and control force, these exercises can be practiced independently and as part of circuit training. Although concurrent task practice is necessary for neural adaptation (Rutherford 1988) and learning to occur, in very weak patients small changes in lower limb strength gained by nonweightbearing exercises may produce relatively large changes in motor performance (Buchner et al. 1996).

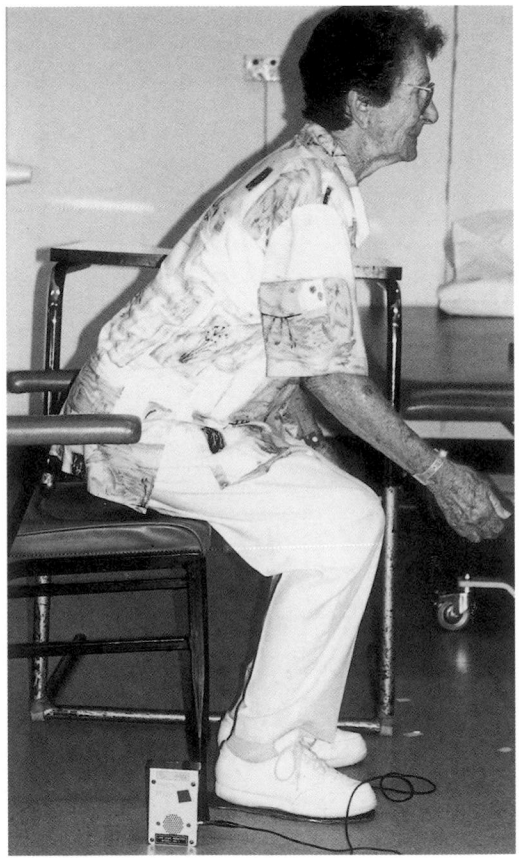

Fig. 5.19 Semi-supervised repetitive standing up and sitting down practice. The patient gets feedback from a pressure-sensitive device under the foot and records the number of repetitions on a counter in her left hand to compare with how many repetitions she did yesterday.

> **Guidelines for Strength Training**
> - Encourage patient to exercise as intensively as possible.
> - Grade the amount of resistance and number of repetitions to the individual's ability.
> - Utilize resistance from body weight, free weights, elastic bands, isokinetic dynamometry, exercise machines, or inclined treadmill.
> - Vary body weight resistance, step height, chair height, weight of object being lifted.
> - As a general rule, a maximum number of repetitions should be performed (up to 10) without a rest and repeated in three sets, with a short break between sets.
> - In progressive resistance weight training the patient attempts 10 repetitions of 60%–80% of the maximum possible load that can be lifted in one attempt.
> - For endurance, a high number of repetitions is practiced at low levels of load; exercises can include stationary cycling, arm cycling, and treadmill walking.
> - For very weak muscles, use methods which facilitate muscle activation and force generation, and include simple exercises, biofeedback, mental practice, and functional electrical stimulation.

Strength training is designed not only to improve force generation but also sustainability of muscle contraction and speed of force buildup (power). To be effective, strength training should transfer into functional improvement. Sharp and Brouwer (1997) found a correlation between increases in strength and in gait speed after a strength training

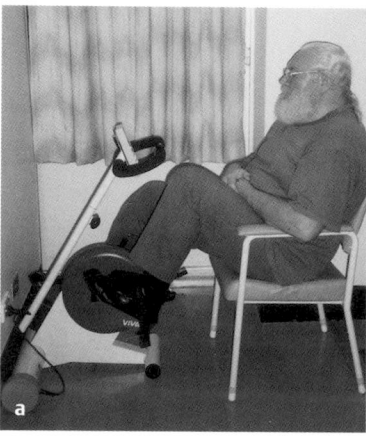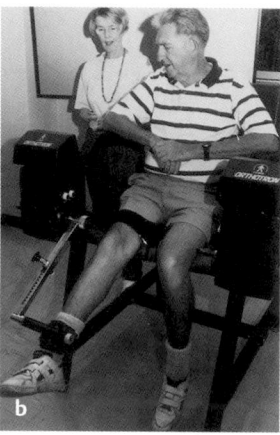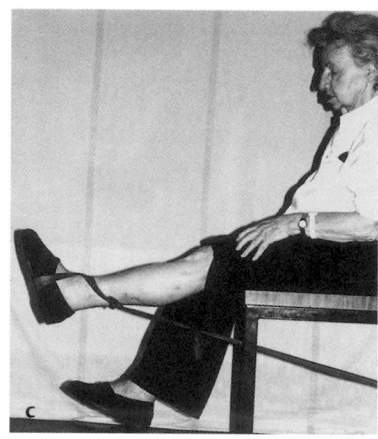

Fig. 5.20 a–c Circuit training stations:
a The MOTOmed provides resistance or assistance in response to the individual's performance *(Reck, Betzen-weiler, Germany.)*
b Exercising on a dynamometer strengthens knee extensor muscles concentrically and eccentrically, or isometrically. This patient's target is to exercise his quad-

riceps at 60% of his 1RM load. He is getting feedback from the monitor. Muscles that act as stabilizers are also being exercised. *(Reprinted with kind permission from PRO-ED Inc, Austin Tx, USA.)*
c The elastic band should be under tension throughout the movement.

program. They reported significant increases in concentric muscle strength and motor performance after concentric strength training in chronic stroke. Weightbearing and nonweight-bearing exercises such as those described above can result in significant increases in:

- Gait speed (Dean et al. 2000, Eng et al. 2003, Teixeira-Salmela et al. 1999, 2001)
- Muscle power and function (Foldvari et al. 2000)
- Walking endurance and the step test (Dean et al. 2000)
- Ability to balance, speed of standing up and muscle strength (Weiss et al. 2000)
- Ability to balance while moving, reduction in falls (Lord et al. 2007, Sherrington and Lord 1997, Sherrington et al. 2008)
- Number of stand-ups during the day and loading of paretic limb when standing up (Britton et al. 2008)

■ Active Muscle Stretching

Due to weakness and subsequent inactivity, the natural tendency is for soft tissues to become stiffer and shorter. Increased stiffness in the paretic plantar flexors has been reported to occur as early

as 2 months (Malouin et al. 1997), although it is likely to occur much earlier as shown in both animal and able-bodied human research. Slow-twitch muscles, such as the soleus, seem particularly vulnerable if they are rarely exposed to active and passive stretch.

Preservation of functional length of muscles, in particular of soleus muscle and hip flexors, requires active stretch during practice of exercises that make similar length demands to those of functional activities. It is particularly important to practice repetitive standing up and sitting down with feet placed behind knees as early as possible after stroke as means of preserving length of the soleus muscle. This muscle shortens rapidly if the person is inactive, and once it is short many actions such as standing up may become compromised. It is natural for muscle length, stiffness, and strength to adapt to an individual's needs, and when our needs change, it is typical for us to stretch and exercise to improve our flexibility when we plan to play an unaccustomed sport. There is evidence that active stretch during repetitive exercise can increase range of motion (Miller and Light 1997, Teixeira-Salmela et al. 1999).

Repetitive practice of functional actions is not only necessary for regaining skill but also preserves the necessary muscle length for performance of the skill. However, passive methods of length preservation in the very early stages may be necessary for some patients. If practice of standing up modified by a raised seat height is not possible, standing on a tilt table with the foot on a wedge for 20–30 minutes will maintain a passive stretch on the soleus muscle (**Fig. 5.21**). It is active stretch, however, that is necessary for preserving functional length.

Increased range of motion after stretching involves biomechanical, neurophysiological, and molecular mechanisms. Tension in muscle consists of active and passive components. Stretch can affect the active component by altering neural activity (Hummelsheim and Mauritz 1993) and the passive mechanical component by affecting viscous and elastic properties of the muscle. The mechanisms of increasing muscle length and range of motion are not well understood, but may possibly be found in the cellular and adaptive mechanisms of a muscle fiber (De Deyne 2001). One characteristic of viscoelasticity is that tissues respond to stretch and to being held at a constant length with a decrease in tension; this is known as stress

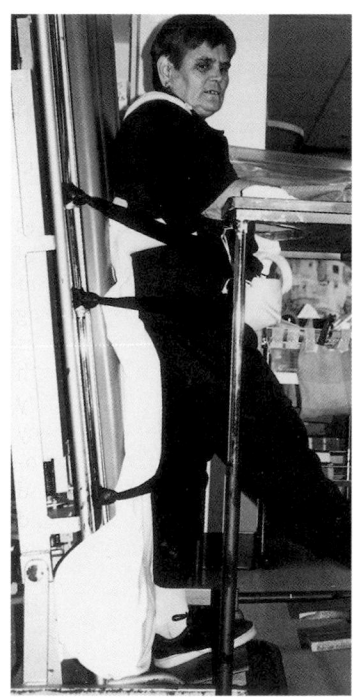

Fig. 5.21 Passive stretch to the calf muscle on a tilt table. Positioning the nonparetic limb on a stool ensures that the paretic calf is being stretched. This position is held for 20–30 minutes.

relaxation. During stretch, soft tissues also undergo progressive deformation and can be progressively extended with a constant force. This is called creep (Herbert 2005).

■ Maximizing Muscle Endurance and Physical Fitness

The extent and time course of change in exercise capacity during rehabilitation has not been studied extensively in the early poststroke period. Similarly, the intensity of exercise and the extent of cardiovascular stress induced during rehabilitation have received little attention (Kilbreath and Davis 2005). The results available suggest that contemporary stroke rehabilitation programs may not be sufficiently vigorous to prevent physical deconditioning. Sustained physical inactivity induces a reduction in aerobic capacity (aerobic capacity is the product of the capacity of the cardiorespiratory system to supply oxygen, i.e., cardiac output, and the capacity of the skeletal muscle to utilize oxygen; Pang et al 2006a), limiting the performance of activities of daily living, and increasing the risk of falls and dependence on others.

Deconditioning may to some extent be a consequence of the relatively static nature of typical rehabilitation programs (Kelly et al. 2003, MacKay-Lyons and Howlett 2005). MacKay-Lyons and Makrides (2002) investigated the aerobic component of physical and occupational therapy for stroke patients by monitoring heart rate (using heart rate monitors) and therapeutic activities biweekly over a 14-week period without influencing the content. The major finding was that therapy sessions involved low-intensity exercise and activity that did not provide adequate metabolic stress to induce a training effect. A disproportionate amount of time was spent inactive. When present, the aerobic component of a typical physical therapy session took less than 3 minutes. Although one might expect progressively higher exercise intensities over time as functional status improves, any increase in hear rate (HR_{mean} and HR_{peak}) did not reach statistical significance.

Implementation of a goal to improve cardiorespiratory fitness by increasing the aerobic component of training during the early rehabilitation period may help to prevent the downward degenerative cycle of decreased physical activity and disability that is frequently reported. Low cardiorespiratory fitness in chronic stroke is said to be secondary to a decrease in exercise capacity, decreased mobility, and increased energy expenditure. The criterion measure for aerobic capacity, peak oxygen consumption (Vo_2), may be as low as 50%–70% of the age- and sex-matched values of sedentary individuals (Eng et al. 2004, MacKay-Lyons and Makrides 2004).

It is well documented that stroke patients have low physical endurance when discharged from rehabilitation, limiting their ability to perform household tasks and to walk outside the home. Loss of independent ambulation, especially outdoors, has been identified as one of the most debilitating of stroke sequelae. Among stroke survivors 1 year after stroke, the most striking area of difficulty was low endurance as measured by 6-minute walk test (Mayo et al. 2005). Subjects able to complete this test were able to walk on average only 250 m, equivalent to 40% of their predicted ability and not far enough for a reasonable and active lifestyle. The detrimental effect of low exercise capacity and muscle endurance on functional mobility and resistance to fatigue can be compounded by the high metabolic demand of adaptive movements. Endurance is likely to decline further after discharge if follow-up exercise programs are not available. Furthermore, low aerobic fitness is a significant determinant of poor bone health (specifically osteoporosis) in individuals with chronic stroke (Pang et al. 2005).

Although it can be difficult to test fitness after stroke, MacKay-Lyons and Makrides (2002) used a treadmill with 15% body weight support in a maximal exercise test. Submaximal tests such as the 6-minute walk test can also be valid. There is some evidence that exercise trainability early after stroke can be both feasible and safe if appropriate screening by medical practitioners (see American College of Sports Medicine 2000) and monitoring of heart rate and blood pressure are used (MacKay-Lyons and Howlett 2005). Training is initiated at conservative intensities. Early indications suggest that walking speed, mobility, and balance improve with such programs.

There are several reports of improved aerobic capacity in chronic stroke with appropriate training such as bicycle ergometry (Potempa et al. 1995), graded treadmill walking (Macko et al.

1997), and a combination of aerobic and strengthening exercises (Teixeira-Salmela et al. 1999). As might be expected, the effects are exercise-specific. Generalization occurs, however, in the improvements noted in general health and wellbeing that impacted on performance of activities they considered meaningful. Teixeira-Salmela and colleagues (1999) assessed the general level of physical activity of their subjects on the Human Activity Profile, a survey of 94 activities that are rated according to their required metabolic equivalents. The results indicated that subjects were able to perform more household chores and recreational activities after strength and aerobic training. These quality of life gains appear to be critical factors for stroke survivors' reintegration into society. A recent systematic review provides good evidence that aerobic exercise, at 50%–80% of heart rate reserve, 3–5 days a week for 20–40 minutes, should be an important component of stroke rehabilitation (Pang et al. 2006a).

The implications are clear. The challenge for clinicians and patients is not only to increase the time spent in physical activity but also to organize time to provide sufficient intensity to induce a training effect. Time spent in therapy is a crude estimate of actual intensity, and does not allow an estimate of the effort and energy that was expended during training. Intensity and aerobic content of training need to be addressed specifically and early after stroke in an effort both to increase exercise capacity and to minimize poststroke deconditioning.

The remainder of this chapter provides clinical guidelines based on contemporary scientific understanding and where possible on evidence from randomized controlled clinical trials. Balance is described first—the ability to make adjustments to the body mass over the base of support as we interact with gravitational and other forces underlies the performance of all motor actions. Next are guidelines for training standing up and sitting down, walking, reaching and manipulation—major actions that are the primary focus of rehabilitation. Outcome data are critical to this process of developing evidence-based (www.pedro.org.au, www.cochrane.org/reviews/clibintro.htm) recommendations for stroke rehabilitation. At the end of each of these sections is a list of measures in common use and the chapter ends with an appendix providing a list of measurement tools that are valid and reliable.

Training Guidelines: Balance

Balance is the ability to achieve, maintain, and restore equilibrium by controlling the center of body mass (COM) over the base of support. Balancing is a complex sensorimotor skill necessary for and part of all activities of daily living in a gravitational environment.

Movement involves modifications of postural alignment. Balance is not based on a fixed set of reflexes but is an integral part of the task undertaken and the environment in which the task is performed, and it becomes more effective with training and experience (**Fig. 5.22**). The idea of equilibrium reflexes as the basis of balance adjustments that has been influential in physical therapy reflected an older view of balance as essentially reflexive and reactive. For several decades this view has diverted clinical practice away from the task-specificity of the muscular and biomechanical characteristics of balance adjustments and their anticipatory and ongoing nature. It is now clear that balance is learned along with each new task and becomes more effective with training.

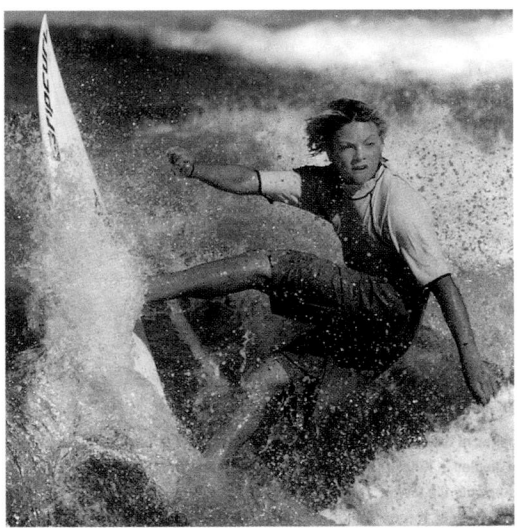

Fig. 5.22 Balance is normally learned during practice of a new task and continued practice of a skilled activity.

Balance is maintained through a complex interaction of the various components of the vestibular, visual, and somatosensory systems that provide information about the body's position and movement with respect to the environment. Sensory inputs critical to the action are coordinated in a task-relevant way. Vision appears to be particularly important, assisting us to orient ourselves vertically, pay attention to relevant features in the environment, and predict upcoming perturbations to avoid a fall.

Evidence suggests that cognition also has an active role in preserving balance and postural control. Paying attention to environmental cues is particularly important when balance is threatened. Focusing on an external visual cue rather than on internal balance control is likely to lead to better performance, allowing balance to self-regulate (Guadagnoli et al. 2002).

The mechanical problem of remaining balanced as we move is a particular challenge for the central nervous system. Ghez (1991) has described a family of adjustments needed to maintain a posture and to remain balanced while moving that has three goals:

- Support the body against gravity
- Maintain the COM aligned and balanced over the base of support
- Stabilize some parts of the body while moving others

Biomechanical Description of the Effects of Task and Environment on Balance Mechanisms

The forces that disturb balance are gravitational and other forces that arise from interaction between segments as we move. These gravitational and interactive forces must be controlled for balance to be maintained. In quiet standing, small movements of the body, called postural sway occur, even when we take a breath. Highly skilled individuals such as ballet dancers may have a relatively large extent of sway, while others, such as highly skilled pistol shooters, have a minimal degree of sway as they prepare to pull the trigger.

Anticipatory Postural Adjustments

The performance of all actions, even simple acts such as raising an arm in standing, are preceded by precisely timed anticipatory postural adjustments, before the action as well as during the movement, to minimize the destabilizing effects on balance caused by the movement itself (Eng et al. 1992). Leg muscle activity (Belen'kiĭ et al. 1967) and small segmental movements (Zattara and Bouisset 1988) are part of the action since they are highly specific to that action. They vary with speed and support conditions. Anticipatory and ongoing postural adjustments ensure the body's COM stays within the base of support.

Specificity of Postural Adjustments

It is clear that postural adjustments are an integral part of an action, adapting to the task and the environment in which it is performed. The experiments illustrated in **Fig. 5.23** clarify the specificity of muscle activity. Subjects interacted with the handle in four different ways: (A) Standing unsupported, they pulled on the handle. The challenge to balance resulted in activation of a postural leg muscle (gastrocnemius) prior to the pull and to the activation of the arm muscle (biceps brachii). (B) Support was provided at chest height. When the handle was unexpectedly pulled away from the subject minimal leg muscle activity occurred since, with the body supported, active maintenance of a balanced position was not necessary. (C) When this support was removed, however, early calf muscle activity was again evident. (D) When subjects held the stabilized handle and the support platform under the feet was unexpectedly moved forward, the arm muscle turned on before a small contraction of the leg muscle. In this latter case, arm muscle activation was crucial in preventing balance from being lost since the hand was grasping the only object that provided stability. It is therefore not always lower limb muscles that play a balance-preservation role in standing.

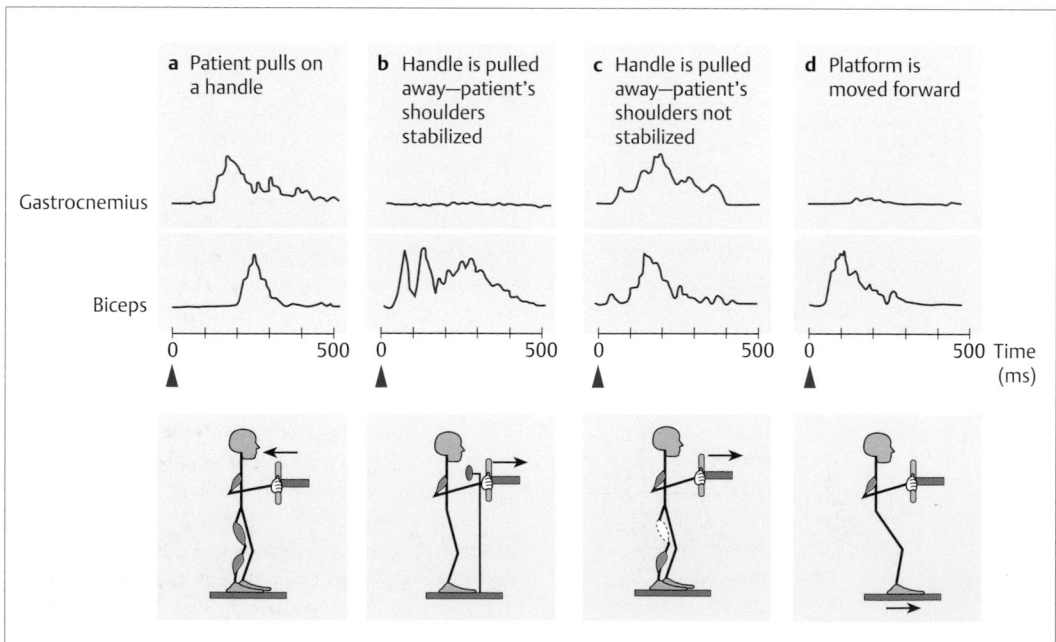

Fig. 5.23 a–d   An example of the specificity of postural adjustments. An arm muscle (biceps brachii) and a leg muscle (gastrocnemius) were monitored.
a Subject pulls on handle.
b Unexpected movement of the handle with the shoulders braced.

c As in B but subject is free standing.
d Unexpected forward platform movement.
(Adapted from Nashner 1983 with permission.)

Taking a Step/Raising One Leg in Standing

Several studies have examined a group of actions in standing in which the body mass shifts laterally to free one leg from support in order to raise it; for instance, to initiate gait (Kirker et al. 2000) or to place one foot on a step (Mercer and Sahrmann 1999). The point to be noted is that in these actions both limbs are involved. Data showed that the foot's center of pressure (COP) shifted first toward the limb to be raised. This occurred milliseconds earlier, and reflected the shift of COP over to the support limb. These postural adjustments in the mediolateral direction occur primarily in the shank/foot linkage (inverter and evertor muscles) and thigh/pelvis linkage (abductor and adductor muscles) (Winter 1995).

Variations in Task and Context

Balance is challenged when walking in a dark room or crossing the street. It has to adapt to walking on ice, on sand, or when stepping on and off a moving footway—a situation increasingly encountered in shopping centers and airports. Balance is challenged when turning the head while walking and in quiet standing (**Fig. 5.24**). The visual system plays an important role in identifying changes in the environment that are likely to affect balance.

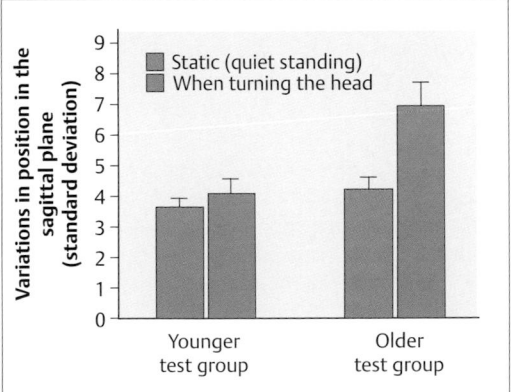

Fig. 5.24 Postural sway in a sagittal direction in quiet standing during head turning with eyes open in a group of elderly compared with young individuals. *(Adapted from Koceja et al 1999, with permission.)*

Unexpected Perturbations

Studies of postural responses to stumbling while walking and to support surface perturbations, provide information about the mechanisms of reactive balance responses which form the emergency back-up system when our predictions fail (Huxham et al. 2001, Patla 1995). Stepping and grasping are the preferred options even when perturbations are relatively small. The responses are rapid, directionally specific, and focused on distal musculature linking the shank and foot. Even rapid responses are adaptive to context. Avoidance strategies in walking, for example, include adaptations to step/stride, increasing ground clearance to avoid an obstacle, changing direction, and stopping. We lose balance only when unexpected events occur and we fail to respond quickly enough.

Reaching for Objects in Sitting

Sitting balance requires the ability to balance on different types of seats while performing a variety of tasks, frequently at more than arm's length, in both the sagittal and frontal planes. We extend the distance reached forward by flexing at the hips and dorsiflexing at the ankles, an integral part of the reaching movement (Dean et al. 1999a, 1999b). The lower limbs play an important role in supporting and balancing the body mass when reaching beyond arm's length both at fast and slow speeds (**Fig. 5.25**) (Crosbie et al. 1995, Dean et al. 1999a, 1999b). In sitting, lower limb muscles are involved in anticipatory, ongoing, and reactive postural adjustments. It is more difficult to reach rapidly beyond arm's length when the feet are hanging free, such as over the side of the bed, than when the feet are supported and providing stability (Chari and Kirby 1986).

Age-Related Changes

The effect of aging on balance is complex, multifactorial, and unclear. Increasing age is associated with a reduction in lower limb muscle strength and an increased risk of developing pathologies, all of which may be exacerbated by physical inactivity associated with a sedentary lifestyle. Loss of ankle joint mobility and reduced strength in the dorsiflexors and plantar flexors are particularly significant for balance control (Vandervoort et al.

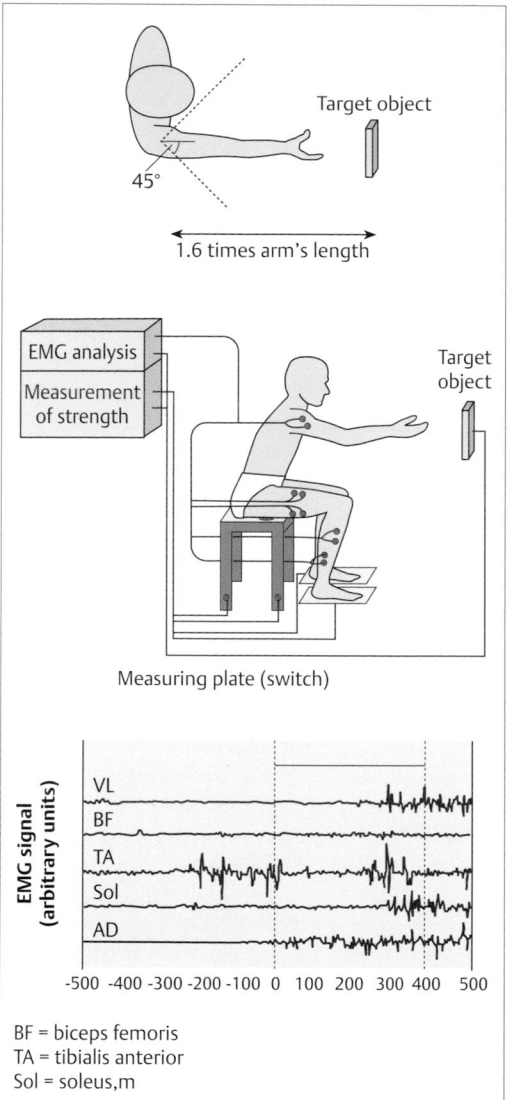

Fig. 5.25 Fast reaching to a target (160% arm length) with the right arm. Trial from one subject showing typical EMG traces from ipsilateral vastus lateralis (VL), biceps femoris (BF), tibialis anterior (TA), soleus (Sol), and anterior deltoid (AD) in a forward direction. Note, TA is the first muscle to turn on and it turns on before the focal muscle AD. Fast reaching beyond arm's length is an effective way to activate TA.

1992). Based on current evidence from 44 randomized controlled trials, exercise programs that are effective in prevention of falls include a combination of challenging and progressive balance exercises performed in weightbearing positions

that minimize the use of upper limbs for support. Resistance, endurance, and flexible training may provide additional benefits if combined with the balance exercises (for analysis see Lord et al. 2007, Sherrington et al. 2008).

Functional Problems—Experimental Findings

Individuals poststroke with muscle weakness and poor motor control have difficulty loading the paretic limb in both sitting and standing and therefore lack effective and efficient anticipatory, ongoing, and responsive postural adjustments. The ability to load the paretic limb and transfer weight from limb to limb are critical for functional mobility and prerequisites for walking and stair climbing (Eng and Chu 2002). Goldie and colleagues (1996) reported that the individuals they studied could shift only 55% of their body weight on to the paretic limb when standing with the paretic limb in front, and only 65% of their body weight in a lateral direction with feet parallel. It is also common for stroke patients to stand up with less weight on the paretic limb. Below are findings from several other studies of balance after stroke.

Standing and Body Transport

- *Support surface perturbations in standing.* Muscles of the paretic limb are slow to respond and unreliable; EMG results have shown increased latencies of muscle onsets, decreased magnitude of activation response, and, in some subjects, absence of muscle response (Di Fabio 1997, Horak et al. 1984).
- *Resisting a force applied laterally by pressure to the hip region.* EMG results showed that muscles were slow to respond to the application of force, had impaired ability to sustain activity to resist the external force, and were slow to respond to release of the force (Kirker et al. 2000, Wing et al. 1993).

Note that in the studies reported above, subjects favored the nonparetic limb, a typical adaptation to muscle weakness and deficient motor control.
- *Taking a step or raising one leg in standing.* Difficulty shifting weight from one leg to another in the frontal plane is evident in studies of both actions (Laufer et al. 2000, Pai et al. 1994). Findings have shown that subjects had difficulty

shifting weight to both the paretic and nonparetic limb when performing leg flexion movements with one limb. For example, in attempting to raise the nonparetic limb, failure to achieve successful weight shift sideways on to the paretic limb was primarily due to insufficient displacement of the COM laterally and failure to stabilize the final position. In attempting to raise the paretic limb, individuals poststroke again have difficulty, since shifting weight over to the nonparetic limb requires the ability to activate the abductor and extensor muscles of the paretic limb at the appropriate time and with appropriate force.

A fundamental biomechanical principle in the maintenance of stationary upright stance is that the COM projection has to remain within the base of support regardless of whether standing is through one or both limbs. Approximately 80% of the total horizontal ground reaction force generated to propel the body sideways (in the frontal plane) to raise one leg occurs briefly beneath the foot of the flexing limb on movement initiation. The dynamic role of hip abductor muscles in contributing to the initiation and performance of the weight shift to one side is in addition to their role in stabilizing the pelvis during single-limb stance (Pai et al. 1994). For the patient to have the opportunity to re-establish this mechanism requires practice of exercises involving single-limb loading and practice of stepping with both paretic and nonparetic limbs.

- *Quiet standing.* Both increased and decreased postural sway have been reported. However, postural sway is poorly related to dynamic actions and is not a sufficient measure of postural stability since limiting sway does not necessarily lead to improved stability (Horak 1997).
- *Walking.* Reduced speed and an increase in the time spent in double support are significant problems (Olney 2005).
- *Walking over obstacles.* Whether leading with the paretic or nonparetic limb, patients have difficulty balancing on one leg to step over an obstacle (Said et al. 1999). Further investigations have demonstrated decreased foot clearance when stepping over the obstacle with the paretic limb (**Fig. 5.26**). In addition, both feet may land too close to the obstacle after clearance; that is, the foot is put down too soon (Said et al. 2005).

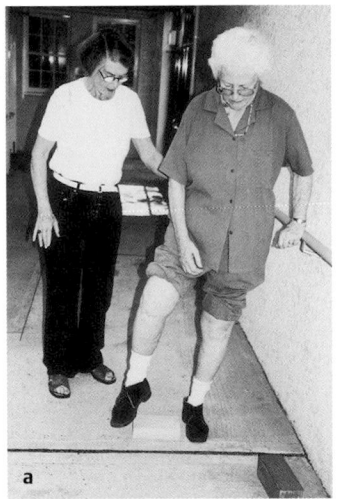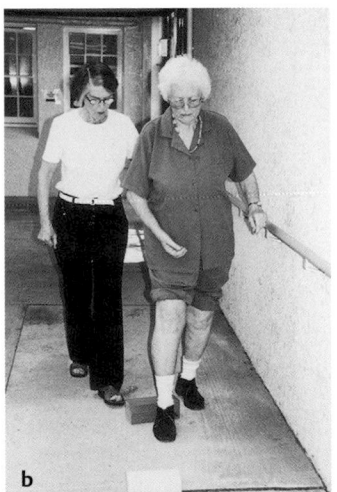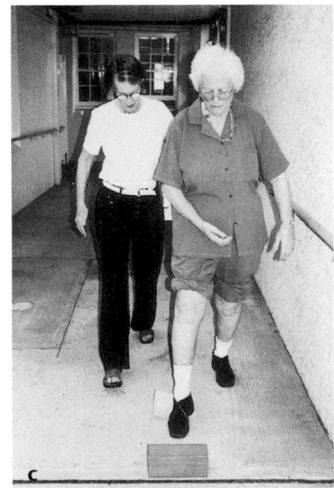

Fig. 5.26 a–c Walking over obstacles.
a On an early attempt, the patient steadies herself on the rail and has positioned her left foot so only a short step is needed. Right hip flexion and dorsiflexion are limited so she adapts by abducting the right hip in an attempt to clear the obstacle.

b She clears the object without needing support.
c She catches her heel on the object. Obstacle crossing provides loading of one limb while moving the body mass forward and controlling step length to avoid catching the heel with the lead limb.

Sitting

- *Difficulty regaining sitting balance early post-stroke* may be a predictor of poor outcome (Loewen and Anderson 1990).
- *Reaching in sitting.* With the feet on the floor, inability to activate paretic lower limb muscles for stability limits the distance and speed of reaching (Dean and Shepherd 1997).

Sensory Dysfunction

Sensory dysfunction can disrupt balance following stroke. Paying attention to relevant information is also important when balance is challenged (Gentile 2000). If one sensory system is dysfunctional, redundancy in the system may allow for compensation (Winter et al. 1990). However, loss of multiple sensory inputs results in balance instability (Di Fabio and Badke 1991, Marigold et al. 2004). The Clinical Test for Sensory Interaction in Balance (Shumway-Cook and Horak 1986) is used to examine sensory adaptation.

Observable Adaptations

When the individual attempts to perform everyday actions, certain predictable adaptations to poor balance can be observed. Adaptive motor behaviors, if allowed to persist, may prevent the regaining of effective balance in different contexts. They include:

- Favoring the stronger, better coordinated and more rapidly responsive lower limb during STS and in activities in sitting, standing, and body transport
- Increasing the base of support in sitting (**Fig. 5.27a**), standing (**Fig. 5.27c**), and walking
- Restricting movement of the body mass to limit the extent of balance adjustments (**Fig. 5.27b, d**)
- Using/relying on hands for support and balance (**Fig. 5.27e**)
- Avoiding threats to balance

Task-Oriented Training

Improving performance and regaining skill in an action largely involves the acquisition of skilled balance control. However, balance cannot be trained in isolation. It is trained simultaneously as part of the training of everyday actions such as walking, standing up and sitting down, or reaching and manipulation. Modifications of the environment or task are made when the person is unstable in order to decrease the balance demands and enable practice of the desired action while still presenting a challenge to stability.

For an individual to regain the ability to balance while being active requires the development of an accurate sense of balance, muscles that are strong enough to support and transport the body mass while keeping the body balanced throughout, and preservation of soft tissue flexibility. After stroke, the patient needs the opportunity to practice a variety of actions in sitting and standing and body transport. As control and confidence improve, the focus changes to maximizing motor skill, keeping in mind the complex environment outside the rehabilitation unit.

Training Balance in Sitting

Establishing sitting balance early poststroke impacts positively on many critical functions (Johansson 2000). For example, in comparison with lying supine in bed, the sitting position provides greater stimulus for gaseous interchange; enables more effective swallowing; and encourages eye contact, communication, and more positive attitudes. Self-initiated movements of the body mass over the base of support (feet and thighs) provide the opportunity to regain the ability to cope with gravity and also to focus attention on people and surroundings.

As soon as vital signs are stable, the patient can sit over the side of bed or on a more stable surface, with the feet supported and close together. In this position the patient practices small shifts of the body mass over the base of support:

- Self-initiated head and trunk movements (e.g., looking over the paretic and nonparetic shoulders)
- Reaching forward, laterally, downward, across the body to touch, move, or pick up an object with one or both hands (**Fig. 5.28**)
- Lifting alternate feet off the supporting surface (**Fig. 5.29**)

To maximize skill, the environment and/or task are changed so that distance to be reached is increased and the person is stretched to the limits of stability (**Fig. 5.30**). Speed can be increased, amount of thigh support reduced, and object

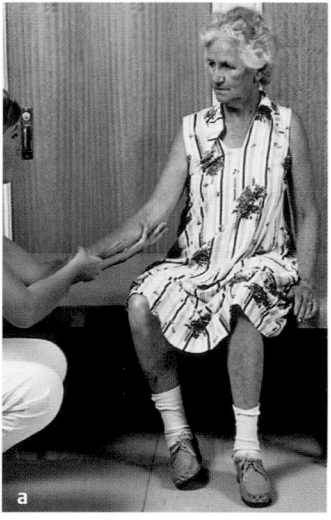
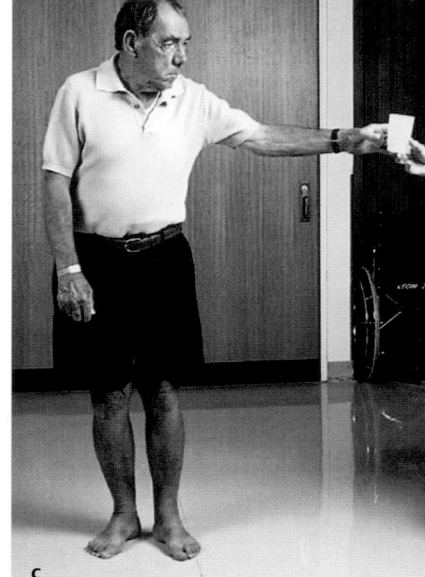
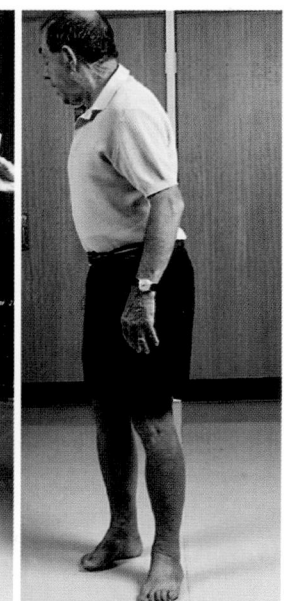
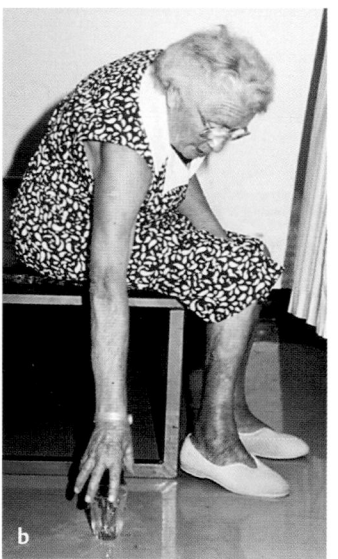
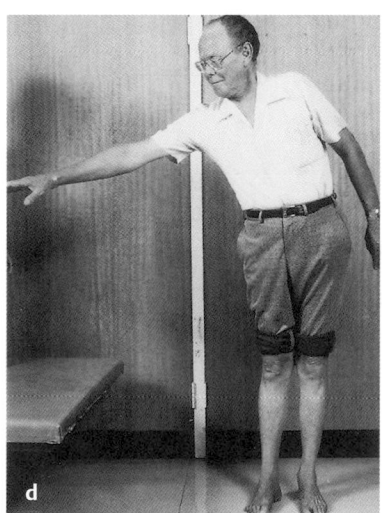
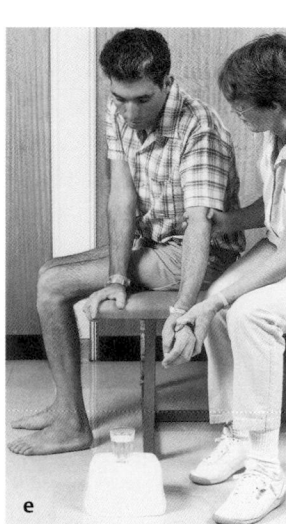

Fig. 5.27 a–e   Typical adaptations to avoid loading and balancing body mass on the paretic lower limb.
a No active support through paretic right lower limb—it abducts at the hip.
b The patient has turned toward the right and leans forward to avoid reaching sideways, which requires more balance ability. She is reluctant to balance over her right foot.

c This patient increases the base of support by externally rotating his right paretic lower limb when he turns to speak to his wife.
d He restricts movement of the body mass over to the right foot as he reaches laterally.
e After his stroke this patient uses his right (nonparetic) arm for support to shift the body mass to the left. This was his first attempt.

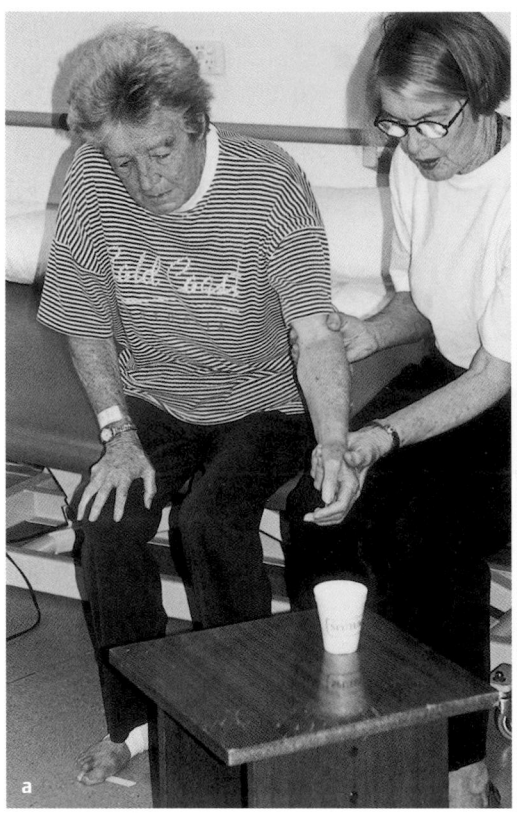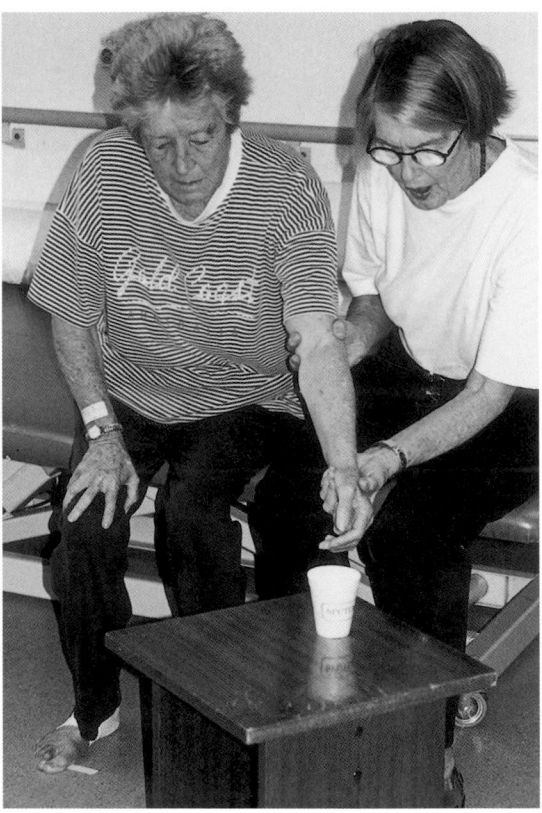

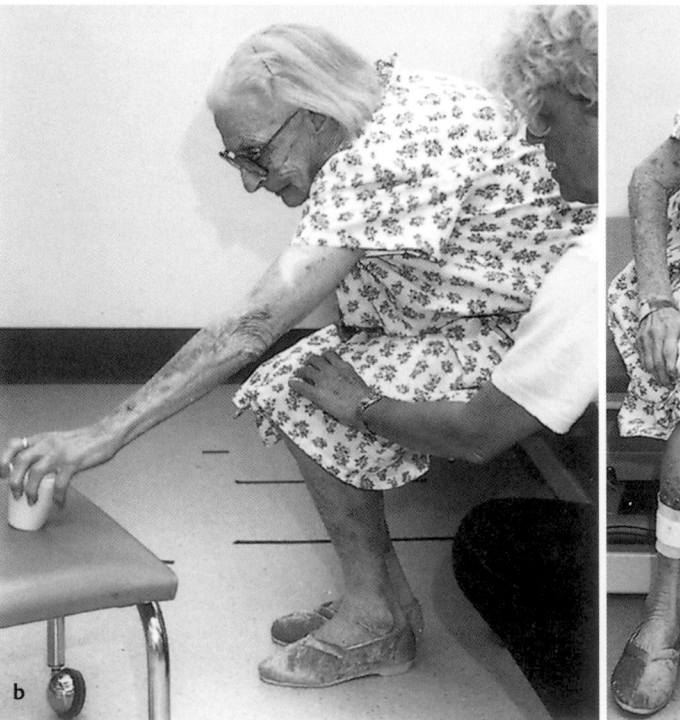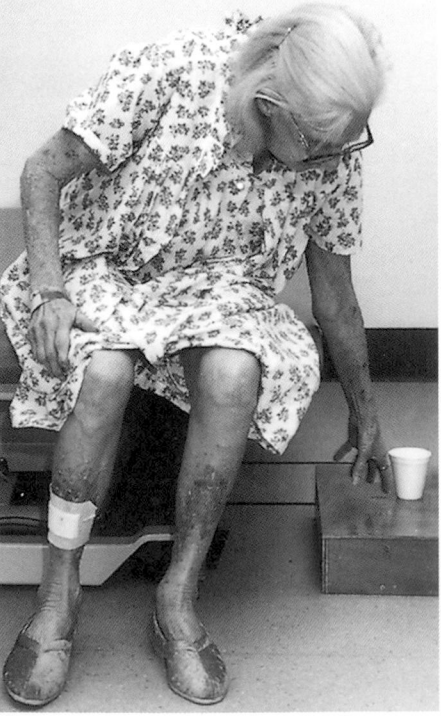

Fig. 5.28 a–c Training sitting balance.
a On her early attempt at reaching the patient is reluctant to move her body mass to the left (paretic) side; some improvement is evident after a few repetitions and she feels more confident in her ability to regain an upright position. The therapist is supporting the paretic arm, the patient is moving independently.
b She is attempting to use her paretic left leg in support and balance as she practices reaching actions.
c Reaching bimanually is practiced also. *(Reprinted with kind permission from PRO-ED Inc, Austin Tx, USA.)*

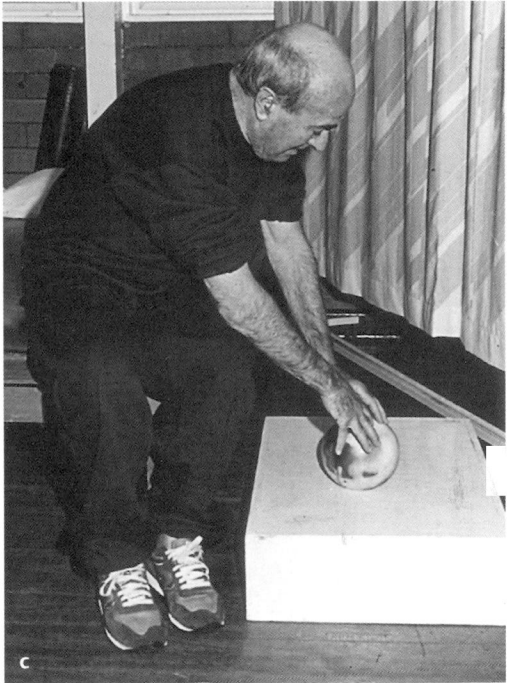

Fig. 5.29 Training loading and balancing with alternate lower limbs to raise one foot at a time off the supporting surface without using the hands for support.

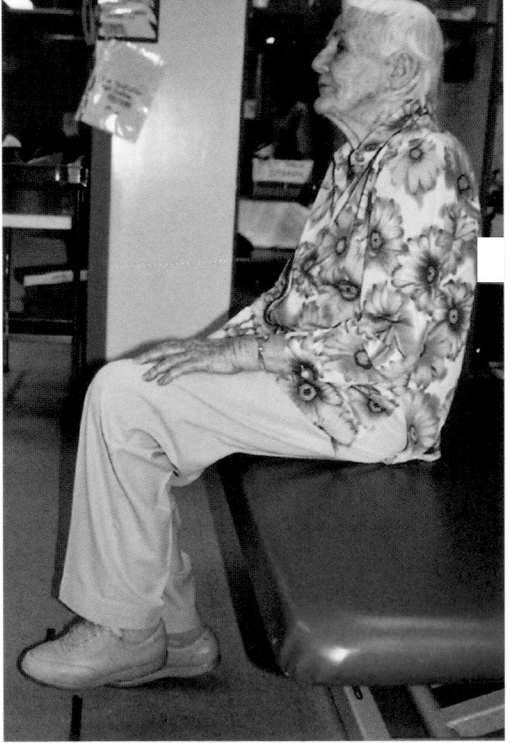

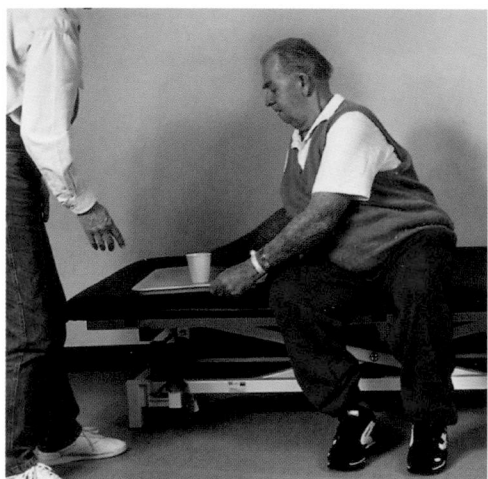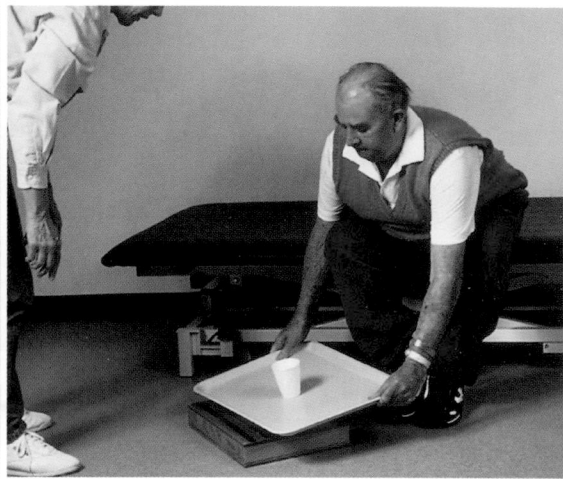

Fig. 5.30   The task is to lift and move the tray without spilling the water or dislodging the cup.

weight and size increased. External demands are increased in actions such as catching a small object and semi-standing up to reach for an object.

In a recent randomized controlled trial, a group of individuals who had a stroke less than 3 months previously participated in a 2-week sitting balance training program that involved practicing tasks that require reaching beyond arm's length. A sham control group practiced cognitive-manipulative tasks in sitting, within arm's length. At the end of the study, the experimental group had increased their maximum reach distance, decreased movement time, and increased peak vertical force through the paretic limb in standing up by 21% of body weight. Furthermore, the gains in sitting ability and standing up were maintained after 6 months (Dean et al. 2007). Each participant in the experimental group completed 230–390 reaches beyond arm's length per session over the 2-week period. Interestingly, vertical force production through the paretic limb in the sham group had decreased at the end of the 2-week training period which included a multidisciplinary rehabilitation program.

The "Pusher" Syndrome (Contraversive Pushing)

Most patients re-establish effective sitting balance soon after stroke, but some individuals experience an altered perception of the body's orientation in space. Evidence suggests that individuals with contraversive pushing have abnormal verticality perception (Karnath et al. 2000). They express a feeling of certainty that their body is oriented vertically even when it is tilted 20° to the paretic side. Affected patients are clearly distressed and fearful when they attempt to move. If attempts are made to move them passively toward the nonparetic side they may respond with active resistance (Carr and Shepherd 2000, Shepherd and Carr 2005).

It is possible that the contraversive pushing behavior sometimes noted by physical therapists may be an adaptation to being moved passively by therapist or nurse. Recent studies have shown that, rather than the therapist moving the patient passively into the erect position, encouragement to visually explore the structure of their surroundings, and to note in particular the vertical alignment of objects, enabled them to align their longitudinal body-axis to earth vertical. They appeared to have a good prognosis when treated in this way (Carr and Shepherd 2000, Karnath et al. 2000). The patient is encouraged to reach toward objects/people on the paretic side and toward the floor on that side, then moving back to the vertical sitting position. This provides a means of actively controlling movements of the body mass toward the side to which the person leans or falls without provoking fear (Shepherd and Carr 2005).

Training Balance in Standing

Supporting the body mass over the feet requires the ability to generate muscle forces that control hip, knee, and ankle joints to prevent the knee from collapsing. Loading the paretic limb is critical to regaining the ability to activate and control lower limb muscles, many of which have multiple roles—to support, balance, and move the body mass over the feet.

An overhead harness makes it possible for even a very weak person to load the paretic limb without fear of falling while practicing small movements of the body mass (**Fig. 5.31**). Use of a belt with grab handles may increase the confidence of patient, physical therapist, and nurse (see **Fig. 5.59**, p. 115). Without such devices, standing actions are likely to be deferred to some time in the future when balance has improved. Balance will not improve, however, unless the person has the opportunity to actively load the limb and practice moving the COM over the base of support, stimulating the necessary adjustments to occur. If the therapist persists in holding on to the patient, the need to make active anticipatory postural adjustments and ongoing corrections is eliminated.

Favoring the nonparetic leg in standing up and in activities in standing is primarily due to inability to generate and control supportive forces in the paretic limb. Loading the paretic limb in sitting and standing, with functional weightbearing exercises for lower limb muscles is, therefore, a major focus in training (Carr and Shepherd 2010) (see **Figs. 5.15, 5.16, 5.17, 5.18, 5.19**, and **Figs. 5.32, 5.33, 5.34, 5.35, 5.36**).

Here are some examples:

- Self-initiated head and trunk movements, looking over the shoulder to both sides, with feet close together (**Fig. 5.32b**)
- Reaching forward, laterally, downward, upward; progress by increasing distance, increasing speed, changing feet to step and tandem positions (**Fig. 5.28** and **Fig. 5.55**)
- Standing up and sitting down (**Figs. 5.49** and **5.53**)
- Semi-squatting to reach for an object on a stool, progress to full squat (**Figs. 5.18** and **5.33**)
- Stepping forward and backward with nonparetic limb, move the body mass forward over the stance limb; with a marked footprint on the floor to indicate how far to step (**Figs. 5.36** and **Fig. 5.58**)

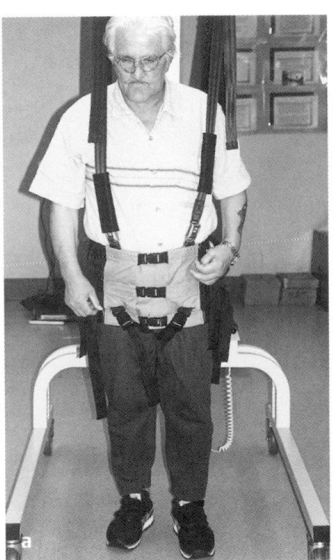 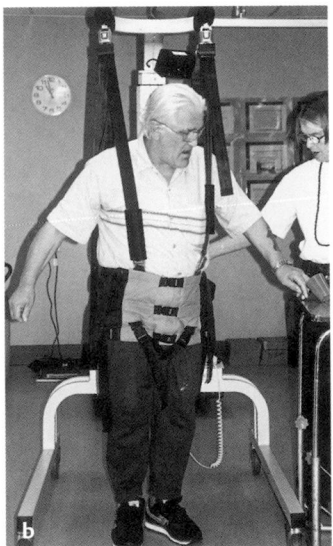 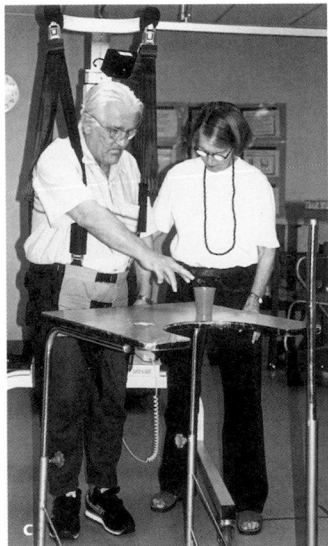

Fig. 5.31 a – c Training standing balance in a harness: **a** Notice that he loads his right lower limb more than the left one.

b Reaching to the cup on his left. As he has to take more weight through his left leg he moves his right arm out in response to a sense of insecurity.
c Reaching across the body requires a greater shift of the body mass over the left foot.

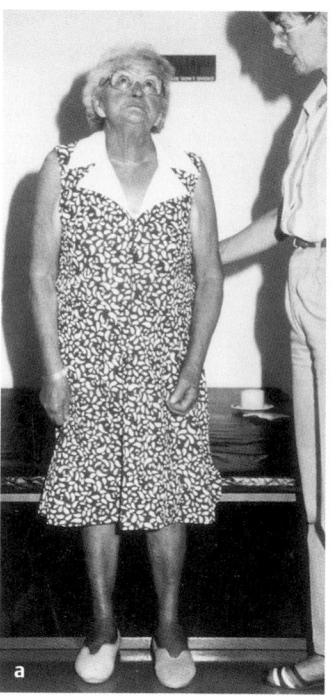

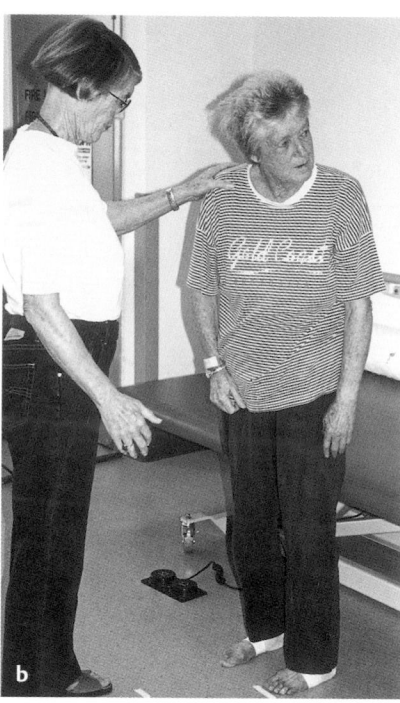

Fig. 5.32 a, b   Exercises practiced when in standing for the first time following a stroke give the patient the idea of balancing in standing.
a This patient practices looking up at the ceiling to locate a target. She needs to be reminded to keep her body mass forward over her feet (hip extension).
b Turning to look over the left shoulder to locate a target. The patient also practices turning to the right. As she becomes more confident, the foot placement can be changed to step standing.

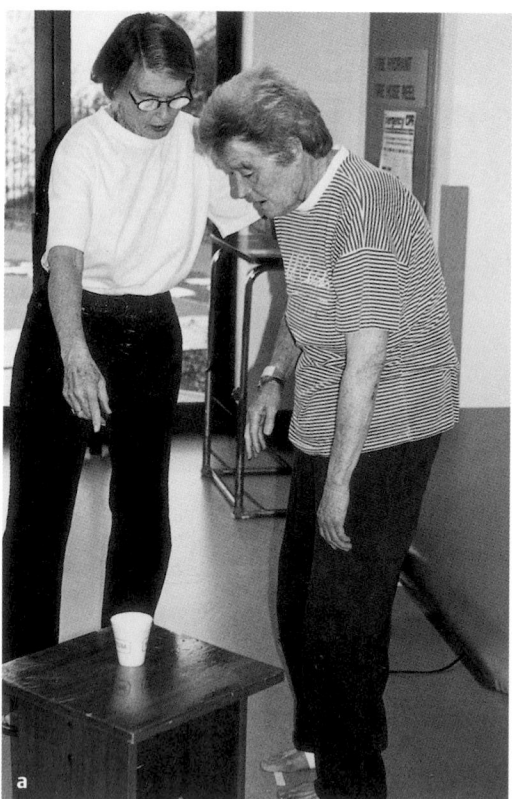

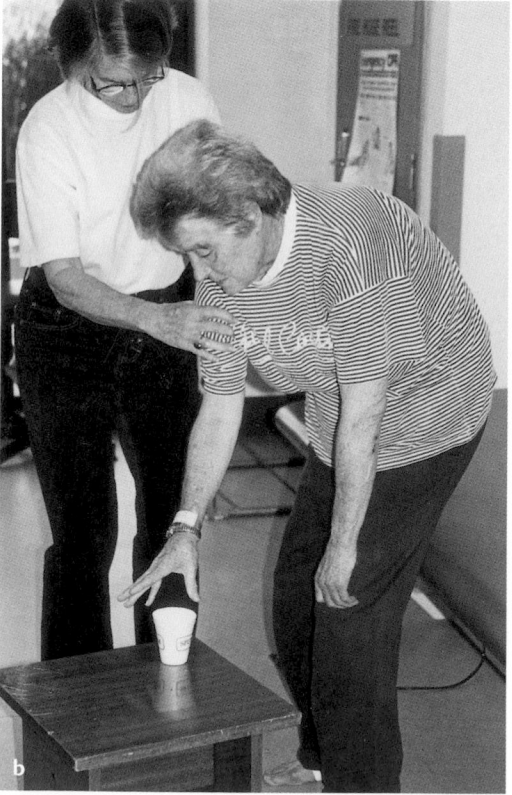

Fig. 5.33 a, b   **a** At first the patient is doubtful if she can pick up the cup, but with stand-by reassurance she succeeds (**b**). Placement of the cup should necessitate a shift of the body mass to the left.

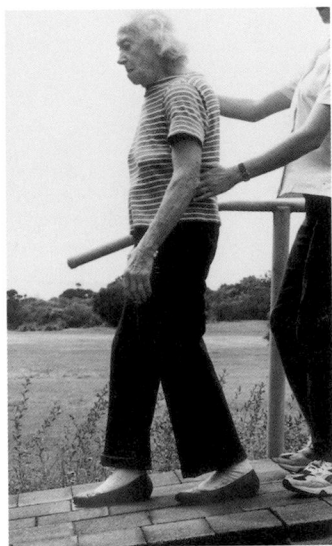

Fig. 5.34 Practice of walking down and up a ramp.

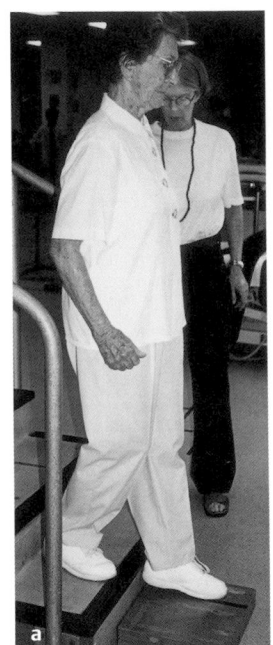

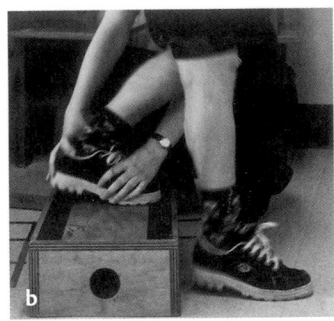

Fig. 5.35 a, b Forward step-downs.
a The task is made easier by modifying the step height.
b The therapist holds the patient's paretic foot to prevent her heel from lifting excessively and to ensure that she controls the lowering of her body mass through that leg.

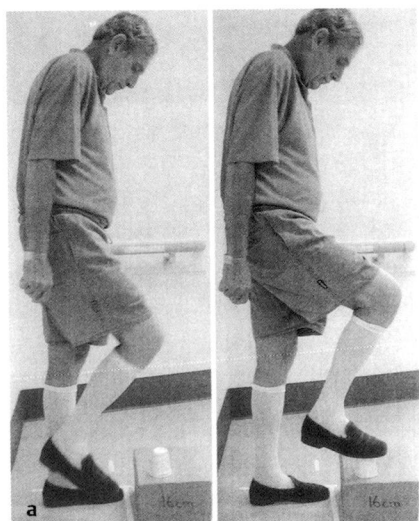

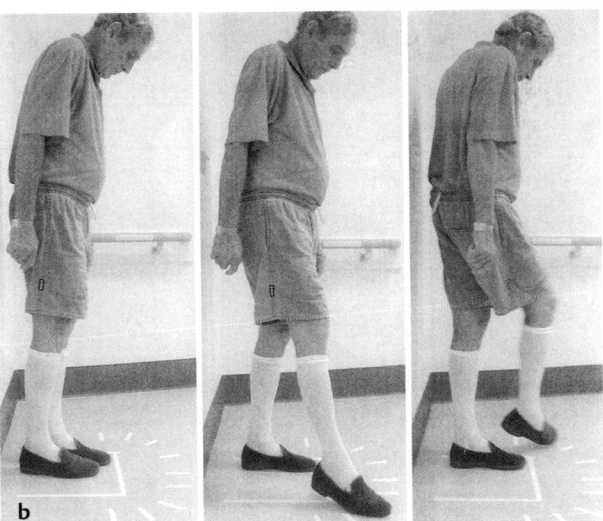

Fig. 5.36 a, b
a Stepping to touch a plastic cup requires careful foot placement while loading and balancing on the paretic leg.
b Stepping across the supporting leg is a difficult action for an individual with poor balance. To improve motor control, these exercises are also practiced with the nonparetic leg. (*Courtesy K Schurr and S Dorsch, Physiotherapy Department, Bankstown-Lidcombe Hospital, Australia.*)

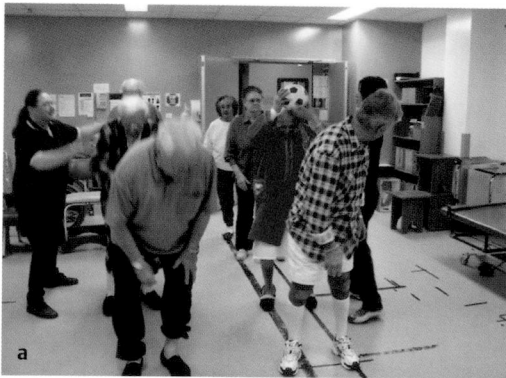 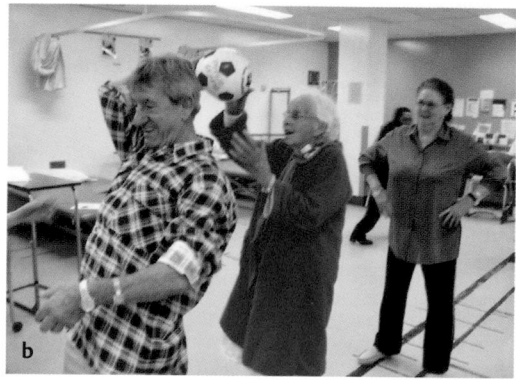

Fig. 5.37 a, b   Having fun and learning to balance and move freely in a group. *(Courtesy K Schurr and S Dorsch, Physiotherapy Department, Bankstown-Lidcombe Hospital, Australia.)*

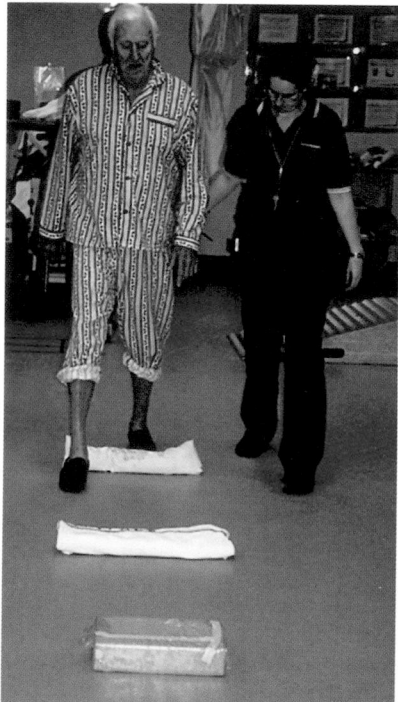

Fig. 5.38   An obstacle course consisting of objects of different heights and widths. Attention is directed toward the object to be stepped over.

- Heels raise and lower (**Fig. 5.17**)
- Walking sideways, forward, and backward
- Walking up and down a ramp, a curb, and stairs (**Figs. 5.34** and **5.35**)
- Marching on the spot

- Dynamic alternate loading–unloading of the paretic limb, stepping forward with one limb to place the foot on a small step about 10 cm from the toes of the standing limb, repeating with the other limb (**Fig. 5.58**)

The therapist provides concrete goals and visual targets for each exercise and discourages adaptive behaviors such as movement of one or both feet to increase the base of support, external rotation at the hip of the paretic limb, and breath holding.

Maximizing Skill

Activities are made more challenging according to their destabilizing effect, with increasingly difficult tasks and more complex environments, like:
- *Stepping to pick up an object.* The object is placed beyond the person's limit of stability, making it necessary to take a step.
- *Stepping with alternate limbs* (**Fig. 5.36**). Increase speed of action to encourage rapid stepping to prevent a stumble or fall.
- *Adding external timing demands.* Play games that require a rapid response and make it imperative to take a step, such as catching and throwing a ball (**Fig. 5.37**), bouncing a ball, kicking a ball.
- *Walking.* Introduce complexity and uncertainty into the environment, for example negotiating an obstacle course (**Fig. 5.38**) and automatic lift doors, walking under and over objects, making sudden stops and turns, walking along a line or footprints on the floor (**Fig. 5.39**), and simultaneously performing two actions such as walking and talking, turning the head, or carrying an object.

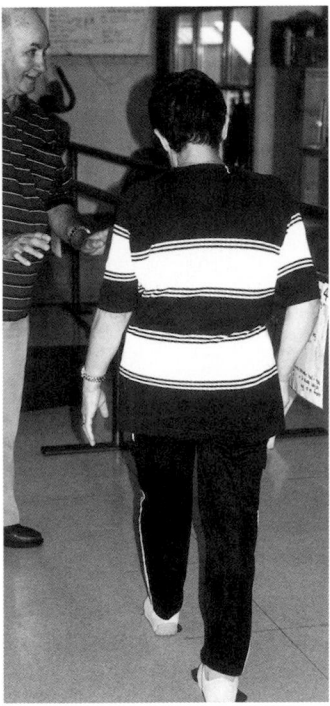

Fig. 5.39   A circuit class station—walking on footprints on the floor. Note: the base is narrow in order to challenge the individual. (*Courtesy of F Mackey, and colleagues, Illawarra Area Health Service, Australia.*)

Measurement

Many tests can demonstrate significant improvements in task performance from which we can infer that balance has improved. There is no single test that can measure all aspects of balance, because balance is an integral part of all the actions we perform. The following is a selection of tests that measure important aspects of balance:

- Functional Reach Test in Standing
- Timed Up-and-Go Test (TUG)
- Step Test
- Clinical Test of Sensory Interaction in Balance
- Obstacle Course Test

Training Guidelines: Standing Up and Sitting Down

Standing up from a seated position is one of the most commonly performed functional activities. The ability to stand up effectively is a critical prerequisite for upright mobility. During standing up and sitting down, the feet act as a fixed segment over which the body rotates to reposition the COM over the feet in standing.

Following stroke, an individual's ability to stand up (STS) from a seated position and to sit down (SIT) from a standing position is affected to varying degrees. Compared with able-bodied subjects, stroke patients may take 25%–60% longer to stand up, put significantly more load on the nonparetic limb than on the paretic limb, and decrease the vertical forces produced under the paretic limb by 20%–25% (Engardt and Olsson 1992, Hesse et al. 1994, Malouin et al. 2004a,b). Similar difficulties loading the paretic limb have been reported during sitting down (Engardt and Olsson 1992, Malouin et al. 2004a,b).

In the early poststroke stage, loading the paretic lower limb may be spontaneously avoided during standing up (**Fig. 5.40**). If this is allowed to continue, the person learns to favor the stronger leg and learns not to use the paretic leg. However, it should be noted that avoidance of the paretic leg is encouraged and reinforced when a patient is taught to pivot on the nonparetic limb to transfer from seat to seat, a common rehabilitation strategy that comes from the belief that the ability to transfer in this way provides some degree of independence. It is likely that this strategy works against the goal of independent standing up and may demotivate the patient. Motivation to use the impaired limb may be reduced because of difficulty loading it in the early days after the stroke and a corresponding increased reliance on the nonparetic limb as a substitute. This self-imposed adaptive behavior may appear to be reasonably effective within the rehabilitation environment with its limited demands. However, failure to engage the available but underused motor system becomes more likely (Kleim et al. 2003). The patient is likely to lose any residual capacity in the paretic limb (Kolb 1995).

Providing appropriate seating for individuals early after a stroke is critical to their ability to learn again how to stand up independently. Seat-

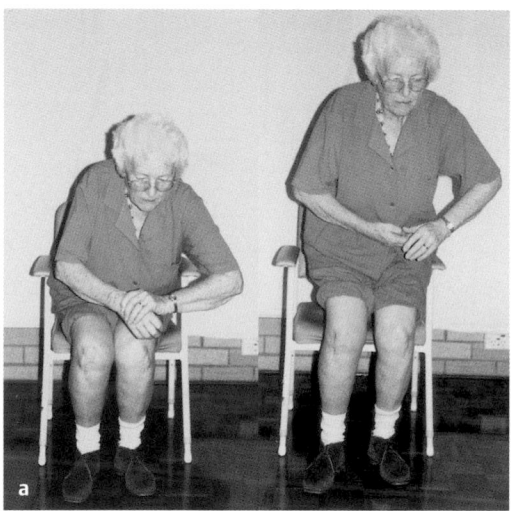 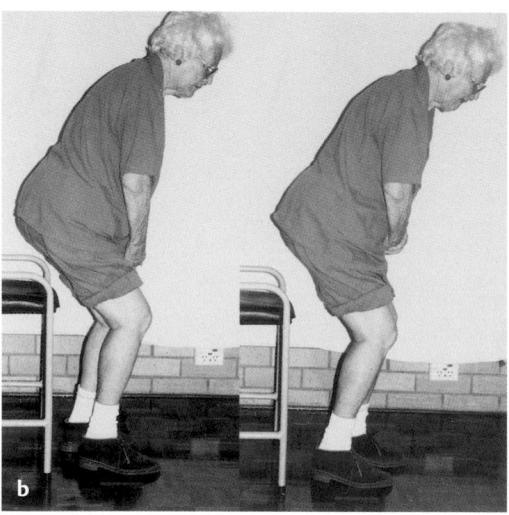

Fig. 5.40 a, b
a Although the patient can stand up independently, she loads the nonparetic left leg more than the right leg. Note that she has moved her left foot back just before thighs-off. If she is not provided with a higher seat and trained to load the right leg, this adaptation will become habitual.

b On her early attempt to stand up from a higher seat, she continued to load her nonparetic limb by moving (on the left) this foot behind the paretic one. The therapist suggests she moves her paretic foot further back and pays attention to loading that limb.

ing for ease of standing up as well as for comfort should be provided throughout a rehabilitation unit. Research has identified several important factors in choosing a chair: it should be height-adjustable with a horizontal seat (i.e., not slanted backward), with no structural block to backward foot placement. In a questionnaire given to people with disabilities, "easy to get out of" was identified as more important than "comfortable for sitting." A raised toilet seat should also be provided. Raising the seat height not only makes it easier for a weak person to stand up, it also makes it easier for a helper to give any necessary assistance and help avoid overuse of the stronger leg.

Success in STS is highly valued by elderly and disabled individuals for whom it confers the possibility of freedom. There is great improvement in morale and lifestyle once a person can stand up unaided. It has been shown that the more a stroke patient loads the paretic limb while standing up and sitting down, the better they score on activities of daily living as measured on the Barthel Index and the Fugl–Meyer Scale (Engardt et al. 1993).

Lack of independence in STS is one of the most likely factors associated with the risk of institutio-

nalization after stroke (Branch and Meyers 1987) and it is a common source of falls. Nyberg and Gustafson (1995) found that many falls among stroke patients occurred during activities in which the patient changed position, in particular when standing up and sitting down and when initiating gait. The greater the difference in loading the paretic and nonparetic limbs, the greater the likelihood of falls (Cheng et al. 1998).

In a study comparing the differences between able-bodied subjects, and poststroke fallers and nonfallers in standing up, Cheng and colleagues (1998) found that fallers stood up more slowly, with a significantly slower increase in the rate of rise in vertical force. In addition, postural sway in the mediolateral direction during STS and SIT was significantly greater in stroke fallers than in both stroke nonfallers and healthy subjects.

Biomechanical Description

Results of laboratory investigations, utilizing video analysis systems, force plates, and EMG, provide biomechanical data on which to base training guidelines and develop a training program.

Standing Up

Kinematics. In STS, the body mass is moved forward over the feet by rotation of the trunk segment forward at the hip joints, and dorsiflexion at the ankle (the pre-extension phase). Note that there is negligible movement within the extended spine as it rotates forward (as one virtual segment) at the hips. As the hips leave the seat, horizontal momentum is transferred into vertical momentum (the momentum-transfer phase). Extension of hips, knees and ankles moves the body mass vertically into standing. The extension phase finishes when the hips are extended. Balance (anteroposterior and mediolateral body sway) must be controlled throughout as a means of gaining stability of the body mass as it moves from a relatively large base of support in sitting to a small base of support in standing (**Fig. 5.41**).

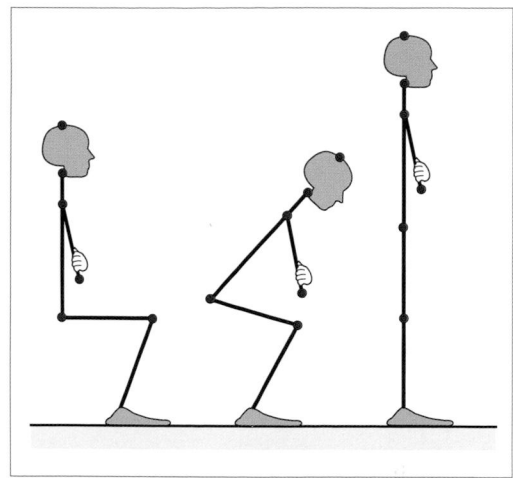

Fig. 5.41 Diagram illustrating the essential kinematic features of standing up in the sagittal plane.

Kinetics. Major force generation (approximately four times body weight) peaks as soon as the lower limbs are loaded at thighs-off, propelling the body mass vertically. Since the feet are on the floor, ground reaction forces play an important part in the movement. Horizontal ground reaction forces are generated in a posterior direction as the body mass is propelled forward, followed by anteriorly directed forces to brake forward momentum as it changes to vertical momentum. Vertical ground reaction forces greater than body weight accelerate the body vertically, peak around thighs-off, and stabilize at body weight when standing is reached (**Fig. 5.42**).

Muscle activity. Principal muscles generating force in the pre-extension phase are hip flexors and ankle dorsiflexors to move the body mass forward and stabilize the ankle. Tibialis anterior is activated early in the action, reflecting its contribution to keeping the foot on the floor, stabilizing the ankle, and controlling the position of the foot COP as it moves just anterior to the malleoli (Brunt et al. 2002). Knee and hip extensor muscles demonstrate peak activity around thighs-off which diminishes as standing is reached. Variability in activity of the calf muscles reflects their contribution to balancing the body mass over the feet throughout the action (Khemlani et al. 1999).

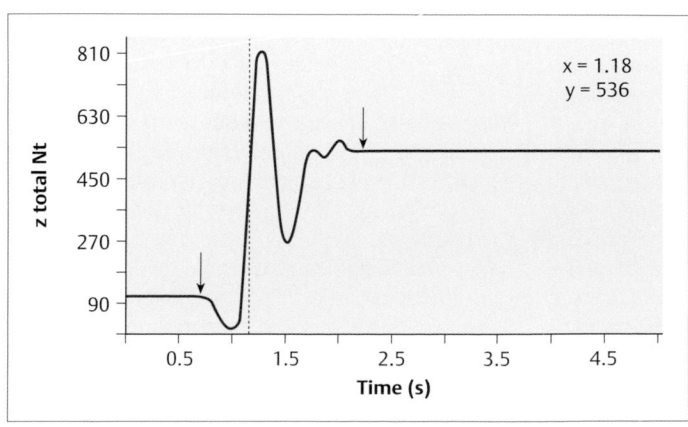

Fig. 5.42 Typical vertical (z) ground reaction force profile of an able-bodied subject standing up at a preferred speed of approximately 1.5 s. The dotted line indicates thighs-off. Arrows indicate movement start and end.

Strength and extensibility of muscles that cross the ankle joint are critical to stabilize the body mass and preserve balance as the body mass pivots over the feet.

Effective STS depends on strength and control of muscles crossing hip, knee, and ankle. These muscles generate and time forces to balance and support the body mass while propelling it forward and upward. The physiological variable most consistently related to success in standing up is lower limb muscle strength, in particular of knee extensors, in combination with ankle plantar flexors and dorsiflexors, and hip extensors (Eriksrud and Bohannon 2003).

Standing Up Under Different Conditions

Flexibility of performance is critical to meet the demands of daily life. We adapt the action to internal (e.g., pregnancy) and external (e.g., seat height) constraints. Although able-bodied subjects can stand up and sit down with weight evenly distributed between the two limbs, in everyday life the motor strategy employed to rise to standing depends on the intention. Loading of the limbs varies as the individual adapts to different task and environmental demands. Below are some of the varied conditions studied.

Standing up to walk. Recent investigations of standing up to walk have shown that the two tasks merge smoothly in healthy subjects (Magnum et al. 1996). When subjects were asked to stand up, forward momentum of the body's COM was arrested in standing. When standing up to walk, however, forward momentum continued while initiating the first step and before the full standing position was reached (Malouin and Richard 2005). Many stroke patients were, however, unable to merge the two tasks, instead standing up first then walking off (Dion et al. 1999, Malouin and Richard 2005).

Mechanical effect of different foot placements. Foot placement relative to knee position specifies the distance the body mass has to move forward in order to stand up. Foot placement is a major factor in force production. Standing up with the feet drawn back and behind a vertical line dropped from the knees reduces the distance the body mass has to move, and requires less force generation across hips and knees when compared with more anterior foot placements, thereby making the action easier (Shepherd and Koh 1996).

Standing up with one foot in front of the other increases the loading of the back limb and decreases the loading of the front limb. Ground reaction forces and the magnitude of EMG activity in quadriceps and tibialis anterior increase significantly in the back limb, with corresponding decreases in the forward limb (Brunt et al. 2002). Stroke patients are spontaneously adapting their standing up when they move only the nonparetic foot back under the seat. This sets up the action to be performed principally by the nonparetic limb and should be discouraged during training.

Timing and speed of trunk rotation. Trunk angular momentum produced as the large upper body swings/rotates forward at the hips is the major contributor to horizontal momentum of the body mass. It facilitates lower limb extension to raise the body mass to the standing position (Schenkman et al. 1990, Shepherd and Gentile 1994). However, standing up slowly, as stroke patients do, reduces momentum, with the result that more force must be produced for a longer period of time (Carr et al. 2002). There is a similar effect when a patient moves the upper body forward, pauses, and stands up from this flexed position. Absence of the facilitating effect of horizontal movement means that greater muscle forces are produced for a longer time.

Seat height. A higher seat results in lower moments of force at hip and knee (up to 60% and 50% respectively). Lowering the seat height increases the need for the generation of momentum, increases the force requirements, and requires greater muscle strength (see Janssen et al. 2002 for review).

Sitting Down

Although sitting down may look the same as STS only in reverse, there are some important differences. Each is performed under different mechanical constraints. Sitting down is performed with the assistance of gravity, and movement from its initiation involves eccentric (lengthening) contractions of muscles that cross hips, knees, and ankles to control descent of the body mass. As the body mass nears the seat, the tibialis anterior works strongly to control the backward path of descent, otherwise the individual would "fall" onto the seat. Maximum shank angle (dorsiflexion) occurs just before seat-on; maximum trunk angle occurs at seat-on (Dubost et al. 2005).

Age-Related Changes

Healthy elderly subjects standing up without arm use have demonstrated motor performance similar to young adults, although they have a tendency toward increased hip flexion resulting in a more anterior position of the COM at thighs-off and increased duration of movement. However, the action can be speeded up when required (Vander Linden et al. 1994). Lower limb muscle force production generally correlates with balance and is the strongest predictor of success in STS for older individuals with impairments (Schenkman et al. 1996). Older individuals sitting down tend to decrease the angle of trunk rotation (i.e., decrease flexion of the upper body at the hips) compared with young adults (Dubost et al. 2005). In frail elderly subjects, sitting down from standing is characterized by difficulty

in movement initiation followed by rapid descent to the seat that is comparable to a backward fall (Dubost et al. 2005). Factors such as joint pain, muscle stiffness, muscle weakness, decreased range of motion, and poor vision can affect performance.

Functional Problems

Although patients vary in their capacity to stand up and sit down, common problems can be observed as the individual attempts to stand up and they provide the focus for training.

* The foot of the nonparetic limb is spontaneously moved backward, but the paretic foot is not (**Fig. 5.43**).
* With the feet parallel, the nonparetic limb is spontaneously loaded, and loading the paretic limb is avoided (**Fig. 5.40**).
* Body mass is not moved far enough forward (**Fig. 5.44**). This may be due to inability to stabilize the paretic foot and fear of falling forward.

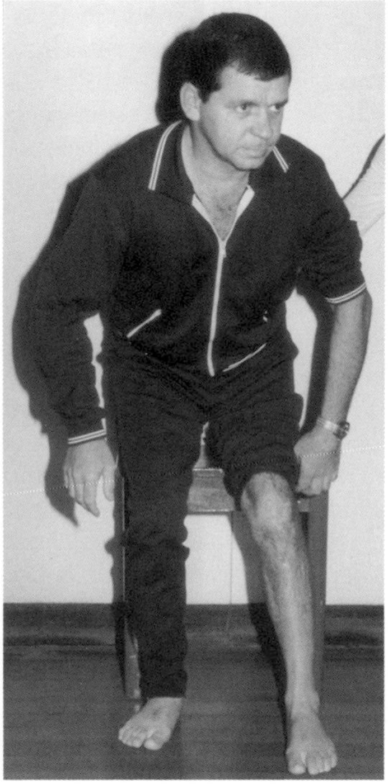

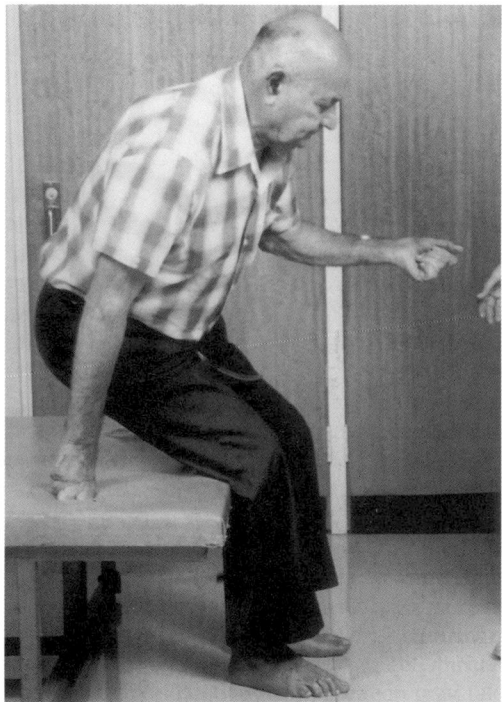

Fig. 5.43 Failure to move the paretic left foot back indicates the patient is favoring his nonparetic right limb. Note the wide base of support.

Fig. 5.44 Failure to move body mass forward (decreased hip flexion and decreased forward movement of the shank–ankle dorsiflexion). Note how the patient adapts, using his arms in an attempt to perform the action successfully.

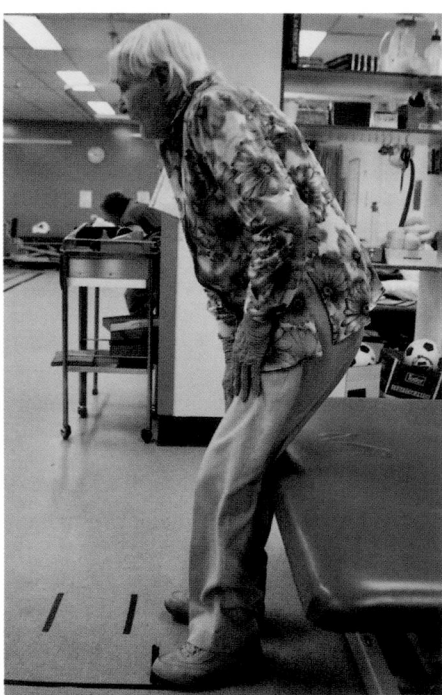

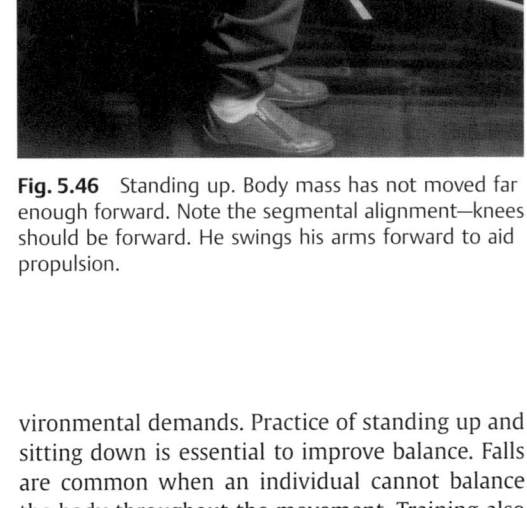

Fig. 5.45 Sitting down. Failure to control segmental alignment during the descent of body mass causes the patient to "fall" onto the seat. Her hips, knees, and ankles should be flexing. Note, tibialis anterior should be working strongly to stabilize the ankle, keeping the shanks/knees forward and controlling the backward path of descent.

Fig. 5.46 Standing up. Body mass has not moved far enough forward. Note the segmental alignment—knees should be forward. He swings his arms forward to aid propulsion.

- Loss of balance at thighs-off in STS, and before thighs-on in SIT that may be due to weakness of knee extensor and ankle dorsiflexor muscles.
- Sitting down—body mass moves back too soon with insufficient shank/foot angle (dorsiflexion) and knee flexion (**Fig. 5.45**).
- Arms are used for support, balance and propulsion (**Fig. 5.46**).
- STS is too slow (25%–60% longer than normal).

Task-Oriented Training

Attention and effort in rehabilitation are directed toward ensuring use of the paretic limb and decreasing overuse of the nonparetic limb. Training involves practice of standing up and sitting down from chairs and seats with different characteristics (different height and shape). This provides opportunities for the individual to learn to adapt to en-

vironmental demands. Practice of standing up and sitting down is essential to improve balance. Falls are common when an individual cannot balance the body throughout the movement. Training also involves exercises to increase strength and motor control, in particular, for lower limb extensors and ankle dorsiflexors. Those individuals who have difficulty activating and sustaining muscle activity require simple exercises to help them get the idea of activating key muscle groups.

Successful standing up and sitting down are critical to the achievement of many different functional goals. Although muscle weakness and lack of vigor may be limiting factors immediately after stroke, training of standing up and sitting down, with other weightbearing exercises to increase muscle strength and endurance, should enable the majority of stroke patients to learn how to stand up effectively and efficiently. For example, Britton and colleagues (2008) examined the effect of a 30-minute daily program over 2 weeks aimed at improving STS performance. Training for the experimental group included repetitive STS and leg-strengthening exercises with a physical therapy assistant. Training emphasized foot placement at the start of the movement, speed of forward movement of the upper body, and weightbearing through the paretic leg. A balance performance monitor gave visual feedback of amount of weight borne through this limb. The control group received an equivalent amount of arm therapy. At the end of the program, the experimental group had increased the number of repetitions from on average 18 to 50, and there was a significant mean difference of 10% body weight through the paretic leg after 1 week of training. In contrast, the control group decreased the amount of weight through the paretic leg.

Critical Mechanical Factors

Several factors from biomechanical research that are critical to successful performance of standing up can be used as "rules" for training and practice to enable even a frail person to actively participate in practice of standing up. These factors are:

Foot Placement

*Both feet are placed about 10 cm behind the knees. This facilitates extensor muscle force production and requires less effort (**Fig. 5.47**). If, however, the patient bears more weight through the nonparetic limb with this foot placement (**Fig. 5.48**), placing the nonparetic foot in front of the paretic foot and increasing seat height enables/forces loading of the paretic limb (see **Fig. 5.40b**).*

Brunt and colleagues (2002) studied standing up in stroke patients to investigate the effects of foot placement on loading the paretic limb. There were three conditions: (A) normal condition, feet paral-

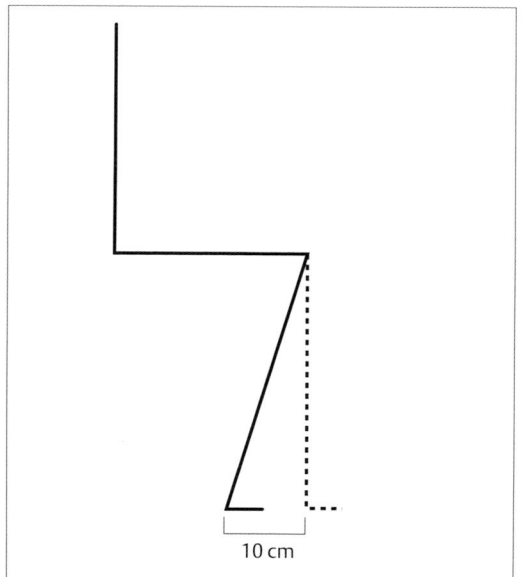

Fig. 5.47 The preferred placement of the feet in able-bodied subjects is, on average, 10 cm from a vertical line drawn from the middle of the knee joint (~75° ankle dorsiflexion). In training STS after stroke, attention needs to be on placement of the paretic foot in 75° dorsiflexion with the nonparetic foot in front.

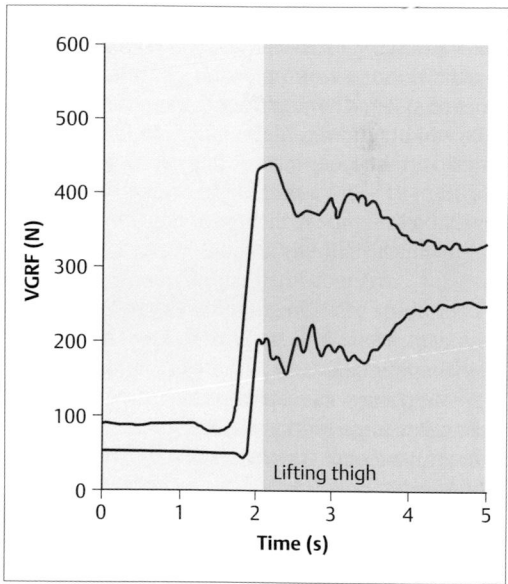

Fig. 5.48 Typical vertical ground reaction force graph (VGRF) of a stroke patient standing up with a force platform under each foot (lower trace shows the hemiparetic limb). Note the difference between the forces produced by the paretic and nonparetic limbs and the fluctuations of the trace indicating difficulty balancing. Compare the shape of the VGRF with **Fig. 5.42**. Vertical line indicates thighs-off.

lel, both knees in 100° flexion; (B) nonparetic limb extended in front of paretic foot with the nonparetic knee in 75° flexion; and (C) nonparetic limb elevated with the foot on a dense foam support height-adjusted to 25% of seat height. The results showed that patients increased loading of the paretic limb in conditions B and C compared with the normal condition primarily because of an increase in peak vertical force under the paretic foot. In addition, EMG activity was increased in the quadriceps and tibialis anterior muscles of the paretic limb, in the quadriceps by 34% in condition B and 41% in condition C, and in the tibialis anterior by 29% in condition B and 51% in condition C. No instructions were given to the patients to increase the use of the paretic limb. The load increased through the paretic limb because the stronger leg was at a biomechanical disadvantage.

A more recent study measured the vertical ground reaction forces under both the feet and the thighs during standing up and sitting down under four conditions:(1) spontaneous; (2) symmetrical foot placement; (3) paretic foot placed backward; and (4) nonparetic foot placed backward. Asymmetrical loading was present before thighs-off and after thighs-on in both standing up and sitting down respectively. Similar to Brunt's findings, when the paretic foot was placed behind the nonparetic foot asymmetrical loading was reduced. The condition in which the nonparetic foot was placed behind the paretic foot resulted in the greatest loading asymmetry and must be avoided if the goal of training is to prevent nonuse of the paretic limb (Roy et al. 2006). It may help the patient get the idea of bearing weight and pushing down through their feet as they stand up if they focus attention on their feet and on "pushing" them into the floor.

Seat Height
*Adjust seat height if necessary—a higher seat makes it possible to stand up if lower limb muscles are weak (see **Fig. 5.40b**). The seat height is lowered as strength increases.*

Trunk
Starting from a trunk vertical position, flexion of the trunk over the hips and a smooth transfer into movement upward into standing optimizes forward and upward momentum.

Give instructions to speed up the action so that forward momentum merges smoothly and continuously into upward momentum.

Training Standing Up
Patient sits on a firm flat surface, trunk vertical, feet flat on the floor (feet placed 10 cm behind the knee), swings head, shoulders, and trunk forward and stands up.
- Directing vision and attention toward a target during STS/SIT provides an external focus for erect body alignment by affecting the path of head and shoulders forward and up. Target is placed 2–3 m in front, at eye level.
- Therapist places paretic foot back if necessary so standing up is practiced from an optimal starting position for loading the paretic limb.
- Therapist can stabilize the paretic foot by pushing down and back along the shank to ensure loading and to keep the heel on the ground at thighs-off. Guiding the knee forward along a horizontal path may help the patient move the body mass forward—do not block the knees from moving forward (**Fig. 5.49**).
- Discourage use of hands.
- Encourage an increase in speed.
- No rests after each performance—continue for prescribed number of repetitions.
- Do not block the movement forward by standing too close.
- Give instructions that identify the body part to be moved—"Swing your shoulders forward and stand up."

Standing up is one of the most common daily activities we perform, and the average person does it about 90 times each day. The patient can record the number of repetitions during a training session and throughout the day with an ActivPal single axis accelerator to provide feedback and incentive.

Training Sitting Down
Patient inclines the upper body forward at the hips, flexes hips and knees, and dorsiflexes ankles to lower the body mass downward and backward toward the seat without losing balance.
- Assist initiation of knee flexion by moving the knee forward.

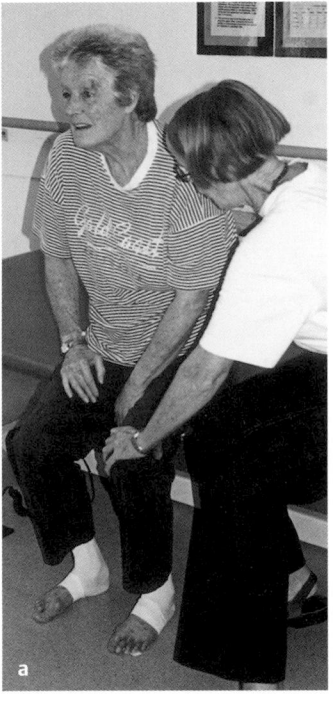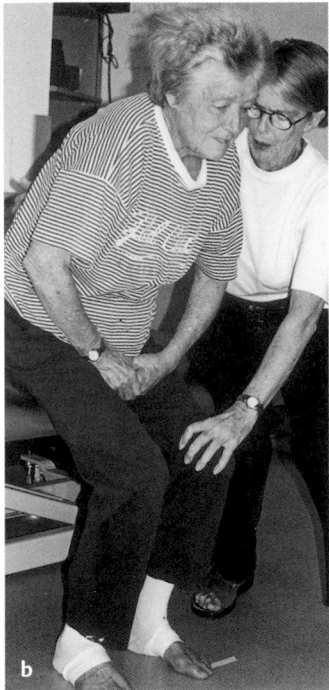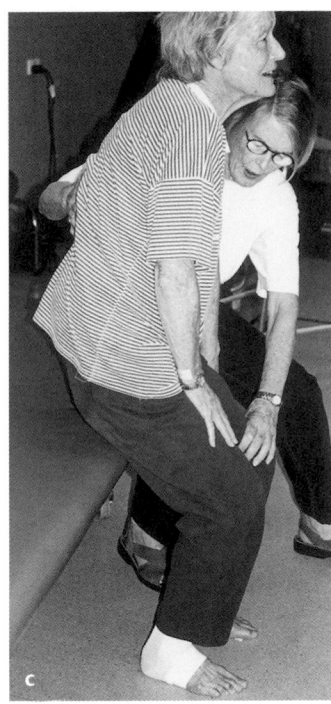

Fig. 5.49 a–c   Practicing standing up and sitting down.
a Therapist stabilizes the paretic foot on the floor by
pushing down and back along the line of the shank to
force loading and to keep the heel on the ground at
thighs-off.
b Therapist holds the patient's body mass to the left to
increase loading of the paretic leg.

c Lateral view shows how the therapist guides the appropriate intersegmental alignment. It is important
that the patient keeps her body mass forward over her
feet as she sits down.

* Stabilize the foot with the heel on the ground to
  assist loading of the paretic limb particularly
  when hips move back toward the seat.

Specific attention to loading the paretic limb is
necessary to ensure an eccentric contraction of
quadriceps throughout the action. Engardt and
colleagues (1993) reported in their study that patients who did not receive feedback about loading
the paretic limb while sitting down did not improve limb loading.

Simple Exercises to Elicit Muscle Activity
*Foot placement backward. Patient sits with feet flat
on floor and practices sliding the paretic foot backward.*
* Therapist palpates hamstrings and gives feedback about muscle activity.
* A line on the floor provides an external focus for
  the patient.

* Resistance from friction from the floor can be
  decreased using a slippery surface or roller
  skate to encourage effective performance (**Fig.
  5.50**).
* Incorporate into STS practice, instructing the individual always to place the paretic foot back
  behind the knee before standing up.

*Moving the body mass forward and backward. Pa-
tient practices moving the upper body at the hips
without flexing the spine; arms resting on a table.*
    Fear of falling forward may be a major barrier to
moving the body mass forward early poststroke.
This exercise enables the patient to get the idea
of the movement so it can be incorporated into
standing-up practice (**Fig. 5.51**).

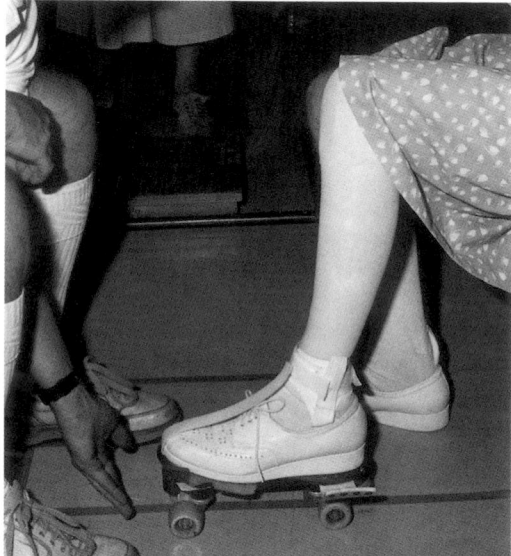

Fig. 5.50 Simple exercises to activate ankle and knee muscles to move the paretic foot back and forward behind the knee. Moving the foot back is a critical feature of standing up.

Training Strength and Motor Control

Effective standing up depends on strength and control of muscles that cross hips, knees, and ankles. These muscles generate and time forces to support and balance the body mass while propelling it upward. Since the lower limbs act as a functional unit, an efficient strength training method is repetitive standing up and sitting down, progressively increasing body weight resistance by lowering the height of the seat, folding the arms (**Fig. 5.52**), and positioning the nonparetic foot in front of the paretic foot. These modifications enable loading of the paretic limb during standing up and sitting down. The earlier section on strength training describes task-oriented exercises to increase lower limb muscle strength, power generation, and control of the lower limbs, using progressive body weight resistance. Engardt and colleagues (1995) found that eccentric training using an isokinetic dynamometer resulted in a greater increase in loading of the paretic leg in STS than concentric training.

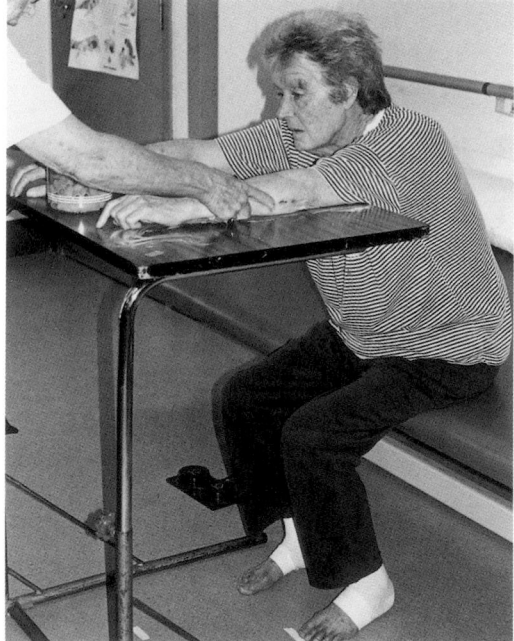

Fig. 5.51 This woman was fearful of moving her body mass far enough forward to stand up. However, with her arms on a high table she can practice reaching to the edge of the table. Concentrating on reaching beyond arm's length, she moves her body mass forward and backward by flexing and extending at the hips. Next, she practices standing up.

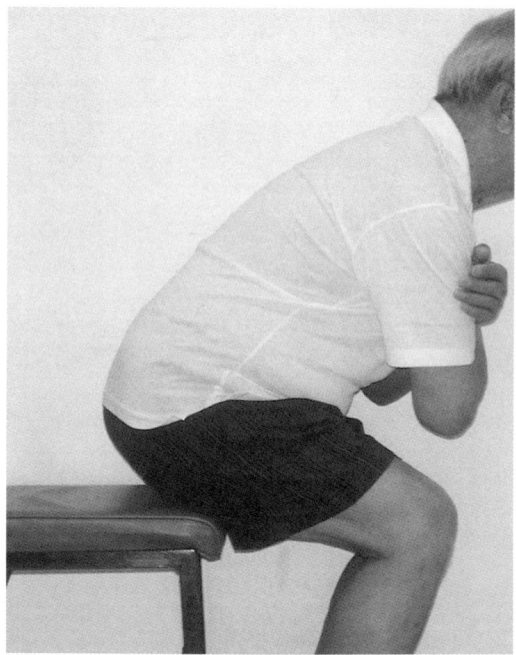

Fig. 5.52 Repetitive practice with arms folded increases production of lower limb extensor force. Focus can also be on increasing speed.

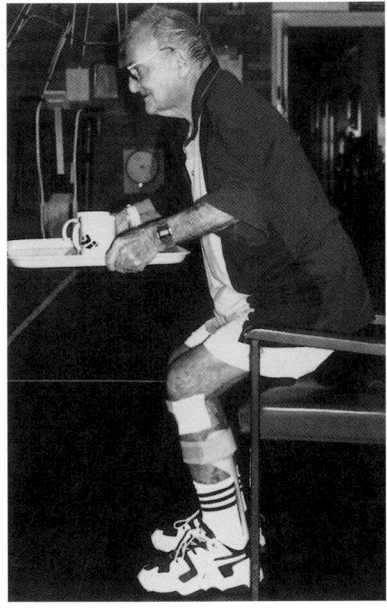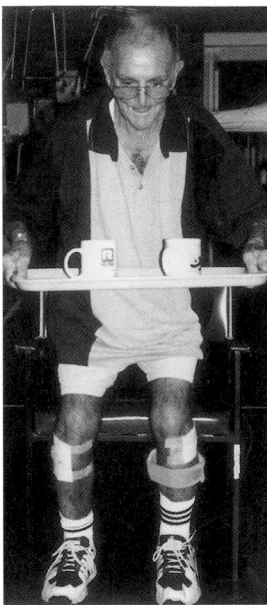

Fig. 5.53 Balancing the mugs on the tray changes the focus of attention from standing up and encourages keeping the body mass forward over the feet at thighs-off.

Mental Practice

There may be several factors that limit the amount of physical practice in the early acute stage, including physical frailty, poor balance, and lack of endurance. In a study of mental practice by Malouin and colleagues (2004a), subjects were trained with mental practice to increase loading of the paretic limb while standing up and sitting down, initially using a visual display of vertical force produced, and then relying on their memory. A single training session of 30 minutes that included seven physical repetitions combined with 35 mental rehearsals resulted in improved loading of the paretic limb. Improvement was retained 24 hours later, suggesting that some learning has occurred. The amount of motor improvement in follow-up was strongly associated with working memory ability, particularly in the visuospatial domain.

Maximizing Skill

As performance improves, emphasis changes from foot placement and speed of trunk rotation to training flexible performance. Practice should provide the opportunity for the individual to adapt to different environmental contexts. Examples include talking while standing up, holding an object, steadying a glass of water on a tray (**Fig. 5.53**), stopping and changing direction without losing balance during sitting down practice (**Fig. 5.54**), reaching far forward (**Fig. 5.55**), and merging standing up into walking.

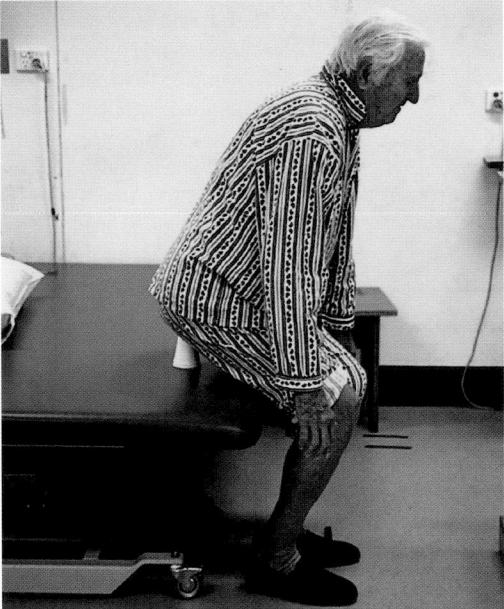

Fig. 5.54 An exercise for improving balance during STS that involves repetitive stopping and changing direction without losing balance. Note the position of the plastic cup.

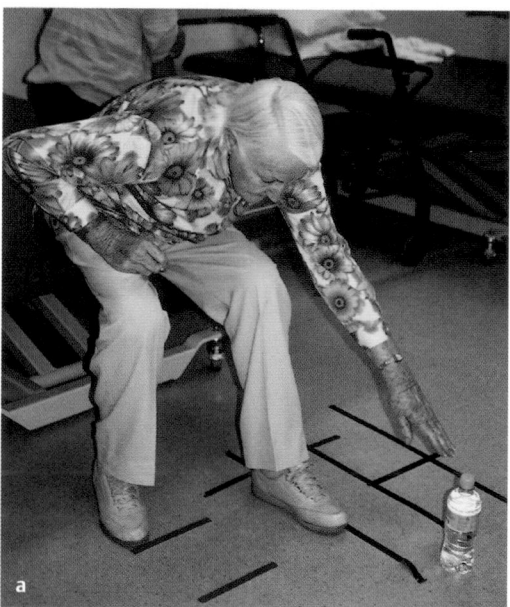 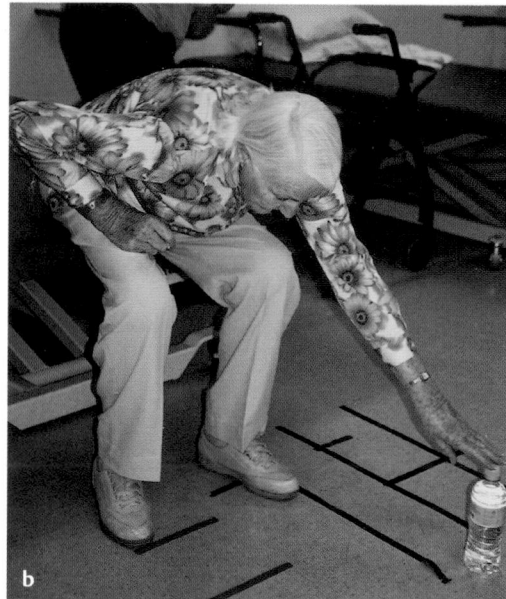

Fig. 5.55 a, b   Reaching beyond arm's length.
a The patient is not loading her paretic (left) leg.

b Foot and object placement encourage her to load the left leg. Note her thighs are about to leave the seat.

Measurement

The following functional tests have been found reliable when performed under standardized conditions:

* Standing Up Item of Motor Assessment Scale (MAS)
* TUG
* Rise-to-Walk Test (RTW)

Quadriceps strength is the variable shown most consistently to relate to performance of standing up (Bohannon et al. 1995, Lord et al. 2002). It is tested using a hand-held dynamometer or spring scale.

Training Guidelines: Walking

Walking is a life-enhancing activity and the most effective way of getting from one place to another. The purpose of walking or running is to transport the body safely and efficiently on the level, or uphill and downhill. Retraining walking is a major goal in rehabilitation after stroke. Walking is not only an important part of day-to-day living but

also needed for participation in recreation. Limited walking ability following stroke restricts the patient's independent mobility about the house and participation in the community, a significant social handicap.

Community ambulation has been broadly defined as locomotion outdoors; for example, to visit the supermarket, shops, or bank. One study reported that only 7% of patients discharged from rehabilitation met the criteria for community walking, which included the ability to walk 500 m continuously at a speed that would enable them to cross a road safely (Hill et al. 1997). A walking speed of 1.1–1.5 m/s is considered fast enough to function as a pedestrian in different environmental and social contexts. Clinical tests of walking ability underestimate actual walking competence. In a recent study of a group of home dwellers, despite good mobility outcomes on standardized measures, nearly one-third of the group did not go out into the community unsupervised (Lord et al. 2004).

Speed is probably the most important variable in competent walking. Slow walking is associated with poor health outcomes (Cress et al. 1995) and disability (Potter et al. 1995). Slow walking disrupts the ease and rhythm of the walking action in both able-bodied and disabled subjects (Wagenaar 1990). If speed is slow, little intersegmental exchange of energy takes place, resulting in a high total energy cost per meter walked (Olney 2005). If a person can be trained to walk a little faster, the energy exchange generated will require less effort as they are walking more efficiently.

Biomechanical Description

Over the past couple of decades there has been a serious attempt to transfer information from research findings in the laboratory into guidelines for clinical practice.

Kinematics

Angular displacements occur in all three planes, but the major displacements occur in the sagittal plane. Since the mediolateral base of support is small in walking, little movement in the frontal plane is required. Kinematic variables such as timing, cadence, joint angle displacements, and linear paths of body parts provide helpful information for observational analysis and can serve to monitor function, but they yield little information about the mechanisms producing the gait pattern. This information requires some knowledge of kinetics.

Kinetics

Muscle forces acting across joints generate the action and are studied as joint moments of force or torques. In actions such as walking that take place with the body supported over the feet, *moments of force* across the three lower limb joints act cooperatively to maintain body support and to prevent collapse of the limb. In this way the limb is controlled as a functional unit (represented biomechanically as the *extensor support moment of force*) that is independent of the motor pattern at individual joints.

Anatomically and functionally, the kinetic variable known as *power* describes the magnitude and direction of the flow of energy into and out of muscles. Without these well-defined patterns of energy generation and absorption we could not walk effectively. Energy is added with each concentric contraction and is absorbed with each eccentric contraction. Maintaining a constant speed requires equal amounts of both (Olney 2005).

Power patterns (**Fig. 5.56**) may be the most valuable of all the gait variables since they describe the magnitude and direction of the flow of energy into (generation) and out of (absorption) muscles (Winter 1985). The generation of energy by the plantar flexors (A2) (~80% at push-off) to move the body forward is the largest and most important energy burst during the gait cycle. Second to this is the energy provided by hip flexors in late stance and early swing for pull-off (H3). In the third important energy burst (H1), hip extension is dominant in early stance as the hip extends to position the body in front of the stance foot, pushing from behind. These major power bursts provide the propulsive force for forward progression. The shape of power profiles of stroke patients walking slowly is similar to these standard details,

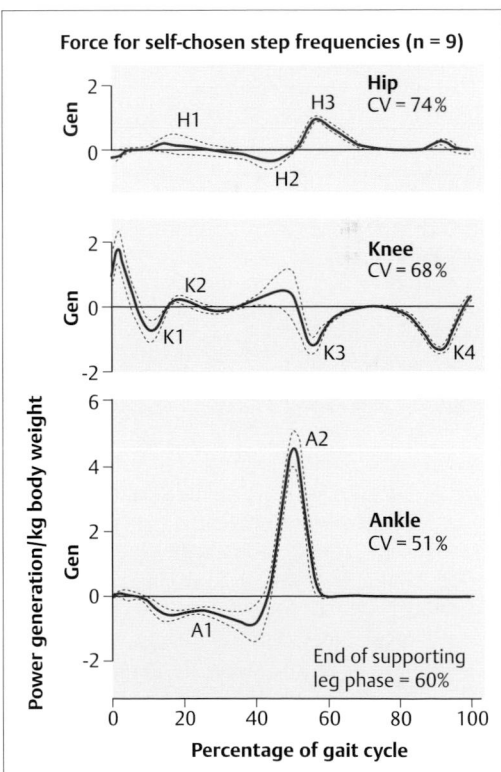

Fig. 5.56 Ensemble averages of power patterns of able-bodied subjects walking at their preferred cadence plotted over the gait cycle for hip, knee, and ankle beginning at initial contact of the foot to the floor. The swing phase begins at 60%. (*Reproduced from Winter 1987, University of Waterloo Press with permission.*)

but the amplitude of power is lower or barely perceptible (Olney 2005).

Muscle Activity

Level walking requires a relatively small proportion of maximum capability of all muscle groups except for the ankle plantar flexors (Olney 2005). The muscle groups that do most of the work are the plantar flexors at push-off, hip flexors at pull-off, and hip extensors in early stance as the hip is extending to pivot the body over the stance foot, acting as a reverse pendulum (Olney 2005).

Biomechanical and behavioral criteria for successful walking (Forssberg 1982, Winter 1987) and, therefore, the focus of training, are:
- Support of the upper body during stance (without collapse of the lower limb)
- Propulsion of the body in a forward direction
- Maintenance of upright posture and balance as the body moves over the feet
- Control of foot trajectory to achieve a safe ground clearance for swing
- Production of a basic locomotor rhythm
- Flexibility—the ability to adapt the movement to changing environmental demands and goals

These criteria depend on strength and control of lower limb muscles.

Functional Problems

After stroke, gait problems arise principally from muscle weakness and disorders of motor control. The most consistent finding is that after stroke patients walk more slowly than able-bodied age-matched subjects (von Schroeder et al. 1995), with speed reflecting the severity of stroke. Walking slowly results from inability of the lower limbs to generate sufficient muscle force concentrically or eccentrically and to time these forces (for further discussion see Olney 2005).

Gait speed correlates with strength of lower limb muscles (Bohannon and Andrews 1990), magnitude of push-off power (Olney et al. 1991), and hip extension angle at the end of stance—the smaller the angle, the slower the speed (Olney and Richards 1996). Speed also correlates with an increase in the time spent in double support phase—the slower the walking speed, the longer the double-support phase (Olney and Richards 1996).

Many scientific studies of walking provide detailed information about movement dysfunction after stroke. Note that in clinical practice, the therapist can observe adaptive step and stride lengths, differences in stance and swing ratios, and differences and deficiencies in joint angular displacements. These kinematic parameters reflect the effects of invisible kinetic forces.
- Decreased vertical ground reaction force at push-off indicating limited concentric contraction of plantar flexors (Carlso et al. 1974)
- Decreased power generation at push-off and pull-off (Dean et al. 2000, Olney and Richards 1996)
- Reduced hip extension at end of stance (Olney and Richards 1996, Richards et al. 1999)
- Decreased endurance—a group of individuals poststroke were unable to maintain their comfortable walking speed over 6 minutes. They walked only about 50% of the distance predicted for healthy individuals with similar physical characteristics (Dean et al. 2001)
- Increased double-support phase is associated with a sense of poor balance and is costly in terms of energy (Olney 2005)
- Decreased adaptability to changing environmental conditions; for example, catching the heel while stepping over objects (Said et al. 1999)
- Asymmetry of step and stride lengths is a frequent observation. However, asymmetry is not itself the problem but is due to the unequal capacity in muscle strength and motor control between the two limbs. These should be the focus of attention in therapy. Asymmetry is corrected as the rhythm and natural speed of walking is re-established.

Observational Gait Analysis

Physical therapists routinely observe gait in clinical practice and there are some encouraging findings that suggest they have the capacity to make accurate judgements under certain conditions. It is particularly important to have at least a basic understanding of biomechanics. An early study suggests that the capacity to make sound clinical decisions relies on the therapist's familiarity with normal biomechanical values (Eastlack et al. 1991). Olney (2005) points out that without understanding the importance of push-off at the end of stance, for example, physical therapists have not known where to look when analyzing their patient's motor performance. In a later study, physical therapists under standardized conditions were able to make accurate and reliable judgements of push-off using observational assessment.

Figure **5.57** gives examples of common problems that can be observed. Readers can check their own observations against the figure captions.

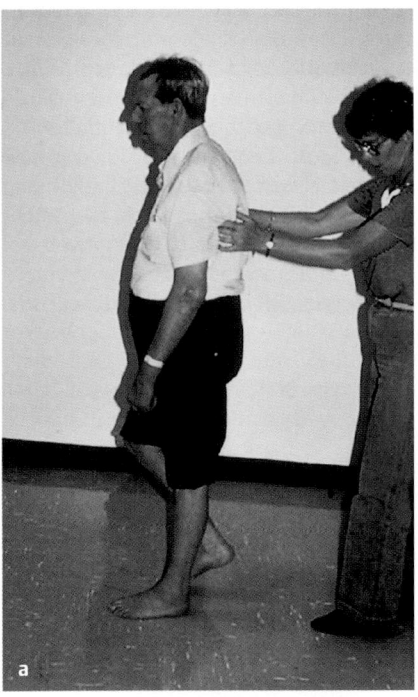
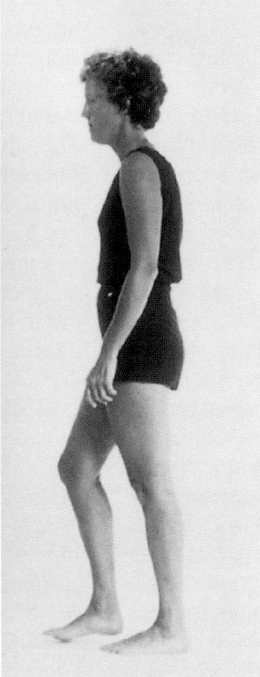

Fig. 5.57 a–c
a At left mid-stance the patient has decreased hip extension and decreased ankle dorsiflexion. Extension at the hip and dorsiflexion at the ankle normally act to move the body mass forward over the stance foot.
b At the start of swing, the patient demonstrates lack of push-off, hip and knee flexion.
c At end of left stance, the patient lacks plantarflexion and push-off.

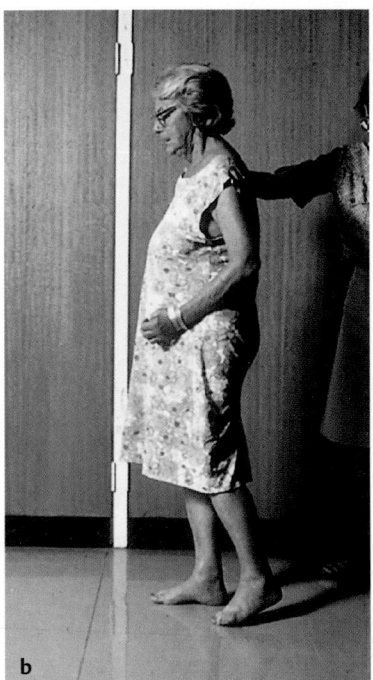
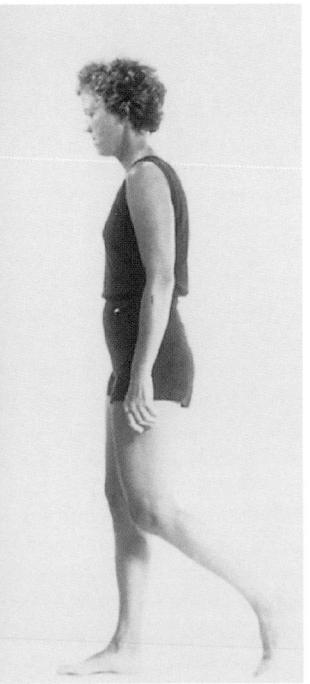
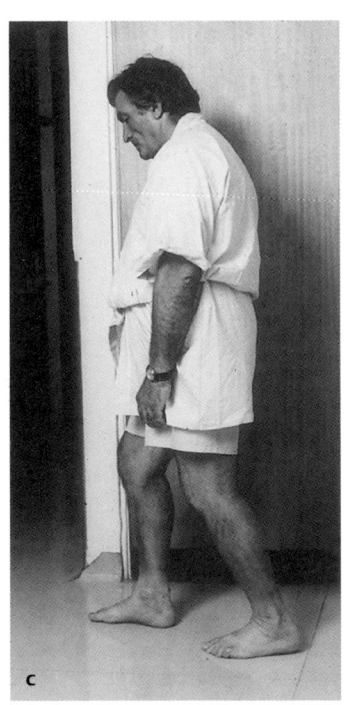

Task-Oriented Training

As soon as the person attempts to walk again in the first few days after stroke, certain gait limitations are evident. They are to some extent predictable, given the typical effects of muscle weakness, lack of motor control of the lower limb, poor balance, and, if the period of immobility has been prolonged, increased soft tissue stiffness or contracture. Training to optimize walking involves:
- Practice of overground and treadmill walking
- Exercises to increase strength and motor control of lower limb muscles, with active stretching of muscles to preserve muscle extensibility
- Training to maximize skill, speed, endurance, and aerobic fitness

It is usual for physical therapy to begin early after stroke, when many patients cannot stand up and walk and some have little ability to activate lower limb muscles. The tendency for the paretic limb to collapse, lack of propulsion for forward progression, and poor balance are common problems in the early stages. These problems are not necessarily a barrier to walking practice.

Weightbearing through the feet appears to be critical for promoting muscle function in the lower limbs, and loading the paretic limb should be the urgent and early focus of attention. In addition, weightbearing exercises using body weight support to train muscle force generation and limb control such as repetitive standing up and sitting down and standing balance activities are trained concurrently with overhead harness support where necessary.

Critical Mechanical Factors

There are several critical mechanical factors that should be focused on in training gait:
- Extension of the paretic limb, to 10–15° of hip extension in late stance. This amount of extension stretches the hip flexors and provides some mechanical advantage to power generation for pull-off, that is, for the initiation of hip flexion at the start of swing phase.
- Plantarflexion at the ankle for push-off
- Knee flexion in swing is initiated by active ankle plantarflexion at push-off augmented by hip flexion. A strong push-off is the most important trigger for knee flexion.
- Flexion at the hip for pull-off
- Taking a longer step with the nonparetic limb. This places the paretic hip in an extended position favoring push-off (**Fig. 5.58**).

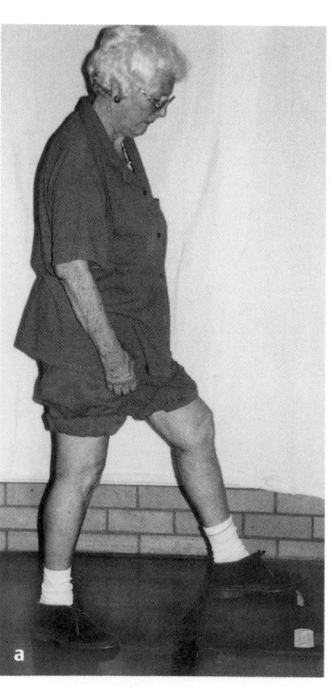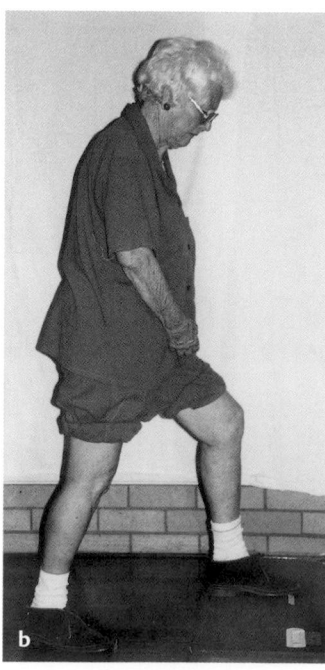

Fig. 5.58 a, b   Exercise to improve control of hip extension. Stepping with the nonparetic leg loads the paretic leg.
a The patient has not moved her body mass far enough forward (decreased hip extension and decreased ankle dorsiflexion).
b The therapist suggests she moves further forward over the left foot. She can repeat this exercise by stepping with the paretic leg.

- Dorsiflexion at the ankle during stance enables body movement forward over the foot (**Fig. 5.58**).
- Ability to change speed and direction as necessary

Overground Walking

Initially it is important that the patient regains a sense of the idea of walking, that is, of the rhythmical, cyclical nature of gait. The individual can be steadied at the upper arm or with a safety belt (**Fig. 5.59**) and is encouraged to initiate walking by taking a big step forward with the nonparetic limb. This places the ankle of the paretic limb in more dorsiflexion, enabling a stronger push-off and a more effective swing forward. Instructions can emphasize that the direction of the push is forward, not upward. This training strategy is par-

ticularly advantageous for increasing the speed of walking, since very slow walking uses more muscle force and energy and interferes with the rhythmic nature of walking and segmental interactions. Suggesting an increase in speed rather than walking very slowly may be counter-intuitive to some therapists who would emphasize slow walking to improve the walking "pattern." However, attempting a faster speed requires less muscle force and less energy.

Treadmill Training with and without Body weight Support

Treadmill training with some body weight support via a harness connected to an overhead support system is a method that is increasingly used in clinical practice (**Fig. 5.60**). The results of a Cochrane systematic review (Moseley et al. 2005) sug-

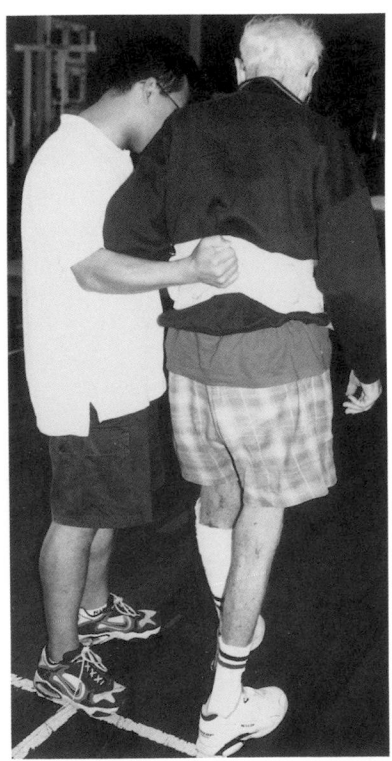

Fig. 5.59 A belt with a grab handle gives reassurance without interfering with the patient's active attempts at balance and walking. The patient's attention is directed to taking a big step with both legs. *(Handi-Lift/Walk Belt, Pelican Manufacturing Pty Ltd, Osborne Park, W Australia.)*

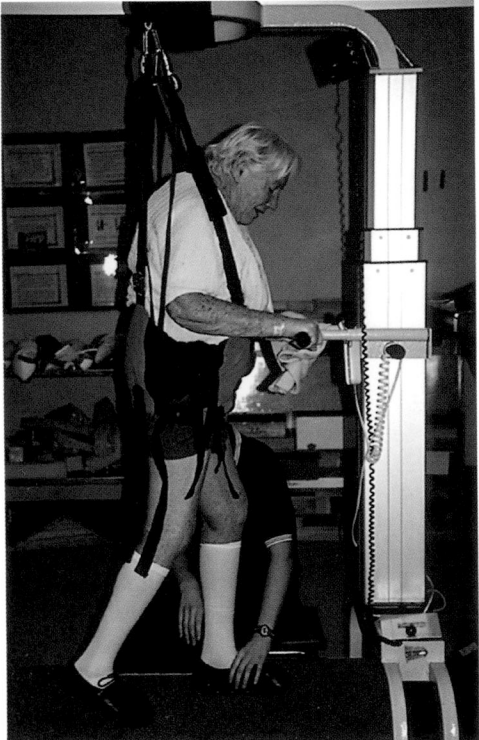

Fig. 5.60 Treadmill walking with body weight support. The therapist may need to assist the trajectory of the foot (toe clearance) and step length during the swing phase of the paretic leg.

gest that treadmill training is a valuable part of gait training in low grade/weak patients, and as a means of increasing gait speed and endurance. Treadmill training with body weight support is well tolerated and effective in the early phase of recovery, and may be the only means of practicing gait for more severely affected, dependent walkers (Barbeau and Visintin 2003). Factors likely to impact on efficacy of treadmill training with or without body weight support are the speed of the treadmill, the amount of body weight support, the amount of assistance provided by the therapist, and the intensity of training. All of these can be adjusted to provide a sufficient training intensity. A Lite-Gait or similar device may help the individual make the transition from treadmill walking to level walking without fear of falling.

Although some physical therapists have expressed concern that treadmill walking is different from level walking, the differences in gait pattern are insignificant. The only real differences are in the visual information received by the individual and the impact of the facilitatory action of the belt on the paretic limb.

The positive effects of a treadmill in walking training may result from the following factors:
- The moving belt stimulates a rhythmic gait pattern, and the harness removes some of the biomechanical and balance constraints of full weightbearing.
- The belt induces a shift toward more consistent temporal phasing and symmetrical gait pattern associated with changes in the timing of muscle activations (Harris-Love et al. 2004, Hesse et al. 1999).
- The belt provides a mechanical stimulus to the hip flexors, optimizing pull-off (Harris-Love et al. 2004).
- Treadmill training has the potential to increase the time spent in practice of walking.

Protocol for Treadmill Walking

Body weight support
- Use the minimum body weight support necessary to maintain active hip and knee extension (<30% of body weight support—Hesse et al. 1997).
- Reduce body weight support as patient improves.
- Encourage patient to reduce hand support.

Speed
- Adjust speed to achieve an optimal step length— if speed is too slow there is little benefit.
- Adjust both speed and inclination of the treadmill to challenge the individual.
- Increase speed.

Initially, guidance from the therapist to assist with foot trajectory of the paretic limb during swing may be necessary (**Fig. 5.60**).

Several studies of treadmill training with and without body weight support have demonstrated effective results, showing significantly better results than those obtained by Bobath therapy/neurodevelopmental treatment (NDT) (Hesse et al. 1995, Richards et al. 1993) or combined proprioceptive neuromuscular facilitation (PNF) and Bobath therapy (Pohl et al. 2002). Furthermore, incorporating principles of sports training such as repetition and training intensity resulted in a dramatic increase in walking speed from 0.6 to 1.6 m/s in a group of stroke patients (Pohl et al. 2002).

When treadmill training is part of an overall task-oriented training regimen, research suggests that such a program is effective in enhancing walking capacity (Dean et al. 2000, Salbach et al. 2004). A closer look at the evidence suggests that a key factor in an effective training program may be the varied and intensive practice of locomotor-related activities that involve functional strength training for both lower limbs, in addition to treadmill training (see Salbach et al. 2004 for description and progression of a training program).

Electromechanical-Assisted Gait Training

New devices for gait training are being developed to increase the time spend in walking practice and to increase the opportunities for individuals to become independent. Two examples are the Gait Trainer and the Haptic Walker for training stair climbing (Hesse et al. 2006). A recent systematic review provides evidence that the use of such devices can have these positive effects (Mehrholz et al. 2007).

Strength Training

Problems with muscle activation are probably the major factors underlying functional disability in gait. It is interesting to note that the results of several recent studies have reported significant increases in motor performance and health outcomes when strength training has been included in the exercise program (Dean et al. 2000, 2001, Teixeira-Salmela et al. 1999). At the completion of a physical conditioning program, subjects are able to generate higher levels of power and increases in positive work by plantar flexors, and hip flexors and extensors (Teixeira-Salmela et al. 2001). An investigation of strength, voluntary activation, and antagonist cocontraction over the first 6 months following stroke demonstrated that stroke patients have the potential for increasing voluntary strength that should be addressed during rehabilitation (Newham and Hsiao 2001). It is possible that many stroke patients maintain significant gait disability because rehabilitation has not targeted strength or endurance as a result of the dogma relating to spasticity. With our present understanding this is a serious clinical error.

An examination of the relationship between muscle torque generated by muscles of both lower limbs in level walking and stair climbing shows that weakness of the nonparetic limb also contributes to dysfunction and should be addressed in training (Kim and Eng 2003). An efficient and functionally relevant way to increase muscle strength and control is to practice weight-bearing actions against body weight resistance. Free weights, dynamometry, and other nonweight-bearing strengthening exercises may also be included. However, these exercises need to be accompanied by functional training of lower limb activities such as walking and stair climbing to enable carryover to function.

Activating Weak or Paretic Muscles

Patients who are unable to generate and sustain sufficient muscle force to support the body in standing and propel it forward require strategies to elicit muscle activity in key muscle groups. Interventions may include:
- Functional electrical stimulation (FES), EMG feedback
- Isokinetic dynamometry (**Fig. 5.61**)
- Taping to assist the patient to activate a muscle; for example, gluteal taping
- Simple exercises (**Fig. 5.62**)

Early after stroke, if the patient is relatively inactive, FES can be used as an adjunct to exercise to maintain the integrity of muscle. It should be

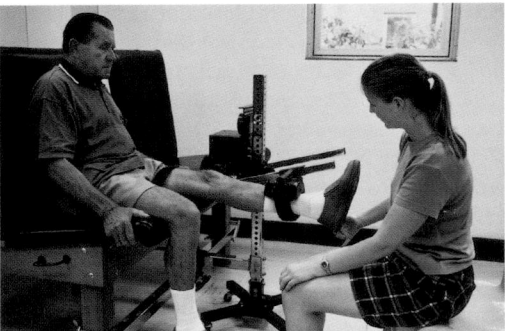

Fig. 5.61 Activating the quadriceps, initially with an eccentric contraction, followed immediately by a concentric contraction. The therapist assists with initial knee extension and the patient attempts to control the weight of the shank while lowering the leg (eccentric contraction) and raising it (concentric contraction). This exercise can also be performed without the dynamometer.

given to those muscles likely to adapt negatively to physical inactivity (such as ankle plantar flexors and dorsiflexors, quadriceps).

Gluteal taping on the paretic side (**Fig. 5.63**) can lead to an immediate improvement in hip extension at the end of single stance with an increase in step length on the nonparetic side and an overall increase in stride length (Kilbreath et al. 2006). In contrast, sham taping did not improve hip extension compared with the no-tape control condition. McConnell (2002) has hypothesized that this taping technique may alter the orientation of muscle fibers, increasing the overlap between the actin and myosin filaments and therefore the possible cross-bridge interactions.

Maximizing Skill, Speed, Endurance, and Fitness

The criteria for gait competency in the community include the ability to:
- Walk at speeds fast enough to cross streets safely (at least 1.1–1.5 m/s)
- Walk for a long enough time and far enough to accomplish daily tasks (at least 500 m)
- Turn the head while walking
- Demonstrate anticipatory strategies to avoid or accommodate obstacles
- React quickly enough to accidental slips and trips to avoid a fall
- Negotiate stairs, kerbs, ramps, moving footways; carry objects

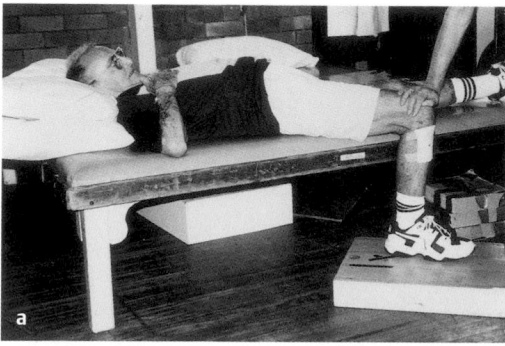

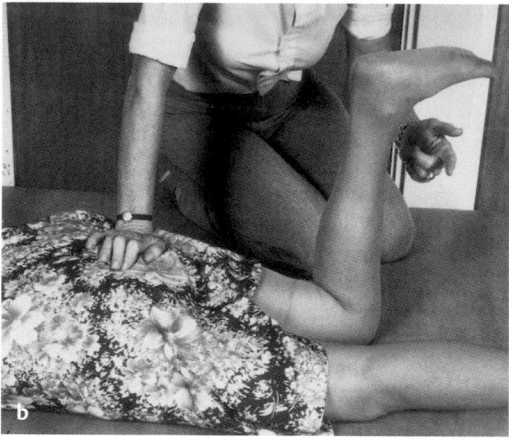

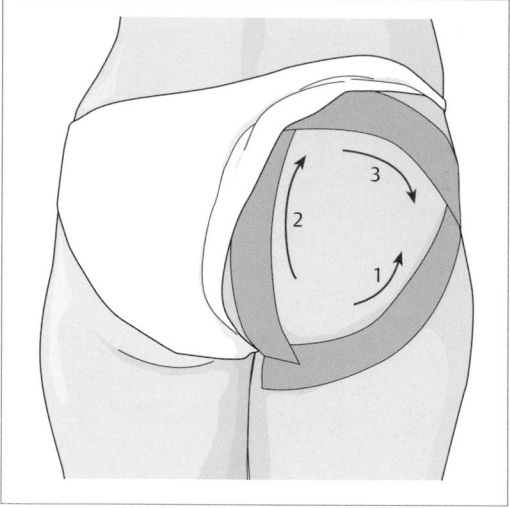

Fig. 5.63   Gluteal taping may improve the patient's control of hip extension during gait. *(Reprinted from SL Kilbreath et al 2006 Australian Journal of Physiotherapy, with permission.)*

Fig. 5.62 a, b   Simple exercises to stimulate muscle activation.
a Pushing down through the heel activates the hip and knee extensors. The therapist may need to stabilize the foot if the muscles maintaining knee flexion (hamstrings) are not strong enough to oppose the knee extension action of the quadriceps. Note that the body is aligned to keep the leg in line with the body.
b The therapist flexes the knee to 90° while the patient attempts a controlled knee extension (eccentric). It may be possible to elicit activity in paretic hamstrings with an eccentric contraction.

Walking should not be a special event that occurs only with the physical therapist. An early goal for the patient could be to walk to the next appointment, or at least part of the way, with the explicit aim of walking further each day rather than being taken in a wheelchair. Verbal encouragement and external cues are given to increase gait speed. A recent study demonstrated that individuals after stroke can increase their level walking speed 2–3 times beyond comfortable levels given instructions to "walk as fast as you can as if you are trying to catch the bus," and encouragement. Fast walking was associated with bilateral increases in joint range and muscle activation, as well as improved symmetry in some spatiotemporal variables, such as increased step length and decreased double-support phase. Quality of life scales indicate that increasing speed results in a greater behavioral repertoire in everyday life (Lamontagne and Fung 2004).

Practice on stairs, walking up and down ramps, hills and kerbs, around obstacles, stepping over objects (see **Fig. 5.38**), marching on the spot (touching knees to hands), carrying parcels, stopping and turning are introduced to prepare the patient for dealing with the complexities of the built and natural environments (**Fig. 5.64**). If practiced with sufficient intensity, these everyday activities can increase strength and control of the lower limbs to support and balance the upper body, and propel it forward.

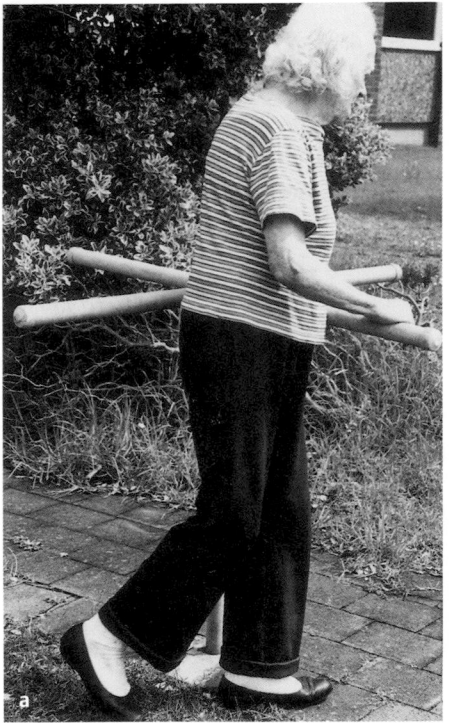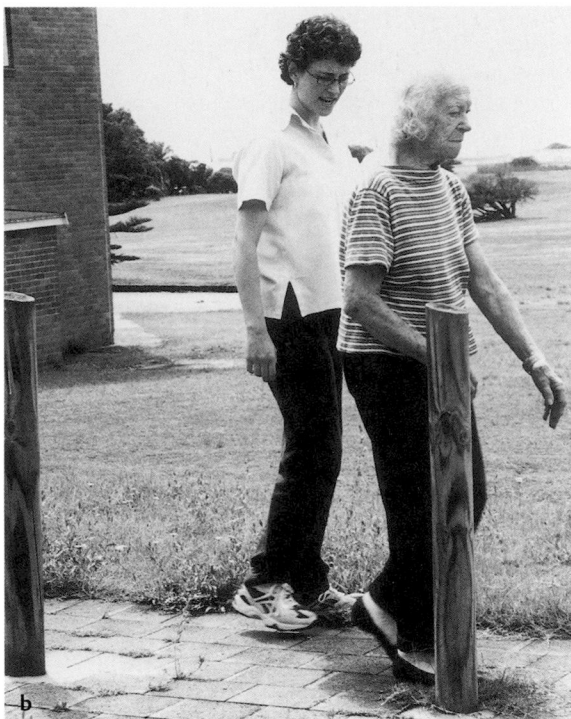

Fig. 5.64 a, b   An obstacle course—walking around objects.

Aids and Orthoses

Walking aids, including parallel bars, a quadripod/tripod stick, a walking frame, an assistant's arm, and a standard stick all rely on support through the upper limb. Only recently have the effects of different types of sticks been compared. Although all walking aids impose some mechanical constraint, a simple walking stick may interfere least with balance and walking while providing some assistance (Kuan et al. 1999).

Research into the potential of ankle–foot orthoses (AFOs) to improve ankle/foot mechanics during gait has produced equivocal results and the issue of whether or not to prescribe some form of orthosis remains controversial. An orthosis that provides mediolateral stability at the subtalar joint, without unduly limiting plantarflexion or dorsiflexion, may be useful for patients with ankle instability. A major consideration in determining the use of an AFO is that constraining motion at one joint necessitates adaptation at other joints, and this may or may not be helpful. Although a rigid AFO holds the foot in some dorsi-

flexion, it imposes a mechanical resistance to plantarflexion for push-off. A recent synthesis of best evidence so far shows no support for the provision of orthoses such as AFOs or hand-held walking aids (Van Peppen et al. 2004). If a device is considered worth trying for a particular person, it is recommended that natural walking speed is measured while using the orthosis or aid, as the patient's preferred speed will give a good indication of the relative merits of the device.

Measurement

Functional tests include:
- MAS Walking Item (performance)
- 10 m Walk Test (speed)
- 6 or 12 minute Walk Test (endurance)
- TUG (balance, skill)
- Step test (strength, balance)

Walking speed may be the most important clinical measure of functional ability. Several critical biomechanical parameters are speed-dependent. For example, as push-off power and magnitude of hip flexion on the paretic side increase, so does speed. The 10 m Walk Test is useful in the acute phase as a guide to progress. However, walking speed over a short distance may overestimate locomotor capacity (Dean et al. 2001). Both speed and endurance need to be measured and specifically trained.

Training Guidelines: Reaching and Manipulation

The upper limb functions principally for reaching, grasping, and manipulation. The arm transports the hand according to task, context, and goal. The distance we can reach is a function of arm length. If the object to be reached is beyond arm's length, movement of the body mass over the lower limbs in sitting and standing extends the distance that can be reached. If the object is judged out of reach, we take a step. Postural adjustments are part of the functional unit and are specific to task and context.

The upper limb is multisegmented, with many degrees of freedom of movement. Nevertheless, the limb functions as a single unit to achieve specific goals. When reaching to grasp, fingers are grouped according to the requirements of the task, environment, and object—how heavy the object, its shape, what is to be done with it, where it is in space, and the object's characteristics (e.g., frictional and deformable qualities). Limb movement arises out of these interactions. The function of the hand is sensory as well as motor, and previous experience determines how sensory input is to be processed, with irrelevant stimuli filtered out. Vision plays a critical role in the control of the hand.

Most actions involve interaction with an object in the environment (e.g., soup in spoon) and many tasks are performed bimanually. In bimanual actions, both arms and hands function as one unit. Effective performance of the task may require coordinated timing of the two limbs performing a similar movement, as in catching a ball, but in many cases performing differently, as in unscrewing a lid from a jar. Reach and grasp may also have to take account of the speed of a moving object.

The dilemma for the patient in rehabilitation is the large number of actions that must be relearned

in the context of returning to an independent life. The patient must be trained to move many body segments as a coordinated unit in functional actions with many different goals, and with a damaged system. However, there is one particular problem to be solved in clinical practice—how to drive the person to use the affected limb when it feels more natural to use the better limb to accomplish the goals of daily life.

Biomechanical Description

Theoretical concepts and data from biomechanical studies of the upper limbs in action provide essential information for clinical practice if the therapist is to be skilled in training individuals to optimize their functional performance after stroke.

Reaching

Reaching to grasp an object is made up of two components—movement of the hand to the object, and manipulation of the object to achieve a goal (Jeannerod 1981). Reaching out with the arm is a ballistic movement. As the hand nears the object the arm slows so final corrections can be made. This component of the action requires visual information and feedback to ensure accuracy of hand alignment and grasp aperture as the hand approaches the object. Manipulation of the object requires visual and tactile sensory feedback. Studies of the relationships between reach and grasp phases show that arm and hand function as one unit. The hand starts to open near the start of arm movement (Hoff and Arbib 1993, Marteniuk et al. 1990) and final adjustment to grasp aperture is made at the end of reach just before grasp (**Fig. 5.65**). Movement of the index finger changes grasp aperture, with the thumb stable in an abducted position (Wing and Fraser 1983). The spatial and temporal relationships between trunk, lower limb, and arm movement in reaching are complex and reflect the degrees of freedom available, the task, and the environmental context (Seidler and Stelmach 2000).

The spatiotemporal organization of limb movement varies according to whether one or both hands are used (Castiello et al. 1992). It takes into account the physical characteristics of the object, for example its shape and fragility, and what is to be done with it (Smeets and Brenner 1999,

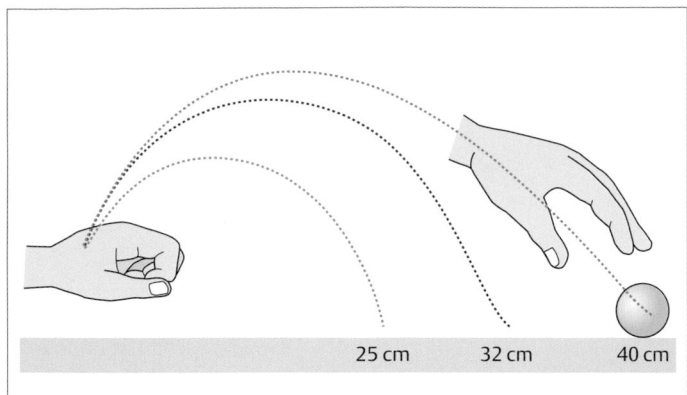

Fig. 5.65 A motion analysis study of reaching toward an object to grasp it. Dots represent successive positions of the hand every 20 ms. The hand slows as it approaches the object. Lines represent the size of the grasp aperture every 40 ms. *(We thank the International Association for the Study of Attention and Performance for permission to reprint from Long and Baddeley 1981.)*

25 cm 32 cm 40 cm

van Vliet 1993). In bilateral actions, aspects of limb movement differ according to whether the individual reaches to grasp with the whole hand or with a fine precision grasp. Castiello and colleagues (1993) studied reaching out to open a can. One hand grasped the can, the other pulled the tab to open it. They found that both hands started and finished the reaching movement together but that kinematic details differed for each hand. The precision hand reached peak velocity earlier and started to decelerate earlier than the other hand. In other words, the hand with the more complex task reached out more carefully than the other hand by changing the relative time spent in acceleration and deceleration phases. A similar result was found for a task in which one hand opened a drawer and the other took out a rod (Wiesendangar et al. 1996).

Cooperation between the two hands and the predictive nature of some tasks are shown in an experiment in which the subject dropped a ball into a cup held in the other hand (Johansson and Westling 1988). The grip force of the cup hand increased in anticipation of the ball's impact—that is, before the ball hit the cup. Due to the complexity of bimanual tasks, it is necessary for an individual to have the opportunity to be trained and to practice such tasks. It is clear that, without specific practice, an individual may not regain the use of both hands together in the same task.

Manipulation

Although the upper limb is involved principally in relatively simple reaching movements, functional hand movements are very complex, involving many joints and muscles. The hand takes on many different configurations in the performance of skilled manipulative tasks, yet control appears to be simplified by certain anatomical configurations, corticomotoneuronal connections, and patterns of force production (**Fig. 5.66**). For example, many tasks involve interactions between object, thumb, and index finger. The thumb abducts and rotates, the index finger flexes, force is exerted on the object through the pads of the digits, primarily by the long flexors of thumb and finger. Each digit is stabilized by a combination of joint geometry and intrinsic muscle action (Lemon et al. 1991). The relative contributions of muscles differ and are task-related.

For some tasks, other grasps are used specifically for precision and power. Bendz (1993) described a locking and a supporting grasp (**Fig. 5.67**). In the locking grasp, the tool is locked into the palm of the hand by the fourth and fifth fingers, flexed at all joints and rotated at the metacarpophalangeal (MCP) joints. The fifth metacarpal is flexed at the MCP joint by hypothenar muscles, with opponens digiti minimi acting directly on the metacarpal. Abductor digiti minimi and flexor brevis flex the metacarpal indirectly through their common attachment to the proximal phalanges of the fifth finger. In the supporting grasp, flexion of the fifth metacarpal enables the little finger to prop up the plate and keep it horizontal. This work by Bendz is particularly interesting as it reminds the physical therapist of the importance of knowing the functional anatomy of the hand. It is clear also that these grasps need specific training with practice of holding, manipulating, and carrying objects.

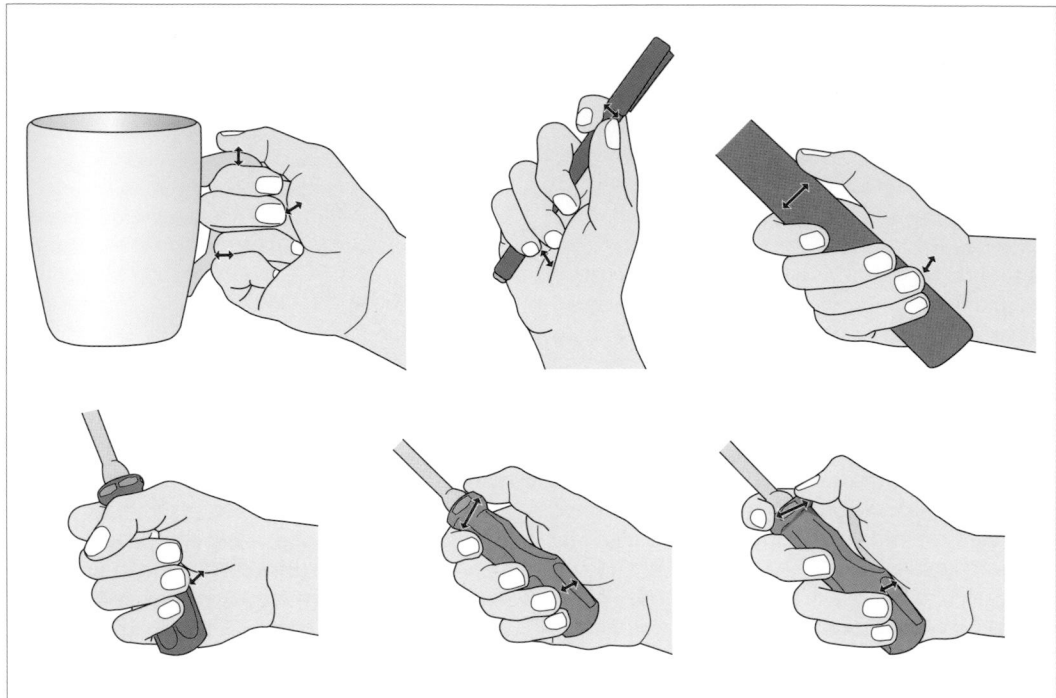

Fig. 5.66   Task- and object-specific grasps showing the different patterns of force production. *(Reprinted from Iberall et al. 1986, with permission.)*

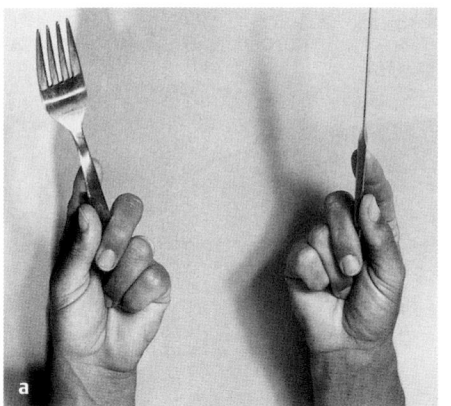
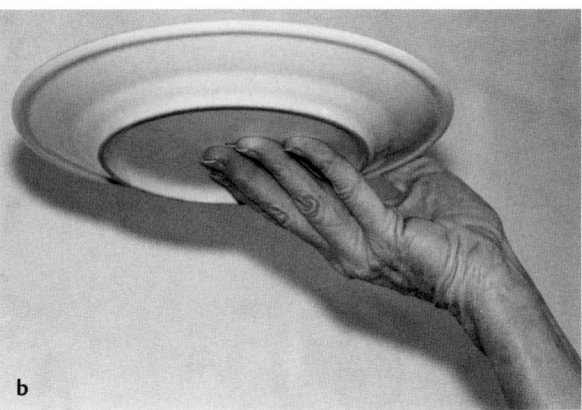

Fig. 5.67 a, b
a Locking grasp holds the knife and fork securely in the palm.

b In this supporting grasp the fingers keep the plate level as well as providing support.

Shaping the hand for different objects and tasks can involve the carpal and metacarpal bones forming the palm of the hand into a concave shape by the combined action of intrinsic muscles. This has been called a "postural set" for the promotion of skilled movement (Lemon et al. 1991). Similarly, when a group of fingers acts as a single functional unit in grasping an object, this unit is called a "virtual finger" (Arbib et al. 1985, Li et al. 1998a, b). When an object is gripped strongly between fingers and thumb, forces are shared cooperatively between the four fingers of the functional unit (Li et al. 1998a). In holding a mug, for example, three functional units, each producing force in different directions, cooperate to ensure a stable grasp (**Fig. 5.66**). Shaping the hand for manipulating an object is partly a function of the anatomy of the hand. It is therefore important from early after stroke to work toward the preservation of the integrity of the natural bony relationships of the hand, by preserving flexibility, length, and whatever contractility of muscle is possible.

Understanding these details of hand function provides information of value in designing an intensive exercise program, in particular for a person who has sufficient muscle activity to move wrist, fingers, and thumb but insufficient motor control to use the hand spontaneously. As both the object and the goal of the person carrying out a task drives the control of the hand, the importance of individuals practicing real tasks with real objects is quite evident.

Practicing real tasks may also aid the individual with sensory impairment, although some individuals after stroke may also benefit from practice of sensory recognition tasks. The role of tactile receptors in the glabrous (nonhairy) skin of the palm has been studied in detail. Johansson and Westling found that tactile signals are used to adapt motor output to the weight of the object (the vertical lifting force) and the frictional characteristics of the object in relation to slip (the slip-triggered grip force) (Johansson and Westling 1984, 1990; Johansson et al. 1992a–c). Sensory inputs from cutaneous touch and pressure receptors in the palm of the hand contribute to movement control. They help us to identify objects and classify them according to properties such as texture, shape, weight, and potential for slipping, and enable motor output (muscle force) to be adjusted as necessary. Changes in grip force also occur in response to inertial forces produced by the movement occurring while the object is being moved. It is quite common after stroke for people to lack this adaptive force control and therefore to have difficulty in maintaining grasp while moving the limb. This ability may need to be emphasized in training and specifically practiced.

Recovery of Upper Limb Function

There is increasing evidence that recovery is minimal in some individuals, particularly those with a severely paralytic limb that persists over the first few weeks (Coote and Stokes 2001, Kwakkel et al. 2003, Nakayama et al. 1994). However, it is also quite common to see individuals after stroke whose spontaneous functional use of the limb is worse than would be anticipated, given that they have active muscles and a degree of motor control. There is increasing evidence of positive effects from certain types of training program that involve task-oriented training of functional actions in an enriched learning environment with emphasis on forcing use of the paretic limb (Davis 2006, Van Peppen et al. 2004, Wolf et al. 2006). A more accurate picture of recovery potential and in particular of the potential effects of intervention is still to come. Studies of recovery have typically not divided patients according to severity of initial paralysis; measures of actual arm use have only recently been reported (Kwakkel et al. 2003) and therapy methods are rarely described in detail.

There may be a group of individuals after stroke who, because of the site and extent of the lesion and comorbidities, are unlikely to regain effective function with the paretic limb. A study testing motor evoked potentials in response to transcortical magnetic stimulation (Pennisi et al. 1999) suggested that individuals with paralysis of hand muscles in the first 48 hours after stroke with an absence of motor potentials were likely to have a poor prognosis.

Functional Problems

Depressed motor output, decreased rate of neural activation, poor timing and coordination of limb segments, and sensory deficits can impact severely on functional performance. Muscle weakness and loss of manual dexterity are often compounded by the development of soft tissue changes, joint pain, and the natural tendency for patients to focus on their nonparetic arm for their daily activities. Muscle weakness and impaired motor control affect motor performance according to the extent and distribution of paresis. There is relative sparing of some proximal muscles that have bilateral innervation, such as the shoulder adductor pectoralis major (Colebatch and Gandevia 1989), while the

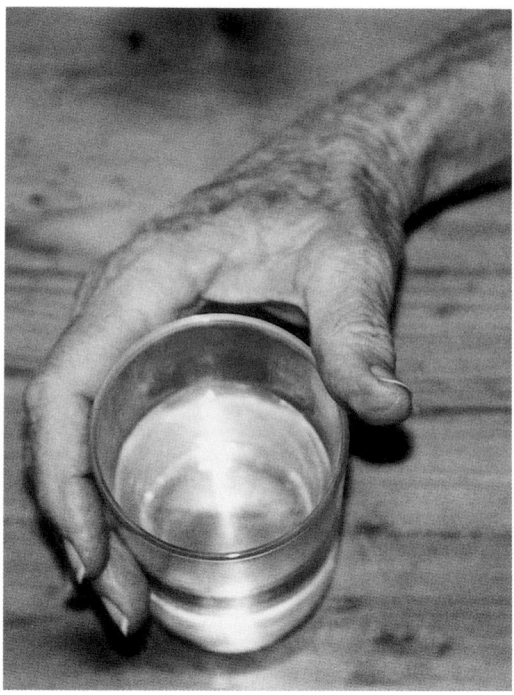

Fig. 5.68 The goal is to release the glass. Extension at the CMC joint and wrist flexion occur adaptively as a result of the difficulty abducting the thumb due to abductor pollicis brevis weakness in the inner range. Thumb abduction exercises are also practiced.

paretic limb preferentially and learned nonuse, and changes to soft tissues due to maintenance of the paretic limb for long periods in internal rotation and adduction at the glenohumeral joint, flexion at the elbow, forearm pronation, thumb adduction, and finger and wrist flexion. The natural resting position of the arm when in sitting, if combined with inability to move the limb, can lead to adaptive changes in shortened muscles that include loss of muscle extensibility, contracture, and pain. Adaptive movement patterns reflect paresis, imbalance between muscles acting over a joint, and soft tissue inflexibility. The person's adaptive movement represents the best attempt possible given the impairments and the biomechanical possibilities of a multisegment system (see **Fig. 5.5** and **Fig. 5.68**). For example, if it is difficult to flex the shoulder and extend the elbow to reach forward for an object, reaching distance is typically increased by moving the upper body forward at the hips. When shoulder flexors (deltoid, supraspinatus) are paretic, an attempt to reach may involve lateral flexion of the spine and elevation of the shoulder girdle. (For more detailed discussion of the factors leading to the development of shoulder pain, see Carr and Shepherd 2010.)

Causes and Prevention of Shoulder Pain

The development of shoulder pain can have a negative effect on functional recovery. The presence of pain may make training, exercise, and practice of upper limb activities impossible.

Clues for the therapist and other rehabilitation staff as to the contributing causes of shoulder pain come from clinical research. For example, the occurrence of a painful shoulder is statistically related to decreased range of external rotation of glenohumeral joint, weakness of glenohumeral abduction and external rotation, and joint stiffness (Bohannon 1988, Rajaratnam et al. 2007). Immobility and persistent positioning of the arm in internal rotation and adduction are major causes of pain from adhesive capsulitis (Ikai et al. 1998). Contracture of muscles linking humerus and scapula, by impeding scapular-shoulder movement, may cause small soft tissue tears. In addition, older adults have an increased chance of having abnormalities of capsule, bursae, and humeral head (Peat 1986), and degenerative change prior to stroke.

antagonist deltoid muscle seems to have direct corticospinal connections (Colebatch et al. 1990). Slower recruitment times of flexor and extensor carpi radialis longus, biceps, and triceps brachii and difficulty sustaining a contraction have been reported (Sahrmann and Norton 1977). These findings help to explain the slow movements commonly observed.

Sustaining and controlling grip force while grasping and lifting objects is a common problem. Force produced during gripping can be slow to build up, difficult to stabilize at the required level for a specific task, and characterized by irregular force changes (Hermsdörfer and Mai 1996). Deficits in interjoint coordination are evident during reaching actions, with difficulty in making smooth, continuous, and accurate movements (Cirstea and Levin 2000, Trombly 1992).

Adaptations to immobility and disuse, and shoulder pain, frequently add to the disability. Adaptations commonly include use of the non-

The likelihood of adaptive shortening and other disuse changes occurring in muscles around the shoulder, particularly glenohumeral internal rotators and adductors, is magnified in individuals who spend most of the day with their arm in a sling. A sling that is in common use holds the paretic limb in adduction and internal rotation. It is probable that it prevents the wearer from attempting to use the limb, as well as predisposing the limb to the negative adaptive changes referred to above. In addition, accidental trauma may occur to a joint that is unprotected due to muscle weakness and disuse, and may lead to pain (Wanklyn et al. 1996) and to inflammatory conditions such as adhesive capsulitis or tendinitis. Trauma can occur by pulling on the arm while helping a person stand up. People who need most help in getting out of bed or from a chair are particularly vulnerable.

Overextensibility of glenohumeral capsular structures triggered by prolonged position with the paretic arm hanging dependent by the side may lead to glenohumeral joint subluxation. There is a high incidence of subluxation in those with little or no muscle activity around the shoulder (particularly of supraspinatus and posterior deltoid); it is much less common in those with recovery of muscle activity within a month of stroke. There appears to be no relationship between subluxation and pain, although the two may be present at the same time. An increase in active range of shoulder abduction and significant motor recovery is associated with decreased subluxation (Zorowitz 2001).

Severe and persistent pain should be investigated and appropriate intervention given, as would occur in a nonstroke population. Preventive procedures should be instigated in the early stages to ensure that no potentially damaging events take place, and that there is sufficient exercise for the paretic arm. Task-oriented training and exercise to increase shoulder muscle activity and joint mobility needs to start early, and be frequent with emphasis on active movement into flexion, external rotation and elevation (see **Fig. 5.70**). In addition, the arm is positioned during the day to avoid soft tissue length changes (Carr and Shepherd 2010).

Shoulder Pain Prevention Program

- Active exercises to train reaching-for external rotator, abductor, and flexor muscles; plus shoulder shrugging exercises.
- Positioning for at least 30 min each day sitting at a table, glenohumeral joint in external rotation and abduction (**Fig. 5.69a**), can prevent contracture (Ada et al 2003).
- Positioning in wheelchair, arm on gutter in mid-forearm rotation (**Fig. 5.69b**).
- Avoid prolonged glenohumeral joint internal rotation/adduction. There is no evidence that a sling prevents pain or subluxation (Van Peppen et al 2004).
- FES to deltoid muscle.
- Avoid damaging events–passive range of motion, pulling on the arm.
- Strapping to the shoulder provides some support to glenohumeral joint.

Task-Oriented Training

Rehabilitation for motor disorders of the upper limb after stroke is a challenge for therapists and patients. In the last few decades, however, several

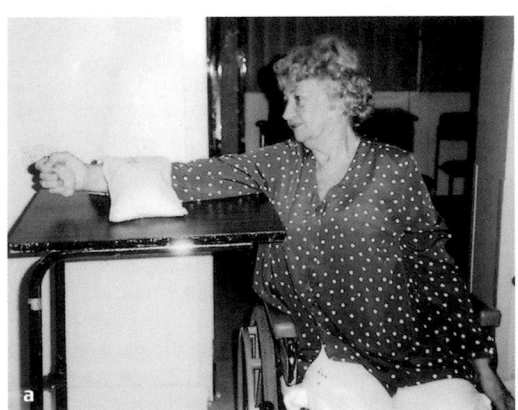
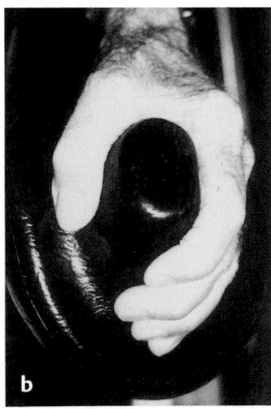

Fig. 5.69 a, b
a Positioning to prevent contracture of glenohumeral adductor and internal rotator muscles.
b Arm gutter on wheelchair has been adjusted to hold glenohumeral joint and forearm in mid-rotation. The hand is prevented from rolling over at the wrist.

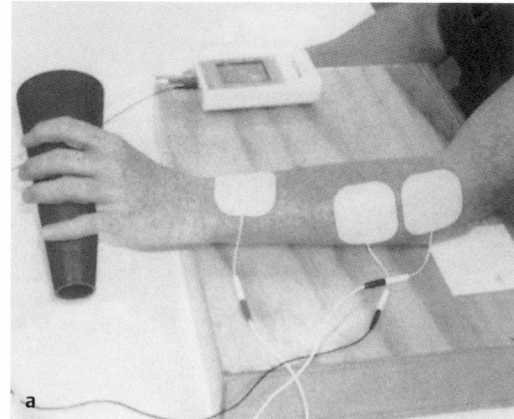

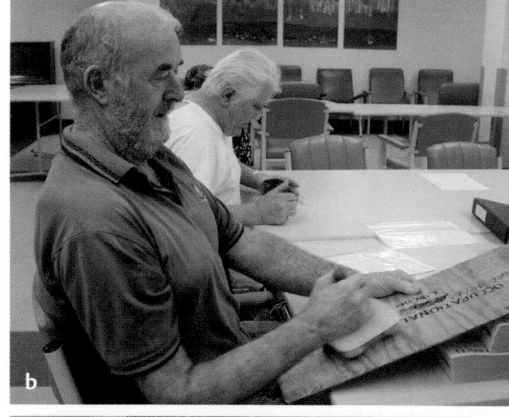

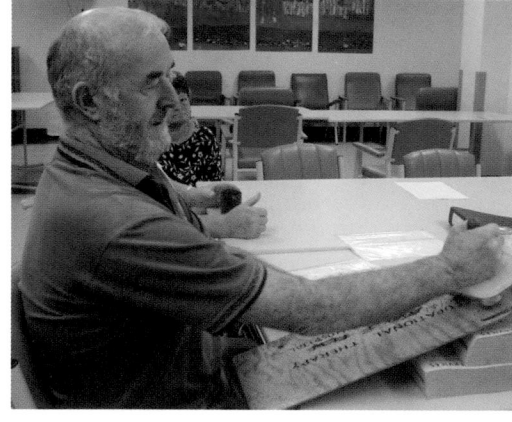

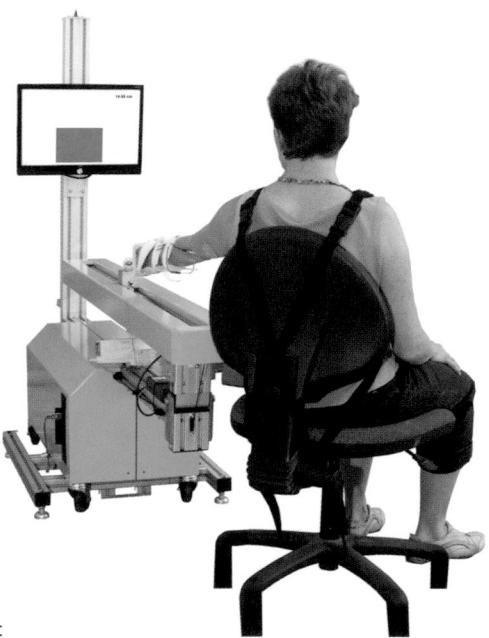

Fig. 5.70 a–c
a Demonstration of EMG-assisted FES to paretic wrist and finger extensor muscles. *(Courtesy of Dr. R Barker, James Cook University, Townsville, Australia.)*
b Hand class: Repetitive shoulder flexion and extension to improve strength and interjoint coordination. When muscles are very weak, using a simple device for early training. His goal is continuous smooth and rhythmic movement. *(Courtesy of S Dorsch, K Schurr, Physiotherapy Dept, Bankstown-Lidcombe Hospital, Sydney, Australia.)*
c A nonrobotic device, the Sensorimotor Active Rehabilitation Trainer (SMART) arm (Neurotrac 5, Verity Medical Ltd) for training reaching. Positioning of the device allows for changes in arm position. *(Courtesy of Dr. R Barker, James Cook University, Townsville, Australia.)*

biomechanical and physiological studies have taught us more about the kinematics and kinetics of reaching, grasping, and manipulating objects, and given us insights into how the limb is controlled in complex actions.

From this increase in scientific understanding, new methods have been developed and clinical studies testing these methods have been performed. We now have available a group of rehabilitation strategies that are based on our current scientific understanding and also have been shown to be effective. The following paragraphs outline these methods, which should form the major part of rehabilitation after stroke. References are provided for the reader to obtain more detail.

Training of active movement should start early. Training reaching and hand use is practiced in sitting at a table. Emphasis is on tasks that may elicit activity in key muscles, prevent development of adductor/internal rotator muscle contractures and painful shoulder, and preserve integrity of soft tissues. Reaching exercises in different directions and with the shoulder elevated may be the key for the patient to regain some muscle activity (see **Fig. 5.70a, b**).

As a general rule, the action to be acquired must be practiced in its entirety. The biomechanics of linked segments ensure that one component of an action is to a large extent dependent on preceding components. Normally movement is organized to ensure that the functional goal is achieved. For this to occur requires that muscles spanning several joints must cooperate throughout the action.

Many investigations of task-oriented training for the upper limb report positive results (e.g., Blennerhassett and Dite 2004, Duncan et al. 2003, Harris et al. 2009, Lin et al. 1998, Winstein et al. 2004, Wu et al. 2000). Some report positive results from a task-oriented circuit-training program, in which reaching and manipulation were trained at one of the work stations. Winstein and colleagues (2004) tested patients after stroke. Each patient received one of three different therapy methods: (A) Bobath therapy, (B) functional training, (C) strength training. Groups B and C performed significantly better than group A on functional tests. At 9 months, the less severely affected patients in the functional training group had continued to improve.

Simple Repetitive Exercises, Electromyographic Feedback, FES

Simple exercises may elicit muscle activity and increase force-generating capacity. For example, reaching on a table top; glenohumeral external rotation with elbow flexed, arm at side, hand moving on table; thumb and fingers extension and flexion; wrist flexion and extension in mid-rotation and pushing a glass; gripping exercises. These exercises give the opportunity to improve muscle contractility in the early stage. **Figure 5.70b** illustrates a simple device that enables repetitive practice of shoulder flexion and elbow extension as part of an upper limb class. A more complex device (**Fig. 5.70c**) is currently in development for

use with EMG-triggered electrical stimulation for individuals with severe weakness (Barker et al. 2008).

FES and EMG biofeedback may be useful in the early stages, as part of reaching, grasping and manipulation training, as a means of assisting the patient to activate very weak muscles. Periods of EMG-triggered FES can be performed during the day to key muscles for a particular task (e.g., wrist and long finger extensors, palmar abductor of thumb, deltoid, supraspinatus) (**Fig. 5.70a**). Electrical stimulation can preserve muscle fiber contractility, can be done with minimal supervision, and is a way to increase time spent exercising muscles. There is some evidence that electrical stimulation can be effective under certain conditions (Faghri et al. 1994). A meta-analysis (Ada and Foongchomcheay 2002) showed that FES given early after stroke can prevent the development of inferior glenohumeral joint displacement.

Training Reaching

It is preferable to practice reaching tasks in sitting with the arms resting on a table, with the goals of reaching to a target (**Fig. 5.71**), and in standing.

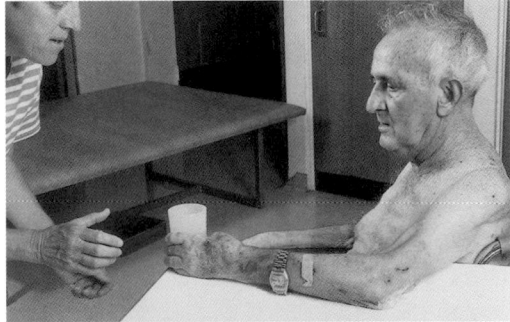

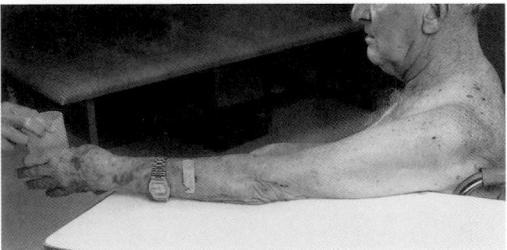

Fig. 5.71 As his shoulder flexor muscles are very weak, the patient cannot raise his arm forward in sitting. However, with his arm supported on the table he is able to reach forward.

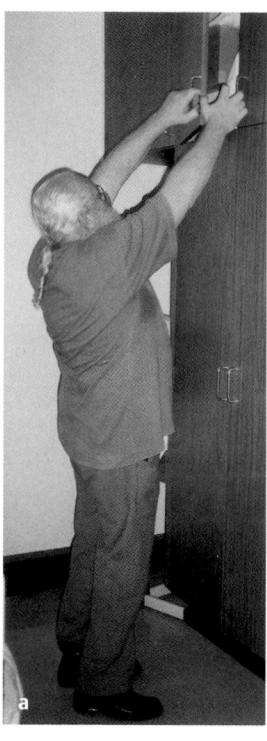

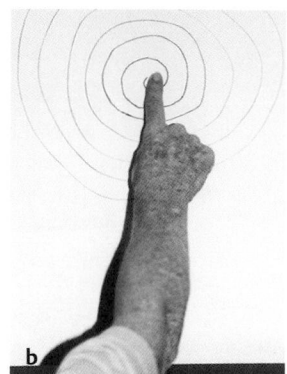

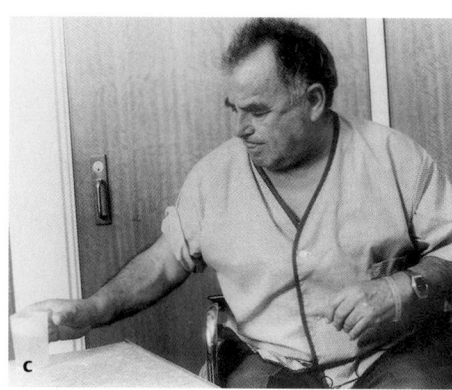

Fig. 5.72 a–c
a Practicing reaching up to open a cupboard and take out an object. *(Reprinted with kind permission from PRO-ED Inc, Austin Tx, USA.)*
b Tracing a circle with finger or pencil without touching the lines.
c Reaching to pick up a glass. The glass has been placed to "force" external rotation of the glenohumeral joint.

Reaching and balancing the body mass are also practiced in sitting (see **Figs. 5.5** and **5.28**). Actions such as pointing to targets on the wall and reaching above shoulder height can be done with the aim of building up endurance in performing a variety of tasks (**Fig. 5.72a, b**).

Training Manipulation and Dexterity

There are many activities that can be used to increase speed and precision of movement and, as a result, skill. Here are some examples:

Sitting at a Table
- *Tapping tasks*, e.g., touch each fingertip to thumb in sequence as rapidly as possible (do a given number of sequences within a given time); tap the table with single fingers.
- *Hand cupping tasks* to train opposition of radial and ulnar sides of the hand; e.g., hold seeds in palm and pour into dish, scoop coins from tabletop into palm of other hand and the reverse.
- Pick up different objects for different purposes, with different grips between thumb and finger (s), between thumb and fourth or fifth fingers,

with a palmar grip (**Fig. 5.73**). Pick up, hold, and move large and small objects. Use target lines on tabletop. Pick up a glass of water and drink from it. Other tasks include: typing on a keyboard, playing a computer game using a manipulandum, drawing, turning door handles, turning the pages of a magazine, and walking while carrying a glass of water.
- Finger tracking exercises, practiced intensively, have been shown to be effective in improving hand control; the results were associated with ipsilesional cortical reorganization in the affected hemisphere (Carey et al. 2002).

Training involves checking performance throughout practice: using pads of thumb and fingers for grasping, not the lateral surfaces; wrist should be in extension in most of these tasks; all opposition movements should take place at carpometacarpal joints.

Bimanual Training
In everyday life, actions performed bimanually are more common than unimanual actions (Kilbreath and Heard 2005). Bimanual training should prob-

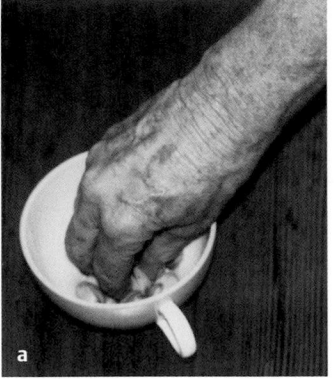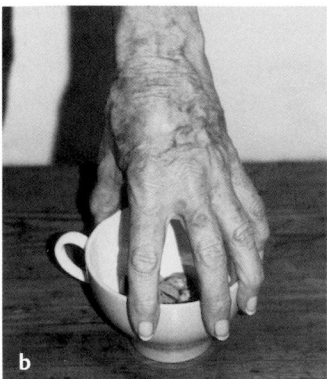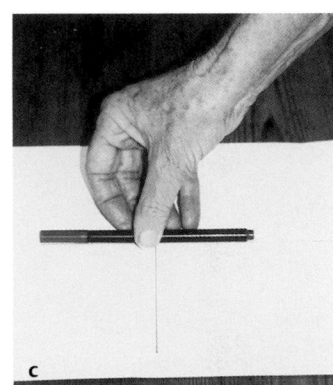

Fig. 5.73 a–c Grasping tasks to train coordinated movement of fingers, wrist and forearm: **a** picking up small objects from a cup; **b** picking up a cup; **c** rotating a pen through 180°.

ably begin early, as soon as the patient has the ability to control simple movements with the affected limb. Exercises include arm cycling, push-ups against the wall, rolling or folding a towel, scooping coins off a tabletop into the other hand, removing lids from jars and cans, pouring from one polystyrene cup to another without deforming the cup, pouring from jug to cup, reaching up to a cupboard (**Fig. 5.74**). Findings from several clinical studies report positive effects of structured bimanual training (Mudie and Matyas 2000, Whitall et al. 2000).

Forced Use of the Paretic Upper Limb

Many of the studies of task-oriented training reporting positive findings included constraint of the nonparetic hand in their program. The results show that a combination of meaningful task training, practice, and a strategy to enforce movement of the paretic limb is effective in individuals who have some ability to actively extend the wrist and fingers. Constraint prevents the nonparetic limb from taking over and may overcome the conditioned response by creating a real necessity to move. Contrast this with the typical hospital and rehabilitation setting, which makes only limited demands on a patient, thus providing little incentive to use the affected limb. The patient may manage by using the nonparetic limb while an in-patient, and with the help of staff. Common clinical practices may, however, have effects opposite to those intended. For example, a wheelchair to be propelled by the nonparetic arm and leg may be provided, and it is still common for patients to wear a sling constraining the paretic arm in internal rotation and adduction for a large part of the day. These two methods encourage use of the nonparetic limbs, encouraging the person to favor these limbs and discouraging attempts to use the paretic limbs.

In several studies of small groups, motor function significantly improved after a short period of intensive, functionally oriented task practice plus constraint of the nonparetic arm (Kunkel et al. 1999, Miltner et al. 1999, Page et al. 2004, Taub et al. 1993, Wolf et al. 2002). In some studies the arm is constrained by a sling or a mitt for most waking hours. Benefits can last for at least 6 months (Miltner et al. 1999). Most important is that many of these studies have shown dramatic improvements in the amount of use of the affected limb in real world environments (e.g., Kunkel et al. 1999, Taub et al. 1993). Another study by Taub and Wolf (1997), in which a half glove (fingers free) was used, showed similar benefits, the patient being taught to use the glove as a cue not to use the nonparetic arm. Individuals appear to tolerate the constraint. Dromerick and colleagues (2000) report that no subject withdrew from their program or lost independence as a result of not being able to compensate with the nonparetic limb. Positive effects of treatment on the control of grasping forces produced during the performance of a key-turning task have been reported (Alberts et al. 2004).

Compelling evidence in support of constraint plus intensive, meaningful exercise and practice also comes from studies of brain reorganization

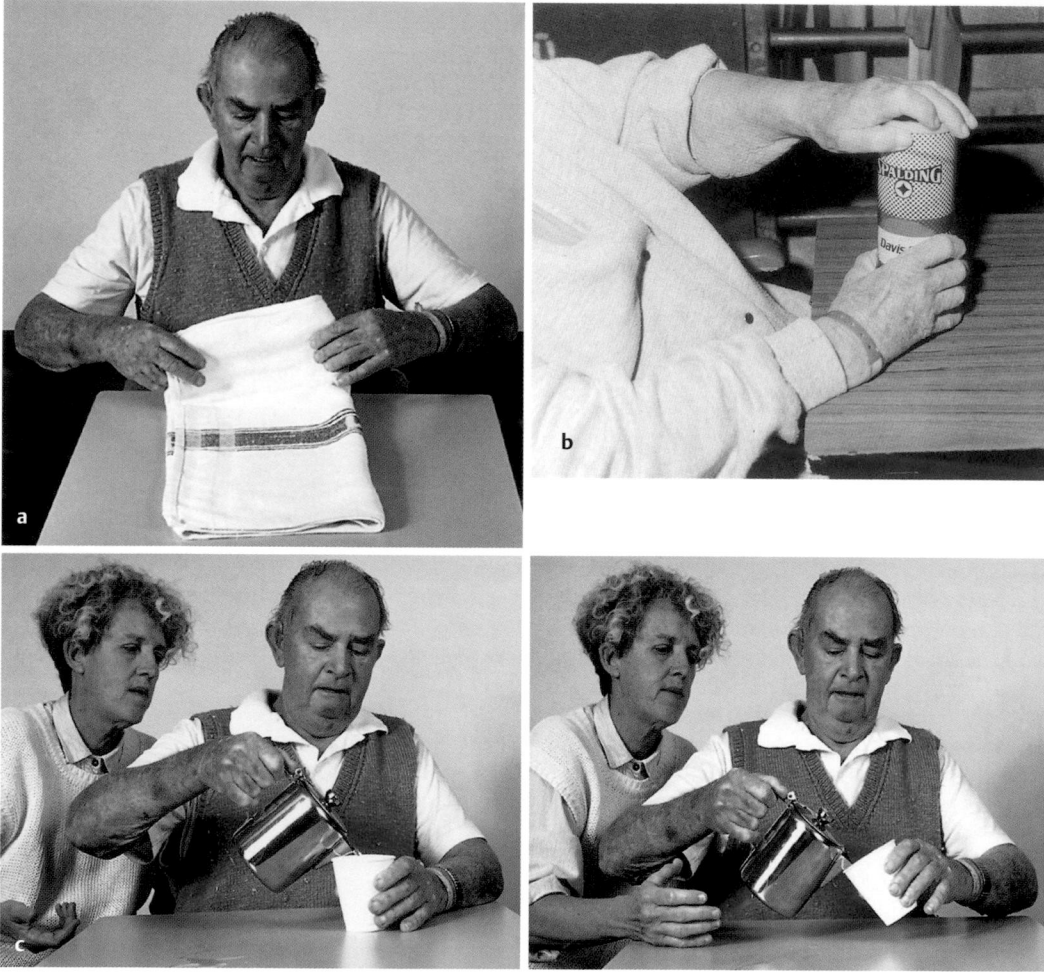

Fig. 5.74 a–c   Practice of bimanual tasks:
a folding a towel;

b removing the lid from a can;
c pouring water.

after stroke. These studies have shown an association between increased use of the affected limb, improved motor performance, and brain reorganization (Liepert et al. 1998, 2000, 2001).

The results of a multicentre clinical trial of CIMT were published in 2006 (Wolf et al. 2006). Experimental subjects, who had had a first stroke within the previous 3–9 months, underwent a program in which they were asked to wear a restraining mitt on the nonparetic hand for 90% of their waking day. They performed a standardized program of repetitive task practice of functional activities and training (behavioral shaping) of the paretic limb every weekday for up to 6 hours per day.

The program lasted 2 weeks. In this large group of participants, the program produced statistically significant improvements in functional performance and paretic arm use compared with the control group who received usual and customary care. Improvement persisted for at least a year. These changes were measured using the Wolf Motor Function Test, a test of performance on timed and strength tasks, and the Motor Activity Log. The latter is a measure of real-time use of the limb, administered to patient and carer who rate how much the paretic arm was used spontaneously to accomplish 30 activities of daily living outside the rehabilitation center. The Stroke Impact Scale, a quality of life scale, showed a significant improvement in use of the paretic hand.

Patients for whom this intervention should currently be provided are those who pass certain "minimum motor criteria" (Taub and Wolf 1997) but who do not use the affected limb in daily tasks despite having the ability to move the limb voluntarily. This is the group of patients reported to benefit so far. It is important to ensure the individual's understanding of and compliance with the constraint by:

- Teaching the individual how to put on and take off the constraint independently
- Making a behavioral contract with each patient, working from their daily routine to decide which activities to carry out with constraint and which require two hands
- Organizing a diary to be filled in to enable monitoring of patient's activities outside therapy time

In the protocol below (**Table 5.1**) we have outlined a methodology similar to that used in testing CIMT outcomes and using methodology developed by Taub and Wolf. This protocol could be followed for 2 weeks initially, followed by tests of functional use. Task practice should be continued for longer if necessary, depending on results and discussion with the individual.

Strength Training

It is likely that all patients who regain the ability to generate muscle force can benefit from strength training, particularly for muscles used in tasks performed at shoulder height and above, and those involved in gripping, holding, and lifting objects. Hand grip strength has been found to correlate significantly with upper-extremity functional tests more than 1 year after stroke (Boissy et al. 1999). Examples of exercise types include:

- Gripping exercises using grip force dynamometer, spring-resisted gripping device, clothes peg, jar with lid, plastic putty
- Using progressively heavier objects in reaching, lifting, and manipulating tasks
- Pushing and pulling exercises, with:
  - Weightbearing exercises for hand or forearm —modified push-ups on a table, against the wall
  - Weightlifting exercises with hand weights

The amount of resistance and number of repetitions are graded to the individual's ability but must always progress, e.g., increasing weight, number of repetitions. As a guide, a maximum number of repetitions up to 10 should be attempted, performed in sets of three. Progressive resistance elastic band exercises can be practiced (Thielman et al. 2004) (**Fig. 5.75a, b**), and arm cycling is another exercise the patient can practice independently (**Fig. 5.75a**).

A self-administrated program of arm exercise (GRASP, www.rehab.ubc.ca/jeng/Our_Exercise_-Manuals/GRASP.htm), recently developed and tested in Vancouver (Eng et al. 2009), and based on current scientific evidence, provides an online manual with guidelines to enable patients to exercise independently. The program has been found to be effective in improving arm function, grip strength, and use of the limb (Harris et al. 2009, Pang et al. 2006b).

Table 5.1 Protocol for constraint and task-specific training

Criteria for inclusion	• Wolf's Minimum Motor Criteria: ability to extend wrist at least 20°, IP and MCP finger joints at least 10° • Willingness of patient to attend initially for a training program 5 days/week for 2 weeks
Constraint	• Hand splint with wrist of nonparetic arm in some extension + sling, or mitt/glove + reminders not to use the nonparetic limb • Wear splint for a prescribed number of hours on each weekday for 2 weeks
Behavioral contract	• Seek agreement with patient about activities to be performed without constraint—e. g., bathing, parts of dressing, activities where balance may be an issue, and with constraint—e. g., eating, grooming, toileting, some domestic tasks
Program of exercises	• Prescribed number of hours of task-oriented training and practice for the paretic limb + home practice
Measurement	• Performed before and after 2-week program

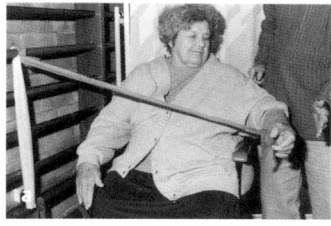

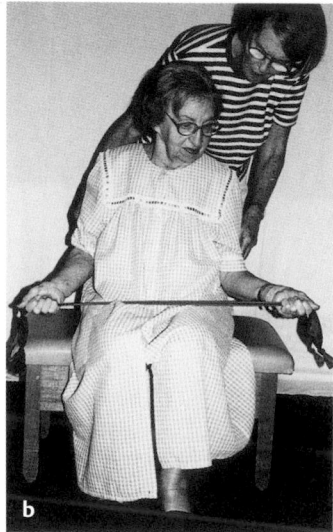

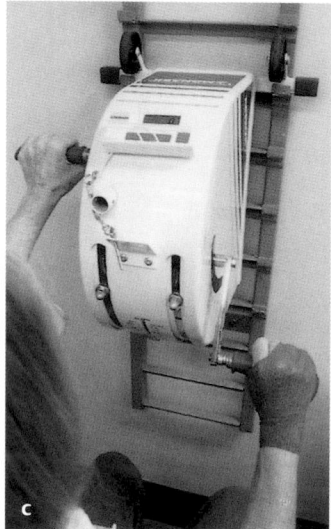

Fig. 5.75 a–c Strengthening and mobilizing exercises:
a for glenohumeral external rotator and abductor muscles;
b for glenohumeral external rotators;
c arm cycling.

Other Training Methods

Mental Practice

Mental practice or visualization, in which simple physical actions are rehearsed in the mind, may assist some patients to focus attention on the action to be performed and to improve performance (Page et al. 2001). Mental imagery may be particularly important for a patient who is unable to practice physically as it is considered to improve ability to sustain attention and plan task performance. A systematic review concluded that there is some evidence that motor imagery can be beneficial for those with upper limb dysfunction.

Object-Specific Training of Sensory Awareness

Sensory awareness and visuomotor function appear to benefit from specific training, and object-specific training, emphasizing exploration of texture, shape, consistency, for example, can be an effective way of improving sensory awareness and functional use of the hand (Carey and Burghardt 1993, Carey et al. 1993).

Computer-Aided Training, Virtual Reality, and Robotic Training

New technologies may have effective applications in rehabilitation after stroke in providing novel training methods and as a means of increasing time spent in useful practice (**Fig. 5.76**). Robotic systems have the potential to increase the number

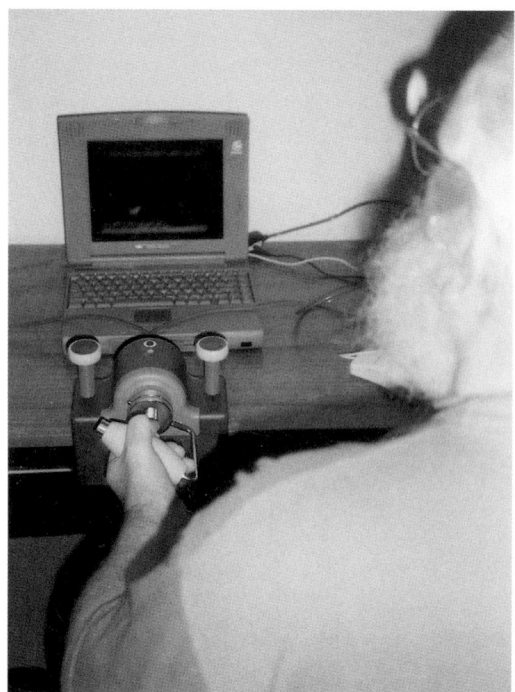

Fig. 5.76   Independent practice of forearm supination and pronation on the Upper Limb Exerciser by playing a computer game. The game, linked to manipulandum, provides motivational and quantitative feedback.
(Courtesy of Biometrics Ltd, PO Box 340, Ladysmith, VA 22501, USA.)

of repetitions of specific actions and thereby aid the process of motor learning. Development of computer-aided training and robotic devices is at the experimental stage.

Improvements in motor activity have been reported in the few studies available; for example, a decrease in hemispatial neglect after a training program using a virtual hand has been reported (Castiello et al. 2004). Overall, results of carryover into improved function are equivocal so far (Gallichio and Kluding 2004, Hesse et al. 2003, Krebs et al. 2002, Lam et al. 2006, Lum et al. 2002, Volpe et al. 2000). However, technical aids may help a patient focus attention, enhance motivation, and provide feedback (Platz 2004).

Splinting

Splinting as it is commonly used may not have the beneficial effects intended by the therapist. For example, no effect of a hand splint on the development of wrist and finger flexor muscle contracture, or pain, was found in a recent study (Lannin and Herbert 2003). In this investigation, the splint was worn for 12 hours at night for 4 weeks. The hand was splinted in the resting position.

Measurement

The following tests have been found reliable when performed under standardized conditions:
- Functional tests:
  - Motor Assessment Scale—three upper limb items
  - Wolf Motor Function Test
  - Functional Reach Test
  - Action Arm Research Test
  - Spiral Test
  - Nine-hole Peg Test
- Real-life arm use:
  - Motor Activity Log—Amount of Use Scale
- Tests of muscle strength:
  - Grip force dynamometer
  - Hand-held dynamometer
- Tests of sensation:
  - Tactile Discrimination Test
  - Proprioceptive Discrimination Test
- Range of motion:
  - Goniometer + dynamometer

Conclusion

In this chapter we set out to illustrate how we can combine theory and practice in rehabilitation after stroke; that is, the process by which we can update and integrate scientific evidence into clinical practice. The methods to be used in neurological rehabilitation should be founded on evidence-based guidelines. We know now that major factors in poor recovery from stroke include the minimal time spent in active exercise and training, and the use of methods that are more passive than active, requiring little participation or effort from the patient. Nevertheless, it is evident that changes are being made in the delivery of rehabilitation and the methods used, with an impetus toward more active and vigorous exercise and training, started earlier, including not only one-to-one therapy but also group and circuit exercise sessions, and with planning for independent, home-based mental and physical exercise.

▪ Appendix

Measurement in Neurological Rehabilitation

Evidence-based practice is important in meeting the ethical imperatives of providing the best possible care for our patients. It is essential in clinical practice that there is a systematic examination of the effects of intervention to document patient progress and to improve outcomes. Physical therapists need skill training to build confidence in their ability to measure patient outcomes using valid and reliable measurement tools (Hill et al. 2005).

Relevant and objective data are collected on the individual's motor performance, under standardized conditions, in actions critical to everyday life. The information gathered enables the therapist to plan, modify, and vary aspects of the training program. Data are collected on commencement of physical therapy, at regular intervals throughout rehabilitation, and in follow-up investigations that should continue into the post-discharge period. These data are used to determine the relative effectiveness of a rehabilitation unit's training programs, and can provide recommendations related to best practice in neurological physical therapy.

Different methods of measurement are used according to the questions being asked. Some valid and reliable measures in current use are listed below. For more detailed information refer to the authors cited and to Bernhardt and Hill (2005), Hill et al. (2005), and Wade (1992).

Global Measures of Function

- *Barthel Activities of Daily Living Index* provides an overview of general status (Mahoney and Barthel 1965).
- *Functional Independence Measure (FIM)* examines the extent of dependence/independence (Granger et al. 1986).

Global Measures of Motor Performance/ Activity

- *Motor Assessment Scale* (MAS) is a valid and reliable scale that measures functional abilities on a variety of everyday motor actions. It is an ordinal scale with eight items graded 0–6 (Carr et al. 1985). It can have a ceiling effect, so a score of 6 should be followed by other relevant tests, such as the Nine-Hole Peg Test, and walking tests that measure distance/time/speed.
- *Fugl-Meyer Assessment* is a lengthy scale of questionable validity since it is based on assumptions about a particular pattern of recovery (Fugl-Meyer et al. 1975). The Motor Assessment Scale has been suggested as a replacement (Malouin et al. 1994).

Gait

- *MAS*, Walking Item
- *10-m Walk Test* The patient is asked to walk at his/her preferred speed or can be asked to walk as fast as possible. To avoid the effects of deceleration and acceleration the subject is timed with a stop watch over the middle 10 m of a 14 m walkway. The results are expressed as time taken (seconds) or speed (meters/second). No importance is attached to quality of move-

ment; however, a progressive decrease in time taken appears to be a valid and reliable indicator of improvement in biomechanical parameters, improved muscle power, and motor control (Wade 1992).

- *6- or 12-min Walk Test* measures the distance walked in 6 or 12 minutes. These tests are used to measure endurance (Guyatt et al. 1985).
- *Stride length measures.* Stride length is measured using foot switches, grids, or a computerized stride analyzer.

Standing Up and Sitting Down

- *MAS*, Standing Up Item
- *Rise-to-Walk Test (RTW)* Time taken to stand up and walk a prescribed distance (Dion et al. 2003, Malouin et al. 2003).
- *Timed Up-and-Go Test (TUG) Test* The patient is required to stand up from a chair, walk 3 m, turn around, and return (Podsialo and Richardson 1991).

Balance

There is no single test that can measure all aspects of balance, and the tests listed below seek specific information.

- *Motor Assessment Scale, Sitting Balance item*
- *Functional Reach Test* is a test of maximum reach forward in standing (Duncan et al. 1990)
- *TUG Test* (Podsialo and Richardson 1991)
- *Step Test* Starting with feet parallel and 5 cm in front of a 7.5 cm high block, the patient steps forward and backward repeatedly as fast as possible for 15 s. The number of steps is counted (Hill et al. 1996)
- *Berg Balance Scale* was originally developed as a measure of balance that is appropriate for elderly individuals. It consists of 14 items that are scored on a scale of 0–4. It has low sensitivity for predicting falls (Berg et al. 1989, 1992, Riddle and Stratford 1999)
- *Clinical Test for Sensory Interaction in Balance* (Shumway-Cook and Horak 1986)
- *Obstacle Course Test* includes obstacles to be stepped over or around and necessitates visual evaluation of size and location of obstacles, and planning of how to best negotiate them (Means et al. 1996)

Upper Limb Function / Reaching and Manipulation

- *Motor Assessment Scale* upper arm function, hand movements, advanced hand movements
- *Wolf Motor Function Test* (Wolf et al. 2001)
- *Nine-Hole Peg Test* measures dexterity and speed (Sunderland et al. 1989)
- *Motor Activity Log—Amount of Use Scale* measures real-life arm use (Taub et al. 1993)
- *Spiral Test* measures coordination of the upper limb (Verkerk et al. 1990)

Impairments

Strength—Muscle Force

- *Motricity Index* (Wade 1992)
- Muscle force is tested using a dynamometer (grip force, isokinetic, or hand-held) (Bohannon and Andrews 1987)

Spasticity

- *Modified Ashworth Scale* was developed to grade "muscle tone" as a measure of spasticity. It is not considered a valid measure as it cannot distinguish between stretch reflex hyperactivity and muscle stiffness (Alibiglou et al. 2008, Ashworth 1964, Pandyan et al. 2001)
- *Modified Tardieu Scale* is an ordinal scale that measures the intensity of a muscle's response to passive joint movement at specified velocities. It appears to be reliable (Gracies et al. 2000, Mehrholz et al. 2005)

Muscle Stiffness

- *Laboratory measures of calf muscle stiffness* are being developed to measure the passive torque in a resting muscle as the foot is passively moved into dorsiflexion. The apparatus consists of a footplate, potentiometer, and load cell. EMG data are collected from calf muscles and tibialis anterior to ensure there is no active muscle contraction. This apparatus also allows a measure of stretch reflex response to movements of different velocities, and can therefore provide an indication of presence or absence of spasticity (Moseley and Adams 1991).

Sensation

- *Nottingham Sensory Awareness Assessment for Stroke Patients* (Lincoln et al. 1998)

- *Tactile Discrimination Test* and *Proprioceptive Discrimination Test* (Carey 1995, Carey et al. 1993a)

Aerobic Fitness and Exercise Capacity

Maximal effort exercise testing requires simultaneous ECG and blood pressure monitoring, and is performed by specially trained staff. A simple method of monitoring exercise level during training is to measure heart rate using a heart rate monitor. Target heart rate (HR) is determined using the following formula:

Maximum age-predicted HR = 220 − age

Target HR = 40%–85% × maximum age-predicted HR

Self-Efficacy

Patient satisfaction has received little attention in rehabilitation until recently. Input can be sought from patients about such issues as their expectations and experiences during rehabilitation. Questionnaires completed anonymously provided an indication of the individual's perception of the value of rehabilitation.

Health-related Quality of Life

- *Medical Outcome Survey Short Form 36. Health Stroke Questionnaire (SF-36)* assesses patient-centered outcomes after stroke (Anderson et al. 1996, Brazier et al. 1992)
- *Nottingham Health Profile* is another short and simple measure of health needs and outcomes (Hunt et al. 1985)

Acknowledgments

Janet Carr and Roberta Shepherd wish to thank the people who so kindly agreed to be photographed for this chapter and their physical therapists from Sydney hospitals who have given us generous support, in particular Karl Schurr, Simone Dorsch and their colleagues at Bankstown-Lidcombe Hospital; Lynne Olivetti and colleagues at War Memorial Hospital; and Fiona Mackey at Port Kembla Hospital, Illawarra Area Health Service, Australia.

The authors of this chapter and the publisher express their appreciation for being granted permission to reproduce Figures as indicated throughout this chapter. Elsevier provided permission for **Figs. 5.2–5.8, 5.10–5.12, 5.15–5.19, 5.20c, 5.21, 5.25–5.27, 5.32–5.35, 5.39–5.43, 5.67, 5.71, 5.73–5.75.**

6 Care of Stroke Patients

Claudia Flaemig

"Why are you shouting at me? I'm not deaf! I understand you perfectly well, but I can't answer you. My language isn't working properly. I'm so afraid—afraid that things will never be as they once were, before I was 'struck'! There is something strange lying in my bed that feels cold and disgusting. When I try to throw it out of the bed, I end up on the floor too, and then the nurses scold me."

(Kellnhauser et al. 2000, p. 1284).

After suffering stroke, patients often experience feelings of horror and dismay, immobility, paralysis, inhibition, and obstruction. The illness appears in most patients completely out of the blue, without any warning signs whatsoever. People who have lived independent lives suddenly find themselves dependent and needing someone to look after them. They are often, with good reason, afraid of never recovering fully. A large proportion of these affected individuals will remain in need of special care for the long term; this presents major problems in the home environment. Care in a specialized institution is thus required, depending on the severity of the illness and the patient's individual care needs. Consequently, patients suffering from this condition are quite often plagued by extreme mood swings, depression, or even feelings of aggression.

This chapter provides an overview of the aims and practice of nursing care for stroke patients during the acute phase of the illness.

■ Care and Treatment Plan

The initial focus of attention in the acute care of the stroke patient is stabilizing and maintaining the patient's vital functions. In some cases, patients require intensive care. Whatever the circumstances, however, treatment in a stroke unit is recommended during the acute phase. The care and treatment plan for each patient is designed according to the severity of the stroke.

Stroke Unit

Definition

A stroke unit is the name given to the intensive monitoring station designed expressly for stroke patients in many hospitals in recent years. Such units consist of specialized in-patient wards in which emphasis is placed on the application of early treatment concepts for stroke patients during the acute phase. For this purpose, specially trained teams are to be found in stroke units, responsible for the comprehensive handling of diagnostic procedures, therapy, monitoring, optimal nursing care, early physical therapy, occupational therapy, and speech therapy.

Specialized equipment similar to that available in intensive care units is also an essential requirement for a stroke unit (**Fig. 6.1**) (Conzelmann and Manz 2003).

As a rule, patients are treated in stroke units for a matter of days, to prevent and treat recurring infarction and alterations in the patient's status that may lead to unstable general condition and health.

Besides the standard medical diagnostic procedures and therapy options available in the stroke unit, nursing care is also enormously significant. To work in a stroke unit, nurses should not only have a strong professional background in general nursing, but should also have a specialized knowledge of the stroke situation, as they are the members of

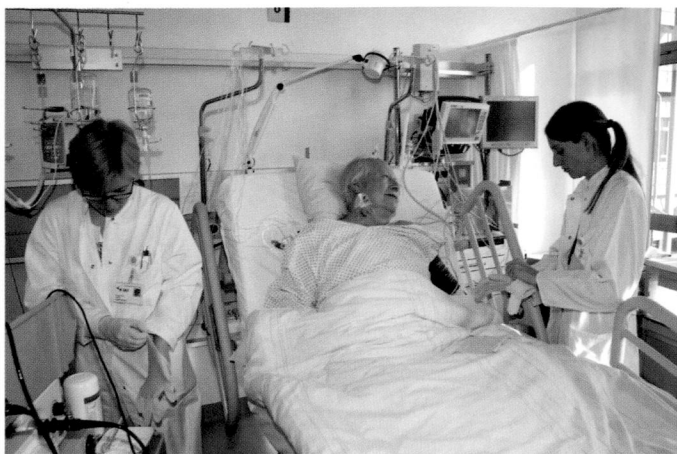

Fig. 6.1   Technical equipment in the stroke unit.

staff who spend the most time with the patients and who thus receive extensive information as to their general state of health. Intensive cooperation between physicians and nurses is crucial; in addition, the constant exchange of information among the other therapists treating the stroke patient (physical therapists, occupational therapists, speech therapists) should be top priority. It is only through this comprehensive treatment that the patient's chances of complete recovery can be maximized (Conzelmann and Manz 2003).

■ Nursing Care during the Acute Phase

Monitoring and Securing of Vital Functions

The following measures must be taken immediately upon admission of the patient to the stroke unit (see also **Table 6.1**):

- Continual monitoring of vital signs (ECG, blood pressure, oxygen saturation)
- Blood glucose monitoring
- Temperature monitoring
- Assessment of neurological status:
  1. Level of consciousness
  2. Pupils
  3. Motor function
  4. Symptoms indicating elevated cerebral pressure
  5. Reversal of existing symptoms, or appearance of new ones
- Fluid balance—insertion of indwelling urinary catheter (according to severity, patient's degree of impairment)
- Assistance with medical and diagnostic measures, for example:
  - Setting up peripheral IV access
  - Accompanying the patient to diagnostic testing areas (e.g., for CT scan)

Table 6.1   Monitoring guidelines for stroke patients (Conzelmann and Manz 2003, p. 57)

Hours	0–2	2–24	After 24	Target value
Blood pressure monitoring	Every 15 minutes	Every 30 minutes	Every 3 hours	140–200 mmHg systolic
Blood glucose monitoring	Every 30 minutes	Every 120 minutes	Every 6 hours	< 160 mg/dl
Temperature monitoring	Every 30 minutes	Every 60 minutes	Every 6 hours	< 37.5°C

Patient Care History and Care Planning

After immediate measures have been taken in the stroke unit, based on the severity of the stroke and following standardized procedures, the patient's care history is recorded and an individualized care plan is subsequently developed in preparation for further in-patient care during the acute phase of stroke.

The patient's medical history is taken using a standardized form. As members of the nursing staff are present while physicians perform the physical examination, they can document the findings directly, in terms of observed symptoms and consequent treatment requirements, and integrate them into the care protocol and plan. Family members generally take part in the documentation of the medical history, as the patients themselves are quite often unable to supply this information, which is of critical importance especially during the acute phase. The information they can provide, for instance, on previous illnesses, medications, accessories (glasses, dentures, hearing aids, etc.), as well as the patient's personal preferences or dislikes, is extremely important when designing an individualized nursing plan.

Taking the patient's medical history is a starting point for the nursing care plan. It serves to collect information and to assess any existing problems, capabilities, or resources, as well as special needs that the patient may have. The medical history protocol includes information relating to the patient's activities of daily living. This aids in arranging individualized care and is a prerequisite for the realization of the care process; it serves as the foundation for optimal care planning and practice. The patient's *care plan* is then designed on an individual basis, according to the hospital's internal care standards.

Prevention and Early Detection of Cardiovascular Complications

Securing a patient's vital functions is always of primary importance. The results of the necessary procedures performed are closely documented so that the staff can respond immediately to any changes that occur.

"During the first 24 hours, close observation, monitoring, and documentation of the patient's blood pressure, pulse, temperature, oxygen saturation, blood glucose, respiration, and level of consciousness (including pupillary reflex) take place. In this time period, the risk of reinfarction is highest." (Conzelmann and Manz 2003, p. 56).

Moreover, during the acute phase of stroke, shock symptoms can occur which may necessitate cardiopulmonary resuscitation.

Surveillance and Safety Aspects of Medical Treatment

When medications, including infusions, are administered, nurses should especially keep in mind the following points:
- The patient must be observed to detect possible adverse effects of any medications administered.
- Blood pressure must be lowered *very* gradually. **Caution:** lowering the patient's blood pressure too quickly also reduces blood circulation in the brain to such an extent that further ischemic events may occur.

Nursing Care during Systemic Intravenous Lysis

The most important nursing care measures during systemic intravenous lysis are:
- Close observation/monitoring
- Hourly assessment of level of consciousness and pupillary reflex
- Continuous monitoring of temperature (by means of indwelling urinary catheter or rectal probe)
- Monitoring of amount of urine excreted (per hour) and fluid balance
- Measurement of blood glucose at least every 3 hours
- Keeping banked blood available at all times
- Observation of allergic reactions (e.g., reddening of the skin), disturbances in level of consciousness, headache, nausea, vomiting, possible seizures, meningism, blood in the stool or urine (Conzelmann and Manz 2003)

When changes occur, a physician must be alerted immediately.

Specific Features of Care: Avoidance of Bleeding

During lysis, basic treatment and care should be planned and performed with the aim of minimizing the risk of bleeding. Attention should be paid to the following aspects, among others:

- Oral hygiene: refrain from brushing teeth, suction only when absolutely necessary
- No wet shaving
- No intramuscular injections
- Bed rest during the first 24 hours
- No puncture procedures
- No removal of indwelling catheters
- Insertion of lines and catheters only if absolutely necessary
- Taking care not to pull on lines and catheters when repositioning the patient
- Ensuring soft stools (i.e., patient should be able to empty bowels without activating abdominal muscles) (Conzelmann and Manz 2003)

Nursing Care during Intra-Arterial Lysis

Local intra-arterial lysis is performed in the radiology department. Preparations for local lysis to be made by the nursing staff in the stroke unit are thus limited to the following:

- Transfer of the patient for angiography, assistance in positioning and repositioning the patient
- Insertion of an indwelling urinary catheter (if possible, equipped for monitoring the patient's temperature)

Observation and Care after Lysis Therapy

The most important points for nurses to bear in mind during the monitoring and observation of patients after completion of intra-arterial lysis include:

- Hourly control of vital signs (time frame 8–12 hours)
- Inspection and control of the bandage in the inguinal region for any signs of bleeding
- Monitoring of pedal pulses in both feet
- Attachment of an oxygen sensor to a toe on the affected leg to monitor circulation status

- Observation of legs: color of skin, appearance, temperature, pain
- **Positioning**: the leg with an open puncture sheath must be kept extended; hip flexion (by keeping the leg raised, or by elevating the upper body more than 30°) should be avoided.
- If possible, patients should be positioned on their backs (soft mattress); if there is an increased risk of pressure ulcers, patients should be placed on their sides, at 30° with the leg extended.
- When possible, patients should be informed of the need to maintain this position; if a patient is uncooperative, the foot or leg must be tied down.
- a sandbag should remain on the puncture site for at least 4 hours.
- **Dressing must be changed** when blood has soaked through the bandage, using aseptic technique, ideally by two nurses.

Other aspects of monitoring and care are the same as for systemic lysis (Conzelmann and Manz 2003).

Implementation of Prophylactic Measures

"Avoidance of complications through the appropriate and adequate care of stroke patients is the main aim to be realized when caring for these patients; this provides the opportunity for the illness to run its natural course during the acute phase. The greatest sources of danger are represented by infections (pneumonia, urinary tract infections), and the fluid balance must also be kept in a stable state. Pressure ulcers and contractures are to be avoided" (Schulz and Enders 2005, p. 18).

During the acute phase of stroke, the following preventive care measures are essential:

- Pressure ulcer prophylaxis
- Pneumonia prophylaxis
- Thrombosis prophylaxis
- Contracture prophylaxis
- Aspiration prophylaxis
- Candidiasis and parotitis prophylaxis in cases of swallowing difficulties or parenteral nutrition

All prophylactic measures should be incorporated into general nursing care procedures, to put as little strain as possible on the patient.

Prevention of Pressure Ulcers (Decubital Ulcers, Bed Sores)

When the patient is admitted to the hospital, their risk of developing pressure ulcers is routinely evaluated over 24 hours with an assessment instrument designed for this purpose. The use of a risk scale with four levels (e.g., the Braden scale) is recommended:

- Low risk
- Moderate risk
- High risk
- Very high risk

According to the result of this evaluation, a care plan is developed for the patient with a view to the prevention of pressure ulcers. The use of special bed equipment, such as pressure-relieving mattresses, is determined on an individual basis. The patient's self-perceptions are nearly always distorted, and support in the form of a firm mattress is required to improve these perceptions. Any type of mattress that is too soft will hinder the promotion of the patient's body perception. The risk of developing pressure ulcers, as well as the patient's body perception, is a factor that plays an important role in the choice of bed equipment. Depending on the patient's individual risk, the interval between changes of position is 2–4 hours. The types of positioning can be determined on the basis of vital signs, needs, and tolerance of each patient. Adequate skin care and selective nutrition, as supplemental measures, also play a key role in the context of pressure ulcer prophylaxis.

Pneumonia Prophylaxis

During the first few days after acute stroke, pneumonia prophylaxis is absolutely essential, as important as any other preventive measures, because of the patient's immobility, circulatory instability, and changes in level of consciousness (**Table 6.2**). Elderly people are particularly at risk. For these

Table 6.2   Causes and treatment options in pneumonia prophylaxis following stroke (Conzelmann and Manz 2003, p. 159 f.)

Possible causes	Possible explanations	Effects	Possible remedies
Breathing through open mouth	Lack of control over mouth muscles	Dried-out mucous membranes	• Moistening of the oral cavity with special mouth care products • Ensuring a proper position so that the mouth can be kept closed • Humidifying the air (inhalations)
Fluid intake too low	Swallowing difficulties, limitations in language and movement	Dried-up secretions	• Adequate fluid intake • Inhalation • Massage with essential oils or ointments

Silent aspiration	Difficulty swallowing and lack of coughing reflex	Foreign material enters the lungs	• Recognizing swallowing difficulties, e.g., food which remains in the cheek, or when patient cannot blow up cheeks, or when the uvula hangs to one side, saliva runs out of the corner of the mouth, or mouth cannot be closed
			• Therapeutic treatment and care:
			  – stimulation of the face and mouth
			  – diet plan may only be formulated by specially trained staff

Inappropriate position, e.g., on back with elevated head	Patient slides down	Patient's rib cage contracts and the lungs receive too little air	• stable sitting position • close control of (re)positioning interval • early mobilization • abdominal position used according to tolerance and vital signs

patients, pneumonia represents a dangerous complication which, if not treated with large doses of antibiotics, may cause such extreme damage to the immune system that the process of rehabilitation is delayed or may even become impossible.

Respiratory Stimulation Massage

Massage is frequently used in daily care as pneumonia prophylaxis.

"This procedure is a rhythmic massage, performed with varying hand placement and pressure, for purposes of respiratory therapy, in the areas of the chest and the back. Through the synchronization of breathing rhythms, communication develops between the physical therapist and the patient which is an excellent means of conveying feelings of heightened awareness, relaxation, and safety.

The aims of respiratory stimulation massage are:
• Psychological stabilization, stress reduction
• Assistance with breathing, encouragement of respiratory rhythms
• Pneumonia prophylaxis
• Helping the patient to fall asleep" (Nydahl and Bartoszek 2000, p. 161)

The basic requirement for the successful completion of these measures is a suitably positive attitude and motivation on the part of the therapist. The time needed to perform the massage alone is approximately 5–7 minutes, during which time any external disturbances should be strictly avoided.

Suggested Procedure for Chest and Back Massage

1. The patient must be positioned so that the therapist can reach his or her back; for example, sitting on the edge of the bed, leaning forward, turned to the side by 135°, if possible.
2. The therapist's hands must be well covered with lotion or oil.
3. Lotion or oil is applied to the patient's back using slow, gentle, downward motions; skin contact is maintained during the entire procedure.
4. When the patient breathes out, the therapist moves their hand, using gentle pressure, a few centimeters along the patient's spine, first

downward, then sideways, in the direction of the rib cage.
5. When the patient breathes in, the therapist's hands return to the spine, using circular movements, this time using less pressure.
6. The patient's back is then rubbed in the direction of the bottom of the rib cage, as described, in spiral movements.
7. The rhythm of the massage is determined by the breathing rhythm either of the therapist or of the patient, depending on the situation.
8. When the therapist's hands have reached the lower boundaries of the rib cage, they are moved back to the patient's neck, one after the other, always maintaining skin contact.
9. It is recommended that this procedure be repeated six to eight times.
10. To end with, the patient's back is smoothed out, as at the beginning, slowly and gently downward, as a way of concluding the session.

Thrombosis Prophylaxis

During the acute phase of stroke, patients should be given appropriate medications (anticoagulants) to prevent thrombosis. Nurses should also keep a close watch on this aspect of patient care, as the patients themselves are often unable to recognize the typical early signs (pain in the calf or the sole of the foot, or overheating) because their body perception may be defective. Meticulous observation is crucial during this phase.

Limitations in mobility during the acute phase result in the inactivation of the muscle pump and thus lead to an increase in blood viscosity. Custom-fitting antithrombotic stockings, leg rubs, regular mobilization/repositioning, and sufficient fluids are all helpful supplementary care.

Aspiration Prophylaxis

The patient will often choke while eating, without noticing that this is happening (silent aspiration). It is therefore important that the patient's swallowing function and protective mechanisms (coughing reflex) are assessed by qualified professionals.

Rules for Administering Nutrition to Patients with Swallowing Difficulties

- Only qualified personnel may administer food to a patient who has a swallowing disorder.
- It is important that the food is specially adapted and selected for these patients (e.g., pureed/soft foods and thickened drinks).
- The patient must be in the correct sitting position, or be moved into a chair, to be fed.
- The nurse should always be on the same level as the patient.
- Food and drink may not be given from too far above or below the patient's level, as this would automatically force the patient's head into an unnatural position.
- There should be no conversation during the meal, so that the patient does not have to chew, swallow, and speak at the same time.
- The patient is only allowed to take very small bites and sips.
- After the patient has swallowed, they should be asked to swallow again.
- The patient's mouth should be cleaned after every meal (special oral hygiene).

A patient who cannot be guaranteed to consume the necessary amount of nutrition because of swallowing difficulties must be fed via stomach tube. If nutrition is administered in this way, the patient's upper body must be moved into a 30° position to protect them from aspirating the food if vomiting or reflux occurs. The tube nutrition may be administered continuously or as a bolus, depending on how the patient tolerates this. Li-

quids may also be given by way of the stomach tube.

■ The Rehabilitation Phase

"Nurses take on the central tasks at all levels of the field of professional care: prevention, acute treatment, rehabilitation, and follow-up care. Nursing care is—and here it differs from the work of other professional groups—very closely associated with patients and their family members for long periods of time. Even though each area of care has its own specific emphasis and its own unique qualities, the care of stroke patients is often, quite simply, rehabilitative care. As part of an interdisciplinary therapeutic team, the nurse aims to promote the independence of the patient and thus ensures the highest possible quality of life for them. The rehabilitation of stroke patients is thus described as rehabilitation from the very first" (Thranberend 2007, p. 105).

In rehabilitative care, various therapeutic concepts are applied during everyday routine practice (**Fig. 6.2**). Nursing care represents a natural continuation of concepts presented and applied during therapy, in terms of carrying out everyday tasks. The basics of therapeutic care often involve the concept of basal stimulation, kinesthetics, and the Bobath and Affolter concepts. It is also important for the practice of nursing care that no single ther-

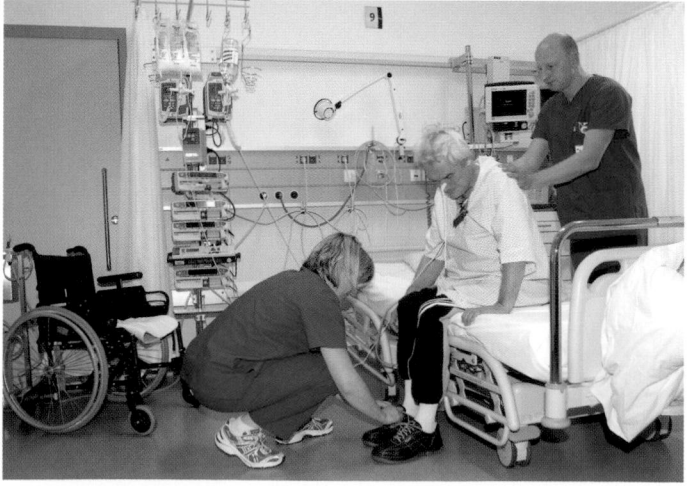

Fig. 6.2   Rehabilitation after stroke

apeutic approach should be viewed as a rigid concept; nursing plans are developed for patients on an individual basis.

Communication Assistance

Stroke patients, especially those with right-side paralysis, experience language difficulties, as the language center is found on the dominant side of the brain (usually the left side in right-handed individuals; in left-handed individuals, sometimes also on the right).

Depending on the location of the damaged area of the brain, different disabilities become apparent:

• Impairments in reading and writing
• Inability to comprehend language, or even to speak

These language disabilities are known as *aphasia*.

A further possible negative effect on communication in patients who have suffered stroke results from the condition of *dysarthria*. When this is present, the patient has a speech impairment. Dysarthria is characterized by slurred speech or a hoarse or nasal voice.

A Patient's Experience

"The words were there in my head; everything seemed to be just as it was before, and they hadn't been injured at all. But when I wanted to use them, it became apparent that they first had to be carried a long, long way.

Along this way, there seemed to be a tunnel that had caved in. When the words reached the tunnel, they tried to squeeze through. But they were torn to shreds and so mutilated as to be rendered unrecognizable when they came out of the other end of the tunnel."

(Thranberend 2007, p. 106)

There are no set rules for dealing and communicating with aphasic patients. However, communication can be greatly facilitated if a few fundamental principles are observed.

Communication with Speech-Impaired Individuals

Principles

The following basic principles should be given due attention when communicating with speech-impaired individuals:

• The affected person should be viewed as an equal conversation partner and treated with respect (aphasic patients are not thinking-impaired).
• Do not talk *about* the patient, but rather *to* him or her.
• Do not speak *for* the patient.

What Can You Do To Understand the Aphasic Patient Better?

• Always allow adequate time for the patient to speak; do not create time pressure.
• Do not suggest words.
• Do not interrupt to make corrections; often the statement makes more sense when the thought is completed.
• Pay attention to nonverbal communication, observe the situation, and try to empathize with the patient.
• Do not discard inappropriate words; use them as further helpful associations.
• Search for the next topic together with the patient.
• Always pay attention to the content; ignore mistakes, do not correct.
• Do not perform word repetition exercises (words have not been forgotten, only blocked).
• Do not ask the patient to read aloud or write, since these skills are also often impaired. (Thranberend 2007, p. 106).

What Can You Do To Improve the Aphasic Patient's Understanding of Your Speech?

• Eliminate any background noise; as few people as possible should take part in the conversation.
• Make use of nonverbal signals, speak directly to the patient, and maintain eye contact.
• Do not raise your voice, use normal word stress, and do not speak too quickly.
• Speak in short sentences and avoid the use of jargon.
• Emphasize important words.
• Avoid a sudden change of subject.

- If the patient does not understand, vary the words (aphasic patients often do not understand individual words, or the meaning of the sentence).
- Ask "yes" or "no" questions; open questions tend to be difficult for people with aphasia.
- Ask the patient what measures you could take to improve his or her understanding. (Thranberend 2007, p. 106).

Language disorders also present a huge challenge to family members in terms of their interaction with the patient. Nurses can be important advisers, giving suggestions on how to deal more effectively with the patient.

Please note that we use the term "nurse" throughout the chapter, although some of the personal care tasks described could also be performed by an occupational therapist, a licensed practical nurse (healthcare assistant), or a family member.

Assistance with Washing and Dressing

Enabling care for stroke patients focuses especially on making the patients aware of their paralyzed side and incorporating it into their daily routine. Here, the concept of basal stimulation is useful.

"The principle of basal stimulation lies in the active perception of the side of the body not affected, in order to apply this to the affected side. Through this awakening of the patient's awareness, sensitivity is carried over to the impaired brain hemisphere and a transfer from the aware to the perception-impaired side takes place, so that the patient feels better oriented in his or her own body and can learn to access things lost or forgotten" (Kellnhauser et al. 2000, p. 1294).

Orientation-Promoting Washing

Preparation

The nurse assesses the condition of the patient, what body position will be most convenient for washing, and whether it is possible for the patient to participate. The head end of the bed should be raised, or the patient should sit in a wheelchair at the sink, to make it possible to see their own body. For washing, the nurse stands on the patient's paretic side.

Procedure

In the first part of the washing procedure the nurse washes the patient's healthy arm, starting with the hand, using strong pressure, and crossing the midline of the body to reach the paretic, non-feeling arm. While this is happening, the patient is requested to follow this motion mentally and to feel it internally. This washing procedure is repeated several times in succession and is always performed by the nurse using both hands. To maintain constant contact with the patient, the nurse moves one hand at a time, with the other hand always maintaining body contact.

Next, the patient is requested to wash his or her chest, starting from the axillary region on the patient's healthy side, over the midline and over to the other side of the chest. The nurse places a washing mitt over the patient's paretic hand, and then guides that hand throughout the procedure.

The direction of washing, from the healthy to the paretic side, is very important. The patient notices how the washing movements feel when performed on the healthy side, and then has to transfer this feeling to the affected side of the body. Similarly, the washing of the legs and back follows this principle of transfer from the healthy to the impaired side.

Dental hygiene, lip care, shaving, and hair grooming should also be done with these principles in mind, if possible (Bienstein and Fröhlich 2003).

Case Study

Mrs. S. is 72 years old and has suffered a massive ischemic stroke. After 5 days, she still has severe language impairment and the right side of her body is completely paralyzed. Through the use of head movements, she is able to respond to requests.

The nurses place her in a stable sitting position in readiness for personal hygiene procedures; this orientation-promoting washing is done once a day. The nurses note that Mrs. S. leans toward her paretic side and follows the washing procedure with great concentration. After another week, she is able to turn toward the paretic side when her position is adequately stabilized.

Dressing

When dressing the patient, the nurse puts each item of clothing on the patient's affected side first. Undressing requires the reverse procedure: articles of clothing are removed from the nonimpaired side first. The patient's own clothes should be used if possible, as this adds to a general feeling of well-being and familiarity.

Therapeutic washing and dressing are extremely exhausting for the patient. Thus, sufficient breaks should be planned immediately after these procedures, before starting the next therapeutic procedure.

Assistance in Self-Help for Daily Activities

Advice on dealing with activities of daily living should follow the **principle of external prestructuring**:

- Choose meaningful sequences of events for activities performed every morning.
- Perform the activities in the same order every morning.
- Pay attention to the patient's individual capacities and be sure to take breaks.
- Keep requests and directions to a minimum, and word them as simply as possible.
- Create a familiar environment (personal cosmetics and clothing).
- Label the patient's wardrobe and personal shelf for toiletries, as well as the bed and the room.
- Encourage positive experiences (praise the patient after each activity performed successfully).

Assistance in Performing Bodily Functions

Stroke patients may have disturbances of defecation or micturition, but the cause of this is not necessarily always associated with the stroke. For this reason, additional causes of the condition should also be sought.

Possible Causes of Incontinence

The following limitations on the part of the patient should be identified and noted as possible causes of incontinence:

- Inability to get undressed quickly enough
- Inability to express need
- Inability to locate the call button to notify a nurse, or find the way to the toilet
- Inability to plan a sequence of events
- Inability to suppress the urge to void
- Inability to recognize the sensation of a full bladder or bowel, due to body perception impairment (Kellnhauser et al. 2000)
- Reduced mobility (in cases of stool incontinence)

Patients experiencing incontinence should be provided with disposable products such as incontinence pants or diapers.

Continence Training for Urinary Incontinence

Measures taken in the case of urinary incontinence, as well as continence training, require a planned procedure in coordination with the attending physicians:

- During the acute phase, urine is drained by means of an indwelling catheter, because of potential urine retention and also in order to assure a more accurate fluid balance.
- The catheter is usually removed after 3 days.
- When the patient has passed urine again spontaneously for the first time, residual urine is measured by means of ultrasound.
- If the volume of residual urine exceeds 100 mL, a new catheter is inserted.
- If the volume of residual urine is less than 100 mL, then the aim is continence training through the procedure of toilet training, according to the patient's degree of mobility and general condition.
- The patient's awareness of the pelvic floor region is to be supported and encouraged, for example, through the correct sitting position in bed, or the proper position when the patient is sitting in a chair. This helps to ensure that the urge to pass urine is sensed early enough.

Toilet Training Procedure According to Set Elimination Times

Patients are taken to the toilet according to a set schedule (the micturition protocol serving as the basis). A running faucet can help stimulate the patient to pass urine. Time intervals of 2–3 hours have proven to be favorable.

During the night, patients receive assistance when they themselves report the need to eliminate. When the patients' mobility is limited, their independence can be preserved or encouraged through the additional use of a special toilet chair, urine-collecting bottle, or similar helpful accessories or equipment (Kellnhauser et al. 2000).

Toilet Training Procedure Based on Asking the Patient to Eliminate

Incontinent patients are requested to use the toilet at regular intervals. Asking patients whether they are wet or dry serves the purpose of drawing their attention to their bladder. Patients are taken to the toilet only when they express the need to eliminate. If a patient initially refuses to be taken, the nurse asks up to three times. When the procedure is successful, or when the patient's incontinence pants are dry, the nurse gives positive verbal feedback (Kellnhauser et al. 2000).

Continence Training for Stool Incontinence

In this case, suppression of the urge to eliminate has to be relearned and trained. This is easiest when practiced in combination with toilet training for urinary incontinence.

Constipation Prophylaxis

To avoid the risk of the patient's developing constipation, attention should be paid to sufficient fluid intake, a fiber-rich diet, and regular defecation. Medicinal treatment involving laxatives, which stimulate intestinal peristalsis, may be administered after careful consideration of each individual case.

Stroke patients often experience "stool smearing." This is often mistakenly assumed to be a sign that the patient's stools are too loose, thus leading to inadequate and inconsistent laxative treatment. This can have the consequence of creating fecal impaction in the rectum through decreased mobility and reduced fluid resorption into the stool. Looser stools exert pressure on the column of hard stool and push it outward, which creates smear marks on the sheets or the patient's underwear. The only effective measures that can be taken in this case involve rectal evacuation and the administration of an enema.

Hemiplegic Shoulder

Many stroke patients complain of shoulder pain.

"This is a complication which arises from inappropriate movement, by the nurse and/or the patient, of the subluxated shoulder with an articular cavity of up to 3 cm" (Kellnhauser et al. 2000, p. 1296).

The following procedures can help to prevent shoulder pain:
- Do not take hold of the patient's arm by gripping the hand; instead, take the weight of the arm through the patient's elbow.
- Never pull on the patient's arm.
- Never take hold of patient by the armpits when sliding them up in bed, or helping them get out of bed.
- Do not move the patient's arm forcefully against any resistance.

When a patient experiences shoulder pain, the pain itself should be treated either by the use of topical medication and dressings or with analgesics. Treatment should be adapted to suit the individual patient and observed over the course of the condition, adjustments being made as necessary.

Being pain-free is a very important requirement for successful rehabilitation. Pain reduces the chances of rehabilitation, because, as a result of the pain:
- The patient avoids active movements and adopts pain-relieving postures.
- Spasticity is increased.
- The patient develops fears about being moved.
- The patient experiences sleeplessness and the relaxation periods become shorter.
- The patient may develop depression, which can reduce their motivation for recovery.

Swollen Hand

Some stroke patients experience swelling and pain in the affected hand. The hand may become overheated and red; alternatively, it may become clammy and bluish. The exact causes of this are unknown, but it is suspected that venous and lymphatic congestion occurs, mainly due to the absence of the muscle pump and damage to the circulation. Further reasons may be tissue damage from IV infusions, or injuries that may occur due to the patient's impaired body perception and ensuing accidents.

To prevent problems with the patient's hand, the following basic principles should be observed:

- The arm should be correctly positioned, allowing venous blood flow to take place along the back of the hand; the wrist must be held in the neutral (0) position.
- The arm should be slightly elevated.
- No infusions are to be set up in the affected arm.
- The affected arm must not be used for measuring blood pressure.

The main task for the nurse in this situation is to check the position of the patient's hand at regular intervals, as it frequently happens that the hand becomes bent at the wrist and comes to lie alongside the patient in bed, or even becomes entangled in the spokes of the patient's wheelchair. The patient may perceive the hand not as belonging to their own body, but rather as a foreign object. It is the nurse's task to reposition the patient gently, to increase the patient's awareness of their hand, and to help cope with this loss (Conzelmann and Manz 2003).

Dealing with Neglect

Neglect, whether visual, acoustic, or somatosensory, is difficult for nurses and other healthcare professionals to treat. The affected individuals are often completely oblivious to their own illness and thus tend to overestimate their own capacities and capabilities.

Nurses must therefore exercise great patience when dealing with these patients. For example, patients should be given clear, concise instructions. It is also especially important to ensure personal safety: for instance, if patients are convinced that they are able to get up alone, bars must be attached to the bed to prevent them from falling out. In addition, the call button for notifying the nursing staff must be moved to the patient's healthy side, so that they are aware of its presence.

All items necessary for personal hygiene (comb, razor, etc.) should be placed in the patients' field of vision. At mealtimes, the entire plate of food should also be placed in the patients' field of vision, as otherwise they may only eat half of it, completely ignoring the rest of the meal. Patients who have dressed themselves or applied makeup irregularly or asymmetrically as a result of neglect should have this pointed out to them as discreetly as possible.

■ Guidance for Family Members

One central area in which nurses work in cooperation with colleagues in other occupational fields is the psychosocial guidance of patients and their family or friends.

The stressful situation resulting from the experience of stroke in the family and its consequences is often very difficult for family members to cope with: suddenly a loved one is gravely ill, can speak only with great difficulty or not at all, and is dependent on others. At this time, the patient's family has a great need for information and clarification. Family members should be offered professional counseling and guidance during these moments when it is "all too much." Taking the time to talk to them is perceived as much-needed assistance and can be a great relief to them. During these conversations, the patient's family members should be advised that they do not have to shoulder this heavy burden alone, and that they will receive help when problems and fears arise.

Visiting hours in the stroke unit should be kept as flexible as possible and scheduled according to the patient's general condition, in cooperation with the multidisciplinary team and in accordance with the patient's own wishes, as well as those of the family members.

7 Ethical Questions Relating to the Care of Stroke Patients

Frank Oehmichen

Trust is a small flame
which makes nothing brighter,
but warms us all the same.

(Éric-Emmanuel Schmitt)

This chapter deals with the medical ethical questions that necessarily arise when dealing with stroke patients, in terms of developing and expanding medical options. Questions pertaining to demographic development and associated changes in morbidity are also considered. In the treatment situation, decisions must be taken that have a positive influence on the patient's chances of recovery and the alleviation of symptoms, but which at the same time accept the natural processes of degeneration and death.

■ What is at Issue?

Stroke is a sudden-onset illness associated with considerable consequences, on an individual level as well as for society as a whole. The mortality in stroke patients is about 15% during the first 3 months; one-fourth of patients survive with severe handicaps. The 30-day mortality of severe strokes, which generally require artificial ventilation, is even higher: one literature review has estimated this figure to be 58% (Holloway et al. 2005). Of these patients who have been so seriously affected, only one-third survive without any severe handicap. In view of these statistics, the question remains as to whether every type of individual or social medical intervention is called for—for example, continuing ventilation in an intensive care unit after the acute phase of the illness has been successfully overcome. Surveys that have been conducted on this topic indicate that it is precisely this long-term care and dependence on machines that represents a price many people do not wish to pay for sustaining a patient's life. If illness-related damage is also associated with loss of consciousness, the acceptability of a type of treatment that produces such results will continue to decrease. Through the explicit expression of the patient's wishes beforehand, by means of an advance directive (e.g., "living will"), the people in-

volved attempt to participate in and to influence treatment decisions.

Especially in stroke patients, it is common for loss of consciousness to occur already during the acute phase of the illness. It is with these patients that health-care professionals perceive decisions pertaining to the aims of treatment as an ethical challenge: should medical considerations suggest each and every possibility for treating a patient, and treatment at any cost? Is every expression of the patient's wishes binding, even one excluding the possibility of survival with severe disabilities?

Case Study 1

A 74-year-old patient has suffered for years from an illness associated with severe developmental and functional disturbances in her blood platelets. The patient's husband finds her in bed, after her midday rest, with her breathing making a rattling, wheezing sound. When addressed, she initially responds by making well-coordinated movements. The paramedic notified decides to have the patient transferred quickly to the hospital. At this point it does not yet appear to be urgently necessary to take special measures to secure the patient's airway. On the way to the hospital, her level of consciousness deteriorates. She becomes increasingly restless; so much so that mechanical ventilation is initiated following oral intubation, in order to secure her vital functions and make it possible to undertake diagnostic procedures immediately upon arrival in the emergency department. The computed tomography (CT) scan shows extensive left-sided hemorrhage with massive bleeding into the ventricular system. The attending internist and the neurosurgeon, together with the anesthesiologists, are confronted with the question of whether the corresponding surgical procedure is indicated in this case. Extreme thrombocytopenia (<50,000/μL) is the most significant pathological value among the laboratory findings.

Case Study 2

On January 17th, an 83-year-old woman falls on the steps on her way to the cloakroom when attending a concert. Up to the time òf the fall, her only known illness has been hypertension. She suffers a cerebral hemorrhage as a result of the fall. An emergency procedure follows, during which operative removal of the blood clot takes place, with subsequent craniectomy to reduce pressure. Due to the presumed need for long-term ventilation, a tracheotomy is performed on January 26th. After a 14-day period of treatment in the neurosurgery department and a further 8 weeks in a specialized rehabilitation clinic, the patient is still ventilated through a tracheal tube, day and night. The patient's consciousness is severely impaired; when spoken to, she responds only sporadically. She opens her left eye sometimes spontaneously, sometimes when requested to do so, and utters incomprehensible, emotionally charged sounds. Upon stimulation, flexion and extension cramping occurs in the patient's limbs; in some instances, a focused pain protection reaction occurs. As the patient is tetraparetic, she cannot exercise even the most minor functions in her right hand. She still has a swallowing difficulty and its degree of severity is unaltered. Her family (two daughters, one son) present the patient's advance directive: "...in the case that I am in a coma, with no prospect of regaining consciousness, I request that any life-extending and resuscitation measures, especially associated with intensive care therapy, not be taken; this includes organ transplantation and artificial ventilation, unless these measures are taken for the purposes of alleviating pain."

Case Study 3

The former manager of a large firm is discovered by his wife one morning lying beside his bed. His left arm and leg are paralyzed; his speech is unclear and almost unintelligible. Diagnostic measures reveal an extensive cerebral infarction. Fibrinolytic therapy proves impossible. Subsequently, the patient's condition deteriorates to the point where he has to be transferred to the neurosurgery department to undergo decompression craniectomy. After completion of acute medical care, neurological rehabilitation is initiated. Even after a 14-week

rehabilitation period, the patient remains completely paralyzed on the left side. The further course of recovery is complicated by occurrences of aspiration and ensuing pneumonia. Despite intensive therapy, severe swallowing impairment persists. The physicians discuss the option of doing a tracheotomy as a means of aspiration prophylaxis. The patient displays only short waking phases lasting 10–20 minutes, during which he communicates partly verbally, partly nonverbally. His sense of orientation is often unclear. Referring to a living will attested by a notary, in which the patient refuses life-prolonging measures in the case of severe and irreversible brain damage, the patient's son expresses his fears that the suggested tracheotomy may not correspond to his father's wishes.

■ Legal Justification of Treatment

Medical procedures require professional and specialized justification, as well as what is referred to as the indication, and are *always* to be viewed as an invasion of the patient's physical integrity. Performing such procedures fulfills the definition of physical injury to the patient; so, to protect the treating physician from committing a criminal offense (e.g., negligence), medical consent is required from the patient, or alternatively from a person representing the patient (Merz 1991). Either the patient him/herself or a court may determine who is to be this advocate or proxy. These rules and principles are an expression of individual autonomy and give patients the potential to devise end-of-life plans according to their own wishes. To make such treatment decisions, a specialist—in this case, the physician—must provide the patient or the proxy with the necessary information pertaining to each individual case. Only after sufficient and proper clarification, or after intentionally abstaining from this, can the patient or proxy consent to a certain medical procedure— or not, as the case may be.

To give legally binding consent, the affected person must be *capable* of giving consent. In such a context, this is defined as the ability of a person to (1) grasp the facts that are relevant to the case in hand, which lead to the patient's consent or decision, (2) judge the consequences or risks associated with the decision, (3) weigh the alternatives of differing modes of treatment, and (4) determine the importance of the different interests or benefits affected by the decision, according to the patient's individual needs. In addition, the patient must be in a position to act according to these expressed views and insights (Strätling and Scharf 2000). In situations where patients cannot give their own consent, they can determine and express their wishes in advance. This can be done through a durable power of attorney, which is an advanced director that allows the patient to choose a proxy to make health decisions for him/her if he/she becomes unconscious or is not of sound mind to make those decisions. The patient's wishes are decisive features for the proxy as well. These wishes may be expressed either in written or in spoken form.

In many cases it is impossible, despite everyone's best efforts, to ascertain the patient's true wishes on the basis of the information provided. In such a situation, it becomes necessary to determine the patient's presumed wishes, considering such factors as the patient's own statements concerning similar circumstances, while accepting a certain latitude on the part of the assessor, and acting according to these presumed wishes. Despite having to make assumptions, with the associated potential danger of misinterpretation, this can be a successful way of coming as close as humanly possible to fulfilling the individual wishes of the patient. Depending on the wording and the actual situation, a written statement describing the patient's wishes may give a clear description of their true wishes, or may only present a partial reflection of the relevant facts and circumstances, and thus only vaguely indicate their presumed wishes. If there is nothing to go by in terms of the patient's presumed wishes, however, the proxy alone must make the decision. In any case, the proxy *must* consider the wellbeing of the person who is incapable of consent when involved in any decision made in this manner.

The loss of a stroke patient's ability to give consent may already have occurred during the acute phase of the illness, which naturally requires the appropriate medical treatment. The patient is, however, sufficiently legally protected from nonaction, as causing bodily injury by omitting appropriate treatment. or causing death by failing to perform the necessary procedures, both come into the category of medical malpractice. If the urgency of the situation does not allow the physicians to ascertain the patient's actual wishes or to question the patient's proxy, then they may act on the basis of the patient's presumed consent. If it is a matter of life or death, one may assume that the patient wishes to live; presuming the opposite requires proof. Justification of medical actions through the emergency exception is also conceivable. But even this legal argument requires the assumption of the patient's basic will to live in unclear circumstances, so that there are no essential differences in terms of handling such legal formulas in actual medical practice. The emergency treatment of a patient incapable of consent is possible with minimal legal risk, even without the assignment or instruction of a proxy.

In summary, it can be established that from a legal point of view, medical treatment can take place only when there is a corresponding indication. Even when there is an indication, except in an emergency, justification for the planned procedure may be obtained only by receiving permission to perform the procedure or treatment method, from either the patient or his/her proxy. In situations with an unequivocal medical indication and a clear wish on the part of the patient or proxy, an equally clear decision can be made as to further treatment. In other situations, however, in which either the indication or the patient's or proxy's wishes are (initially) ambiguous, day-to-day practice requires an organizational approach for problem solving and clarifying any ambiguity. Such unclear situations frequently occur in the case of stroke patients who are experiencing decreased levels of consciousness.

■ Medical Treatment Options

Modern medicine offers a wide range of treatment options with varying levels of invasiveness and is associated with different complications and prospects of success. A highly specialized system has been developed to ensure medical care, through emergency to intensive medicine, general hospital care, and rehabilitative medicine, to further the medical, nursing and therapeutic options aimed at responding to each patient's needs. It is precisely because of the innovative developments made in the field of modern emergency and intensive medicine, in the form of resuscitation and life prolongation through artificial organ substitution, that the chance of surviving severe illnesses exists at all for many patients. As a consequence, situations necessarily arise in which applying technical methods to certain target parameters does not bring about any measurable effects. It is conceivable that theoretically plausible treatment options could prove to be so complicated that they would exhaust the financial resources of society. Lastly, the procedures themselves, or the limitations of the surviving patient resulting from the procedures, may exceed a certain limit that is no longer acceptable with the patient's own idea of what life is. Decisions must be made about necessary and possible treatment options. After basic options have been considered, criteria must be formulated to make understandable and fair choices about further medical and technical options. Here, societal and individual interests may come into conflict. Physicians may significantly influence their patients' decisions, so an initial attempt should be made to describe suitable therapeutic measures to them.

Modern treatment options, including fibrinolysis in the case of acute ischemic insult, various surgical techniques for treating hemorrhage-associated stroke, or surgical decompression procedures, as well as interventional neuroradiology procedures, all share the aim of minimizing the amount of damage and destruction to brain tissue. In addition, intensive care procedures are required to secure the patient's vital functions. These procedures include all forms of therapeutic intervention that may be necessary for diagnosing and treating the patient during the critical phase of the illness, particularly in more complex cases. Thus, intensive care establishes the external criteria for healing the underlying cerebral illness. In particular, securing the airway and ventilating the patient are virtually synonymous with intensive care medicine. In addition, renal dialysis, procedures supporting the circulatory system, the use of antibiotics and blood bank products, parenteral nutrition, and ensuring electrolyte and fluid balance are also important treatment methods in intensive care units. Intensive therapy always involves the expenditure of vast quantities of time and energy on monitoring patients' vital signs in order to detect any disturbances as early as possible. Furthermore, intensive nursing care is a necessary component of patient management during this critical phase. In some cases the treatment will be successful, making complete recovery pos-

sible and eliminating the need for further intensive care. In patients with severe damage, the irreversible course of deterioration cannot be halted despite every attempt made using every available resource, and death occurs due to circulatory or cerebral causes. In still other instances, medical intervention leads to damage reversal, thus stabilizing the patient's condition, either through therapeutic intervention or spontaneously during the securing and monitoring of the patient's vital signs. In this case, patients may display differing degrees of residual damage. Such patients require less acute or intensive medical treatment during the further course of therapy. Thus, circulatory support and the level of ventilation can be discontinued in the short- and midterm. The immediate threat to the patient's life decreases to a minimum.

The further course of severe cerebral disease is often a long-lasting process of healing and adaptation in which freedom from life-prolonging or life-sustaining measures is achieved only very gradually. For instance, in a patient with a history of cardiopulmonary or accompanying vascular illness whose condition worsens as a result of a severe stroke, the oxygen supply may only be guaranteed by continuing ventilation and detoxification through renal dialysis. Long-term use of these life-sustaining procedures represents the only chance for the patient's survival and favorable progression through suitable rehabilitative measures. Many stroke patients in particular experience swallowing difficulties and associated risks and dangers while ingesting food. Accordingly, life-sustaining measures, such as artificial feeding and intensive nursing care, are required over long periods of time.

In this phase of the illness, the importance and role of the mode of access to the patient's respiratory tract can change. Initially, securing adequate oxygenation by ventilation was the top priority; however, protecting the patient from aspiration and guaranteeing a secure mode of suctioning the respiratory tract take on increasing importance during the further course of treatment and thus represent the sole function of the inserted airway after the patient has been weaned from the ventilator. As the length of the treatment increases, the acuteness of the situation decreases, and the patient's condition is no longer life-threatening, the focus of attention shifts to potential adverse events of the treatment, nursing care, physical therapy, occupational therapy, and speech therapy, as well as further rehabilitative aspects. Thus, for instance, oral access to the respiratory tract is switched over to a tracheotomy. This change makes it possible to avoid damage to the vocal cords that is potentially significant when reversal of cerebral damage is taking place; it also makes it possible to secure a permanent mode of entry and to facilitate care. Rehabilitative measures for patients suffering severe stroke take on special significance in terms of structuring the patient's later life: "While the central message of curative medicine is healing or at least prolonging the patient's life, the application of related measures and methods in the area of medical rehabilitation has as a primary goal the preservation or improvement of the disabled patient's impaired quality of life" (Delbrück 1998, Vol.3, p. 179). If there is a swallowing impairment, a safe method of nutrition must be ensured; it may be dangerous or even impossible to give food to the patient in the usual, natural way. Such life-preserving measures must decrease the risk of aspiration. Initially intravenous nutrition is possible, and during the further course of recovery nutrition can be administered via a transoral, transnasal, or percutaneous tube. Only then can the patient attain and maintain a condition of general health, which in turn allows the realization of rehabilitative measures.

Throughout the course of the patient's illness, any existing comorbidities may worsen, or complications may pose a threat to further recovery. Thus, measures taken to treat comorbidities, the treatment of intercurrent infections, and general prophylactic measures for conditions, such as thrombosis and pneumonia, must be considered.

A renewed increase in the need to monitor a patient's vital signs, as well as further intensive care, including resuscitation measures, can also be considered if the patient's condition worsens and if deemed necessary. It may be determined, not only in the initial phase but also during the later course of the illness, that the damage is irreversible. In such a situation, palliative treatment options must be considered, particularly for patients suffering severe stroke: "In contrast to curative treatment, with the aim of actually curing the patient, palliative therapy involves the comprehensive therapy of an ultimately incurable condition… The goal of palliative treatment is to achieve the highest quality of life possible for pa-

tients and their families" (WHO 1990, Hunold 1998, Vol.2, p. 818).

In rehabilitative as well as in palliative therapy, measures and methods that can improve the patient's quality of life represent the main focus of attention. Rehabilitation is patient-centered; in palliative medicine, the focus is not only the patient, but also the quality of life of the patient's family members, which is of equal importance. When the immediate phase of dying is imminent, pain-alleviating (medicinal) measures should be supplements to the general measures taken in caring for the dying.

■ Decisions Made On the Basis of the Medical Indication

Meaning of the Term "Indication"

Medical indication is a necessary but not sufficient requisite for medical action to be taken. It is limited by the wishes of the patient or the patient's proxy. The patient's wishes alone are also not sufficient; medical justification—that is, an indication—is required. The indication is understood as the basis for the initiation of treatment for a disease, which may be based on the knowledge of the cause, present symptoms, or by the nature of the disease (Stedman's Medical Dictionary 199, p. 777). Contraindications are the various conditions or circumstances that preclude a certain form of treatment or procedure that would otherwise be appropriate. In situations associated with immediate danger, a vital or absolute indication is considered to be the exception; here, in some instances, immediate and life-saving measures take precedence over the evaluation of risks and contraindications, or further diagnostic procedures.

"The indication is the well-founded decision to take a particular course of action, but not the action itself. It imposes an intellectual demand consisting of careful thought devoted to the patient's symptoms as well as consideration of this exceptional instance, if necessary, including consultation with other colleagues" (Anschütz 1982, p. 6). Determining an indication appears, at first, to be completely dominated by the diagnosis. "Diagnostic thinking governs … scientific medicine so overwhelmingly that the diagnosis is often viewed as the sole basis for indicated therapeutic procedures .... The diagnostic imperative rules medical thinking" (Anschütz 1989, p. 541). From this limiting perspective, the belief in the actual existence of objective indications arises in parallel to the assumption that a diagnosis can be determined objectively. However, it is not only the diagnosis (and the associated possibility of misdiagnosis), but also an array of other factors, including the prognosis and therapeutic options, that have an impact on the indication. The patient's individual circumstances such as the stage of illness, earlier successful or unsuccessful treatment attempts, and also age and closeness to death, are important factors. With all these determinants for the physician to consider when reaching an indication, it is critically important to bear in mind that the *patient* is the focus of attention. Doctors wish to offer their patients the best possible treatment; patients visit their doctor with the assurance that they will receive the best possible assistance and care. Such a definition of indication, oriented toward the doctor–patient relationship and thus a flexible concept, may in many cases govern the complicated process of the physician's actions, from first taking the patient's medical history to writing the epicrisis, but there are also dangers associated with this. "And it is precisely because of this complexity that we physicians are so easily corruptible when it comes to this governing concept of 'indication'" (Gahl 2005, p. 1155). Thus, through the biased view and emphasis placed on "autonomy," "doing no harm," and "doing good" (Beauchamp and Childress 2001), high performance expectations and, with them, possible indications, can be pushed beyond all reasonable limits.

External circumstances influence factors of the direct doctor–patient relationship that may be medically indicatable; social issues such as the availability of resources, affordability, and fairness should not be ignored, either. It is therefore necessary to rediscover the cultural aspects of these measures in determining an indication (Kirchhoff 2005).

To disassociate the concept of indication from the limiting association of diagnosis, it may be helpful to link it to the treatment aims for a patient in an ideal situation, thus individualizing the treatment. Such treatment aims are often general in nature; they could be, for example, saving a patient's life, healing an illness, prolonging a pa-

tient's life, improving the quality of life in cases of incurable disease, or alleviating pain and providing terminal care.

The further categorization of indicatable medical procedures as being necessary, desirable, helpful, or superfluous is currently under discussion, with the aim of putting the unduly close association of the indication with the doctor–patient relationship into perspective. These distinctions help us to further determine medical indication in relation to the background of socially available, or allocated, resources.

A *necessary* procedure is defined as prevention in cases of avoidable death, healing and amelioration of illnesses, and pain associated with such conditions. Treatment related to the support and control or guidance of natural human life processes is *desirable*, especially in instances of increasing blindness, deafness, or failing memory. *Helpful* procedures include measures taken in nursing care, guidance, health education, and the treatment of minor conditions. *Superfluous* medical procedures are, for example, duplicated tests, exaggerated demand for documentation, long-term medications still being taken but no longer needed, and a violation of the principles of rigor. The individualized treatment indication should be discussed against this backdrop—a treatment indication that results from medical expertise, the patient's own wishes and plans, as well as social circumstances, and which begins to take shape after intensive conversations with the appropriate members who must consider all of the individual factors.

"This balance between such factors as respect for individual findings and the 'mission' to heal, between what is medically possible and what the patient wishes, between individual hope and collective performance, between healing attempts and research projects, between daily results and long-term prognosis, such considerations require standards which must be developed through the process of thoughtful and self-critical observation of medicine and research in the culture and value stability of our constitutional state" (Kirchhoff 2005, p. 239).

Accordingly, perspectives other than merely the medical standpoint, and that of the patient, should also be considered during the communication process. Thus, the indication is ultimately determined by the individual state of illness and the prognosis; collective experience; medical possibilities concerning diagnostics and therapy; and personnel-related, organizational, institutional and economic conditions, or society as a whole. There is therefore no such thing as an "objective" indication. "The indication is decided by the physician, the patient, the patient's family members, and by society with its institutions of health" (Gahl 2005, p. 1157). As a consequence, an indication can only be determined in a decision process that is understandable to all parties involved.

In addition to the inadequately perceived multidimensionality of determining an indication, there is a further problem in connection with the classic concept of indication. The static misperception of the term indication is defined as the excessively strong association of indication with the patient's original, healthy condition (Strätling and Schmucker 2004). As the severity of an illness increases, the prognosis also worsens, and the range of treatment methods narrows. This illness-related change must be reflected by an adequate adaptation of the therapeutic aim. The ultimate consequence of pursuing an unattainable therapeutic aim is "overtreating," which, in turn, is detrimental to the patient.

Meaning of the Term "Prognosis"

To avoid damage in the sense of "overtreating," as well as "undertreating," a detailed assessment of the prognosis and the incorporation of these results into the process of determining an indication are essential. The term prognosis describes a "forecast of the probable course and/or outcome of a disease" (Stedman's Medical Dictionary 1990, p. 1265). Therapeutic action must always be oriented toward an individualized evaluation of the prognosis. The nosological prognosis of an illness is to be distinguished from a patient's individual prognosis (Schäfer et al. 2005, p. 638). This individual prognosis can indeed be derived from the nosological prognosis, but it may be either more or less favorable, depending on subjective factors. When making such an assessment, deviations— sometimes considerable—from average estimations must be tolerated, and the individual prognosis must be adjusted constantly, at times intuitively and subjectively dictated by experience, to fit the course of treatment or the diagnostic find-

ings. Despite all these uncertainties, determining the prognosis and its associated therapeutic consequences is absolutely indispensible. "Either we perform every therapeutic procedure employing maximum efforts and continue these efforts until intervening complications determine the further course to be no longer alterable, or we terminate the therapy after a more or less long course and put up with, inescapably, a good portion of faulty judgments—we can protest as loudly as we wish" (Spittler 1999, p. 45).

A prognosis can be classified with a certain degree of probability as good, uncertain, doubtful, unfavorable, poor, or very poor. Estimating a prognosis only after a specific and finite treatment has been attempted is necessary for the evaluation to have the greatest possible certainty. Uncritical long-term treatment should not be perpetuated as a result of this initial treatment; it is important that unfavorable courses of treatment be sufficiently recognized with a high degree of certainty to avoid applying senseless medical methods and intensive medical care (Wedekind and Klug 2005). Accordingly, it is a medical obligation to make reliable assessments aimed at developing prognostic criteria, and then to incorporate the collected data and results into further decision processes. Medical decisions that do not respect an individualized prognosis are associated with a considerable risk of damaging the patient through erroneously recommended "overtreatment" or "undertreatment."

Evaluating the prognosis requires a professional approach as well as the appropriate emotional distance. In a study of hospice patients, the responsible physicians gave a precise assessment of the patients' life prognosis in 20% of cases; they overestimated the prognosis in 63% of cases; and they underestimated it in 17% of cases (Christakis and Lamont 2000). The prognostic statement became more precise in direct proportion to the increasing amount of professional experience; however, it became less precise as the emotional closeness of the physician to the patient increased. Too positive an assessment of life expectancy may result in the initiation of medical measures and procedures that can cause an unwanted and uncalled-for prolongation of the patient's dying process.

From these results, two problem areas become apparent: first, it seems to be the case that every prognostic assessment has a subjective component. This subjectivity can only be confronted, for the benefit of the patient, if the attending physician examines his/her own standpoint by comparing it with a second opinion. Likewise, this subjectivity must be openly discussed in conversations with the patient, his/her appointed proxy, or family members. In addition, such scrutiny can highlight a special problem involving the medical prognostic procedure: the prediction or determination that the patient has entered a new phase, namely the dying process.

The Dying Process As a Specific Prognostic Responsibility

Speaking about topics such as death and dying can bring about fundamental changes and redefine the nature of social reality as it has always existed for everyone involved in the situation. This type of communication is extremely difficult because it involves planning for the foreseeable future and permanently removing a member from the social group or community (Schneider 2004). The quality of communication sets the stage for further organization of the patient's dying phase and also for the period of grief and mourning for surviving family members. Thus, defining the dying process presents a specific medical and prognostic question, because its introduction is associated with certain social and therapeutic consequences, and, thus, with necessary changes relating to the assessment of the medical indication for treatment options. During the past few years, the American Medical Association, the National Cancer Institute, the German Medical Association, and the British Medical Association have been dealing specifically with these problems, which are of such enormous significance in the practice of medicine.

When treating dying patients, the physician has a specifically defined task, that is, a set of actions specially indicated in such a situation, clearly defined as early as 1979:

"Terminal care is the limitation of treatment to the alleviation of symptoms and the simultaneous abstention from applying life-prolonging measures in the dying patient. It includes the omission or discontinuation of medication as well as technical measures, for example, artificial respiration, oxygen, blood transfusions, hemodialysis, artificial nutri-

tion" (German Medical Association (Bundesärztekammer) 1979, p. 958).

Today, a number of professional medical societies have issued statements addressing the subject of granting basic (nursing care) support to relieve suffering and alleviate distressing symptoms, in addition to palliative treatment (by physicians). This includes providing accommodation under conditions which preserve the patient's dignity; giving the patient adequate attention; caring for personal hygiene; supporting, comforting, and respecting a patient's autonomy; and alleviating pain and suffering (American Academy of Family Physicians, 2011; American Medical Association, 1991; British Medical Association 2009; German Medical Association (Bundesärztekammer) 1998). Supplying the patient with nutrition and fluids may not always be included in this concept of basic care, as it may represent a burden to the dying patient. Still, hunger and thirst are to be alleviated when they are experienced by the patient as subjective sensations.

The determination of the onset of death thus has considerable consequences for what is medically indicated. Because of these existential consequences, the grounds for taking such important decisions must be absolutely clear and understandable, since the end of this process represents the end of a human life. It was established in the German Medical Association's 1979 statement that judging whether the immediate dying process has begun requires a physician's expertise. A dying patient is an ill or injured person for whom a physician has made the decision, on the basis of several clinical signs, that the illness is irreversible, or that there is no hope of the traumatic injury ever improving and that death will occur within a short period of time.

"The dying process begins when the elementary physical vital functions are considerably impaired or completely absent. If these basic life functions are affected to such an extent that the patient is no longer able to be the subject or agent of his or her own functions, that is, to possess any control over his or her own life, and death is imminent due to life-threatening complications, a large degree of latitude is granted the physician to perform what he deems to be necessary" (German Medical Association (Bundesärztekammer) 1979, p. 958).

The first attempt in the United States to define the dying process legally was "An Act Related to and Defining Death," adopted by the state of Kansas in 1970, but it was superseded in 1972 and 1975 when the Uniform Determination of Death Act of 1981 was drafted. In 1979 the American Medical Association drafted its own definition of the dying process in its "Model Determination of Death" statute, and a year later it teamed up with the American Bar Association and the National Conference of Commissioners on Uniform State Laws to draft the Uniform Determination of Death Act. It was approved and signed into law in 1981. The Act specified a distinction between "the existing common law basis for determining death—total failure of the cardiorespiratory system" and "new procedures for determination of death based upon irreversible loss of all brain functions" (Uniform Determination of Death Act 1981). Not to be included in the category of dying patients, however, are patients with neocortical death or those in a persistent vegetative state (Uniform Determination of Death Act 1981). The principles established in 1981 define a dying person as someone who has sustained "irreversible cessation of circulatory and respiratory functions," or someone with "irreversible cessation of all functions of the entire brain, including the brain stem" (Uniform Determination of Death Act 1981). However, the fundamental principles approved by the American Medical Association in the 1981 Act refrain from making clear medical criteria for determining death, allowing physicians the freedom to "formulate acceptable medical practices and to utilize new biomedical knowledge, diagnostic tests, and equipment" for medical procedures and diagnostic tests to determine when those functions cease (Uniform Determination of Death Act 1981).

Although it is necessary to determine when the dying process begins, a great degree of uncertainty remains regarding the precise and comprehensible description of this point in the course of the illness for a specific patient. Dying, as an integral part of life, takes place immediately preceding the death of the individual. Whether severe and irreversible brain damage is already included as a part of the dying process can scarcely be decided on a medical basis. In the literature, attempts have been made to explicate this point further, guided by the distinction between dying in a narrower or in a broader sense. In the broader sense, the dying phase begins when none of the following criteria is fulfilled: there is no realistic hope that the patient will (re)gain his/her own state of consciousness, be able to perceive others consciously and interact with them in a target-oriented manner, maintain a subjectively satisfactory lifestyle, or halt the progression of a severe illness that will inevitably lead to death (Strätling and Schmucker 2004). With respect to treatment in these cases, the authors conclude that there is no longer any indication for life-prolonging measures (e.g., artificial nutrition) during the dying phase in the broader sense, because it will only prolong the process. If any doubts should arise as to whether the dying process in the broader sense has begun, life-sustaining measures may justifiably be taken when a relative indication is present. During the dying process in the narrower sense, there is an absolute contraindication for the continuation of life-sustaining forms of treatment.

Evaluating the onset of death in patients with severe disturbances in their level of consciousness is very difficult. In any case, the genesis of the disease, prognosis, previous and concomitant illnesses, and the patient's age must all be incorporated into the overall evaluation.

As to the assessment of the dying process, "... the perception of and attention to many different phenomena is necessary. It is recommended that the patient's condition be evaluated by experienced physicians from different disciplines" (Eibach 2002, p. 128). According to opinions given by physicians interviewed, dying begins when the patient's life expectancy is only a few hours (6.8%), a few days (50.4%), a few weeks (24.4%), or a few months (7.5%). Altogether, 10.8% of these physicians described the onset of death as being associated with the patient's mental and physical condition and/or the underlying illness. The greater the professional experience of the physicians, the earlier they defined the onset of death. Anesthesiologists and intensive care physicians more often chose the option of "a matter of a few hours"; general practitioners and internists were more likely to choose "days" or "months" (van Oorschot et al. 2005).

In the face of such uncertainty surrounding the determination of onset of death, as well as the consequential therapeutic recommendations by a physician who carries the responsibility of such a decision, the focus is placed not on the enforcement of the "right to die," or a "right to determine one's own time of death," but, rather, it is based on a humane and dignity-preserving plan for the final phase of a patient's life.

"If, however, one were to waive the concrete legal safeguarding and preservation of the patient's life, the danger of arbitrariness and undermining of the patient's life protection would present itself, for instance, when no uniform statutory regulation exists with respect to the definition of 'dying persons'" (Plenter 2001, p. 28).

Such rigorous requirements concerning a uniform legal description of the term "dying" can be overburdening and also have the effect of narrowing down the reality of the dying process to justifiable and measurable arguments. Just as with the description of illness, the perception of dying as a biopsychosocial entity also appears to be necessary. Sporken (1989, p. 1081) emphatically refers to an extended definition: "The dying process as a human event begins when death is bound to occur, irrevocably or in the foreseeable future, and one or more persons from the patient's immediate surroundings are informed as to these happenings." This ultimately social understanding of the dying process elucidates various interpretations in the evaluation of a patient's condition when their level of consciousness is severely impaired. Patients with such forms of damage are certainly to be considered "living persons," but they may also be viewed as "dying persons." How they are described depends on medical, biological, psychological, and social factors, as well as on the severity of the damage, concomitant illnesses, and prognosis. It also depends on the position of the individual concerned and of his/her family members. Assessing whether the dying process has begun can ultimately only take place if actual circumstances and different interpretations or perceptions can be communicated, exchanged, and coordinated. The results of this exchange are only effective in individual circumstances, never for all patients in general.

■ Decision-Making Based On the Patient's Own Wishes

Treatment decisions made on the basis of the patient's express wishes correspond to the executing the patient's right to self-determination. Following the necessary medical information and consent relating to different therapy options, the patient decides on the further course of action, based on his/her own value system and wishes. To make such decisions, patients require information, counseling, and time, so that they are better able to understand what they wish for themselves. Here the affected person may consciously choose not to make his/her own decision, opting instead for a judgment to be made, or actions to be taken, by others on his/her behalf. Whether the patient's wishes can be formulated with sufficient precision depends on the patient and his/her social environment, the course of the illness, the treatment options, and the urgency of the decision at hand. In any case, it is the physician's task to support the patient in reaching a solid decision based on the competent assistance provided. The patient's capacity to give consent also has to be examined and confirmed; the relevant criteria have already been mentioned above. In emergencies, a situation often arises in which it would simply take too long to analyze the patient's wishes. Irreversible damage may take place during the time it would take to come to a decision. In such difficult situations, it must be assumed, when considering the various possibilities, that the patient has a general will to live; as a result, all life-extending measures are taken. The opposite position—that is, that a patient does not possess the will to live—requires actual proof. Therefore, examining the patient's own wishes at a later point remains guaranteed by the fact that the procedure leaves the decision open. This method requires that the consensual procedure be repeated as soon as possible to establish the patient's wishes, allowing the subsequent and immediate enforcement of these expressed wishes.

People may communicate their wishes to others in a variety of ways. Direct oral communication is one possibility; written communication is another. To deal with such forms of expression of the patient's wishes and written advance directives ("living wills"), the British Medical Association has provided the following statement: "Advance [directives] allow competent adults to say what they would like to happen later if their mental capacity becomes impaired. ... Subject to certain criteria being met, refusals are legally binding. Even advance [directives] that fail to meet the legal criteria can provide some insight into the patient's thinking and be helpful in indicating what is in the individual's best interests" (British Medical Association 2009). The living will as a legal document has been discussed more and more frequently over the past few years, and the concept is becoming more widespread. There are, however, no reliable figures that would indicate how often such an advance directive actually forms the basis for medical decisions in terms of the further course of action. In modern society, there are other forms of transmitting the will besides the usual spoken or written modes; for example, various audiovisual techniques. All of these forms have one thing in common: confronting the subject beforehand. This confrontation gives rise to the formation of the patient's own intentions and wishes, which are influenced by different biological, psychological, and social components. The formation of these intentions may vary in length, depending on each individual's consideration of various aspects. In life-threatening situations, decisions must be made by the affected person, and these are decisions that must be seen as existential in nature and that may considerably impede the process of forming a truly "free" will. In such a situation, an intervention by the physician may unduly influence the patient during an already difficult decision. So, in order to reduce the danger of manipulation and increase patient empowerment, physicians should help patients reconsider their refusal of necessary treatment.

In the event of sudden-onset severe stroke, such medical guidance while determining the patient's wishes is often only conceivable when the patient's declaration of intent is formulated in an advance directive. When a patient is incapable of giving consent, the wishes expressed in an advance directive are binding for the physician, in the sense of accepting or rejecting a certain form of treatment (British Medical Association 2007). Situations in which treatment decisions are unequivocally settled by the patient's own wishes do not require a proxy to make a decision. In cases of greater ambiguity or when the patient's wishes have not been expressed, a patient incap-

able of giving consent will need a legal proxy. This proxy may be named by the patient, or may be determined and legitimated by a court decision. A proxy is nearly always required in most cases of severe cerebral damage, which occurs without any previous consideration of the problem, and when there has been no formation of a clear idea of what the patient wishes in terms of treatment, or at least a clear statement issued on the subject. In such circumstances, too, a decision must be taken that considers the patient's wishes for development. Expressing the presumed wishes, which can be defined as the wishes of the patient as he/she would express them if he/she were still capable of good judgment, can fulfill this requirement for the affected person. Information from advance directives, earlier statements, biographical clues and cues, as well as information communicated by trusted persons, all contribute to the overall assessment. Insufficient information would prevent the execution of the patient's will, and any irresponsible interpretation. The proxy and the physician are required to communicate and to respect the patient's wishes—or *presumed* wishes, as the case may be. Here, the patient's statements and wishes must also be considered; his/her general attitude toward life and family also contributes to this process. Family members or friends may present arguments that help reconstruct the patient's own wishes. Likewise, constantly reassessing the situation is essential for determining whether, and to what extent, the patient is able to participate effectively in the decision-making process. This obligation is represented externally, if nothing else, in the substitution of the legal term of "incapacitated" with "care." The legal form allows a large degree of freedom in decision-making and therefore a wide-ranging spectrum of self-determination, in relation to the range and implications of a given medical procedure as well as the patient's corresponding, intact ability to consent. This is also true in cases of severe cerebral damage resulting from stroke, when the patient may produce several different statements.

Operating under the presumption that patients with severe brain damage are human beings whose actions are teeming with "hidden messages" to be deciphered, Tolle (2005) interviewed nurses and relatives with experience caring for patients in a persistent vegetative state. Based on the patients' external behavioral features (muscle tension, eye and head movements, expectoration, types of breathing, utterance of nonsensical sounds, mouth movements, transpiration, hand movements, tear production, reddening of the face, and wrinkling of the forehead) Tolle was able to derive and establish comparable interpretations of the patients' perceptions, feelings, and utterances. Thus, from the associations of the persons questioned, patients' emotions, such as a sense of wellbeing or discomfort, attentiveness, and interest, or the desire for peace and quiet, appetite and hunger or satiation, physical ailments, anxiety and defensiveness, and the need to change positions, could be interpreted. "External" characteristics and reactions should be viewed as the expression of the patient's "internal" perceptions and circumstances. Further differentiation into interpretations of physical, psychological, and social dimensions can then be attempted. It is precisely such utterances that can be interpreted as the only possible mode of communication for patients with severe disabilities. Accordingly, these statements and utterances can be included when determining the patients' presumed wishes and thus, in turn, when determining the patient's wishes to continue or terminate a certain form of treatment. The incorporation of these "updates" through expression of the patient's wishes offers the opportunity to allow the patient maximum participation. But this also carries the danger that the caregivers "… may thus possibly project and transfer their feelings and views onto the patient," thereby giving a false interpretation of the affected person's wishes. "Therefore, opening the eyes, making certain eye movements without focusing, and displaying vegetative reactions such as acceleration of the heart rate, or perspiring, when family members leave the room, for instance, are very difficult to transfer from a subjective interpretation to a universal, objective level of interpretation" (Plenter 2001, p. 248). In spite of these obstacles, the approach does offer the advantage—and the sole opportunity—of incorporating anything the patient says, even the vaguest statements, into the production of his/her presumed wishes, thus allowing a decision to be made that corresponds as closely as possible to the patient's actual wishes. At the same time it poses the danger that the patient's wishes may be distorted as a result of the different versions presented by family members—who represent their own interests—as well as the faulty interpretation of the patient's wishes by caregivers

and attending physicians. Hence, it must be noted that determining the patient's presumed wishes will never be completely free of false interpretations and outsiders taking the initiative. However, these limitations also apply when determining the patient's wishes even in the absence of disturbances in consciousness. One can say that not only the emergence of the patient's wishes, but also the formation of the true, or presumed, wishes of the patient, represents a communicative process that demands the proper management of time and personnel, which must be granted and organized.

■ Communicative Determination of the Individual Indication and Individual Wishes of the Patient

Only in a few rare cases can an individual medical indication be derived directly from generally indicatable medical options. For an individual prognosis, assumptions must be made regarding the patient and any special circumstances, derived from the nosological prognosis, and based on experience and occasionally through intuition. With rare exceptions, patients who are confronted with a special situation, often existential in a medical context, are incapable of forming a precise and realistic statement of their wishes immediately and without further reflection or consideration of their general wishes and attitudes. Moreover, in cases of severe acquired cerebral damage, patients can influence the decision only indirectly; that is, through a previous statement pertaining to their wishes, or by physical reactions interpreted as an indication of these wishes, or by way of a patient's presumed will. In many instances, a proxy must be present. Making a decision requires a serious discussion between all concerned, which demands varying amounts of intensity and time, depending on the individual patient. Describing the organization of such discussions, which often involve persons other than the patient and the physician, plays an essential part in the decision-making process, during which different positions and possibilities are assessed. The particular social context in which an individual lives can influence certain events and decisions. The structure described in the following sections should help make such discussions possible and should be understood as a description of a virtual discussion room, which can and should be altered to suit the individual situation (Oehmichen 2006). It is a setting that may convey a sense of orientation, but not obligation. The decision model consists of a series of steps, a description of the possible levels, and the adaptation to differing requirements depending on the urgency of the decision at hand.

Internal Formation of Decisions

Following a situation analysis, which summarizes the case for the members participating in the discussion, all theoretically available courses of action must be described. The next step involves weighing the different options against the background of the individual situation, as well as consideration of their bindingness. Finally, a decision must be taken and each step must be subsequently documented. This stepwise model gives structure to the decision process independently of the type and the levels to be incorporated, as well as the urgency of the decision to be made.

Decision Model—Steps
1. Situation analysis
2. Description of all possible courses of action
3. Weighing of options and confirmation of bindingness
4. Decision
5. Documentation

Structuring of the decision process independently from the type and urgency of the decision.

In medical decisions, not only many different situations, but also different options for the courses of action, must be taken into consideration. These factors must be analyzed and considered on medical grounds as well as on nursing and therapeutic levels. The patient's own perceptions and views, as well as those prevailing in his/her living environment, are critically important when determining the individual medical indication as well as forming and communicating the patient's wishes. In addition, the legal framework and background conditions must be incorporated into the discus-

sion so that at least the basic social consensus is respected. The different fields of competence that may be needed during the consideration process can be derived at each respective level; these define the possible participants in the discussion and the perspectives that pertain to the decision at hand.

Decision Model—Levels
1. Medicine
2. Nursing care and therapy
3. Patient
4. Living environment
5. Law and ethics

Description of the necessary fields of competency of participants in the discussion, or of perspectives in the evaluation.

Depending on the urgency of the situation, distinctions can be made in a medical context between short-term decisions, such as realistic attempts at resuscitation in the case of circulatory arrest; mid-term urgent decisions, such as initiating or continuing intensive therapy employing ventilation or renal dialysis; or decisions without special urgency, e.g., decisions pertaining to prophylactic measures or artificial nutrition. Depending on the urgency of the decision at hand, different requirements may emerge concerning the necessary extent of inclusion at each level: urgent decisions require minimum consideration at the individual levels, long-term decisions require maximum consideration. In practice, the varying demands that relate to the consideration of the different levels can be realized by specifying the vocational groups and individuals involved in the discussion process.

Decision Model—Urgency
1. Short-term (e.g., cardiopulmonary resuscitation)
2. Mid-term (e.g., intensive therapy, artificial ventilation, renal dialysis)
3. Long-term (e.g., thrombosis prophylaxis, artificial nutrition)

Using this communicative decision model, individualized decisions may be made with respect to the indication for a certain type of intervention as well as the presumed wishes of the patient, if needed. The model described above grants the at-

Formation of Intentions and Individualization of the Indication	
Patient's general wishes and ideas	Fundamentally possible and indicatable forms of medical treatment
Shared communication Reflection and consideration Application to individual cases	
Actual and reflected wishes	Subjective and individual medical indication

tending physician leeway in terms of the medical indication; at the same time, it offers various possibilities according to the patient's wishes. This freedom is only possible if it is jointly exercised by everyone involved in the discussions. Such flexibility allows decisions which justify or reject certain treatment options based on the patient's presumed will and wishes; it also allows decisions that require—or no longer require—certain treatments, determined on the basis of an individualized indication.

The size and range of the discussion space, determined by the proxies of each individual level, guarantees the necessary transparency; at the same time, it is practical and appropriately protects the patient's individuality. A special protected space is thus created for decision-making, a space in which everyone participates in making a shared, medically supervised decision, while allowing room for the patient's wishes as well as objective medical possibilities. This also makes it possible for individual recommendations and opinions from the various experiences and fields of competency of participating physicians, nursing staff, and therapists to be incorporated into the final decision without undue manipulation of the patient or the proxy. The conscious involvement of the different levels mobilizes internal resources for decision-making purposes. Likewise, the model can serve to standardize the decision process, at the same time rendering it more comprehensible.

External Influences on Decision-Making

Situations naturally arise when the communication resources of the treatment team and the patient or the proxy, as well as the family members, are not well developed enough or cannot be sufficiently exploited. In such instances, activating step-by-step external support options is necessary to arrive at a decision.

The simplest form of supplementation is the activation of an external expert consultant who can assess treatment options and evaluate the forms of treatment that have been suggested up to that point. Of course, this consultant may also present further treatment or decision options for consideration.

The decision model suggested here requires excellent communication skills for all those involved, as well as a willingness to communicate. These prerequisites are not always fulfilled, however, or they may become too exhaustive during the course of the discussion. In this situation, it is possible to fall back on the option of having the decision process moderated by an external expert, whose task it is to organize the conduct of the discussions. This could reveal undiscovered resources for the decision at hand and make them more applicable to the decision.

As the next possible step for obtaining external support, a committee, such as a clinical ethics committee, may express a vote according to its own analysis that can then be considered by those responsible for making the decision. This form of external support also serves the purpose of strengthening the ability of the participants to come to a decision and thus enabling them to take over responsibility.

If these various methods of optimizing communication fail to produce the desired results, then a decision must be made beyond the boundaries of the involved parties' responsibility. This decision can only be reached through legal means. Here, the laws of guardianship offer sufficient options. Each of the people involved can appeal to the responsible court and thus come to a decision, or arrange for evaluation of the situation, using legal assistance. This decision process, once legalized, naturally requires a certain time frame to allow the judge to examine the circumstances, and, if necessary, also to allow time to obtain an expert opinion to make a subsequent decision. During this time, the outcome must be kept open by the use of medical and nursing measures, possibly even against the patient's will, as may be confirmed afterwards. Such a solution may be chosen not only when communication among the parties participating if the decision fails completely, but also when external communication proves unsuccessful. It should be understood as an *absolute* exception, being the most extreme step in an approach to arriving at an individual indication for treatment and the patient's subjective wishes, which has up to that point proven unsuccessful. It should, however, also be viewed as a pressing need to secure legal precedence in cases of establishing boundaries in medicine. Furthermore, the control and sanctions of the criminal law remain intact here; they represent additional safeguards against irresponsible decisions, in the patient's best interests.

External Support for Decision-Making
1. Second opinion for suggested procedure: Expert professional consultants
2. Moderate the discussion: Ethics consultants
3. Vote on the decision: Ethics committee
4. Resolution when communication attempts fail: Judicial clarification

---

As indicated above, many decisions may be realized without the assistance of a court, in the protected environment of a "discussion space" for the participants in the decision process. This space remains sufficiently transparent for the decision makers who function as proxies of the individual levels according to the decision model, and, at the same time, the space offers adequate security through legal means—a security that represents sufficient protection against misuse, thus setting the stage for amicable decision-making by everyone. This model supplies quality criteria for decision-making in complex medical situations. It is suitable for clarifying the essential action-determining steps, levels, motivation, and reasoning in a retrospective assessment of the decision.

Course of Events in Case Study 1
Before the patient undergoes imaging procedures, she is intubated to secure her airway and placed on a ventilator. The CT scan reveals such an extensive cerebral hemorrhage that, according to the neurosurgeon's assessment of the situation, an extremely unfavorable prognosis is expected even with surgical intervention. The previously diagnosed hematologic illness, responsible for the patient's greatly reduced platelet count, presents a further risk factor. The surgeon and the anesthesiologist determine that the risk of bleeding during surgery is very high. From the internists' point of view, no long-term treatment option for the patient's long-standing thrombocytopenia can be suggested. Together, the participating physicians confirm that surgical intervention would produce no successful results. The patient is admitted to the intensive care unit. After presenting her medical situation and the possibilities still available, the senior physician suggests terminating the intensive treatment, which was considered to be futile from a medical point of view, and recommends palliative treatment. During the following night, the patient dies in the presence of her husband and their daughter.

Course of Events in Case Study 2
During discussions about further treatment options available, attempts are made to determine the patient's wishes. The attending physician decides that the patient has not yet reached the level of unconsciousness described in her living will, and, as a result of this interpretation, no clear statement of the patient's wishes is available. The patient's children attempt to describe their mother's thoughts in greater detail: "Unconsciousness means more than a dictionary definition, more than the loss of wakefulness and the ability to respond to stimuli. Consciousness, according to our mother, would be defined as follows:
- that I can perceive my surroundings with my sensory organs.
- that I can communicate, in whatever form necessary; that is, I can express my wishes.
- that I am aware of myself as a person, my condition, and my situation and can express my will.
- that I can experience emotions and am able to feel a certain degree of enjoyment.

Would the formulation of '*fully* regaining consciousness' perhaps have been clearer?"

Based on the presumed wishes of the patient, the patient's family and the multidisciplinary team (i.e., attending physician, senior physician, nurse, physical therapist, and social worker) come to the unanimous decision to forego all further intensive care measures. Neither ventilation nor placement of a tube for purposes of artificial nutrition is deemed necessary. The family, together with the social worker, makes arrangements for palliative care to alleviate pain and discomfort in the patient's home. Eight days after her discharge, the patient passes away. In a telephone conversation, the daughter reports: "Without nursing care we wouldn't have managed at all. It is possible that she took in some of what was going on …, that gave us strength, since we were not doing it for ourselves, but rather for her, or mainly for her …, We sang to her often …, The nights were very difficult; we had to suction a lot. Our mother didn't need any morphine. We fed her from a cup with a spout. We spent the final twenty-five minutes at her bedside, and this brought the whole family so close together."

Course of Events in Case Study 3

The interpretation of the patient's actual wishes causes great difficulties for the people who are with him during the course of the illness. On one hand, the advance directive was written by a man who was a highly active and influential person in his former state of health and who had made it clear that he rejected a state of dependency. On the other hand, he gives the impression of still being able to experience a certain amount of pleasure in life. He agrees to all nursing, therapeutic, and medical procedures. The possibility of a tracheotomy is explained to him during a conversation, and he appears to accept this. The various assessors involved have differing views of his ability to consent. A discussion ultimately takes place, during which the patient's wife and son, an attorney (a friend of the family), the attending nurse, the physical therapist, the occupational therapist, the attending and senior physicians, and the patient are all present. The result is the opinion that the patient is unable to give his consent for complex decisions; however, a positive statement of his wishes concerning the tracheotomy has become clear. The tracheotomy was carried out as a prophylactic measure to prevent aspiration. Since that time the patient has been living in a nursing care center.

■ Discussion

The most important organizational structures for treating ethical questions in hospitals and other care institutions were conceived during the last third of the 20th century. The spectrum of possibilities ranges from the ethical discussion of the case at the bedside to the ethics committee of the organization. Top-down and bottom-up models can be distinguished as ideal-typical models in the context of organizational ethics (Steinkamp and Gordijn 2003, p. 128). According to these models, the suggested solutions to ethical problems are presented one level at a time. The top-down model assumes that recommendations, guidelines, and overall concepts are developed at the top level and can then be carried down to the lower levels. The bottom-up model postulates that the decisions are made primarily within the context of the doctor–patient relationship, and the organizational environment does not take on independent significance. In practice, however, such ideal-typical models rarely occur. Often, mixed forms are created, e.g., a clinical–ethical interaction model (Steinkamp and Gordijn 2003, p. 146). In this model, a centrally appointed ethics committee presents recommendations and organizes ongoing training, thus allowing decentralized ethical case discussions.

The model introduced in this chapter is also a mixed type, but it clearly emphasizes that the parties responsible for the patient's care should undertake the decision-making. This does not require the involvement of an ethics committee. With no central guidance, it is necessary for individual occupational groups to make active arrangements for appropriate training courses and make use of relevant ethical information, recommendations, and guidelines that are available from many external sources. If there are no ethics advisors or ethics committees at the institution in question, then external resources must be mobilized as required. Hence, the model is particularly well suited for smaller organizations. Problem areas in this model include the lack of uniform recommendations and insufficient support of such initiatives through the leadership of the organizational unit; however, these drawbacks appear on the whole to be of lesser significance. The model focuses on enabling the participants to incorporate significant aspects of the issue at hand into a predetermined —but at the same time sufficiently flexible—sequence of events. Just as with other measurement tools for bioethical practice, central questions in the decision process are predefined and function as an orientation point for the participants in the discussion. However, clinical experience is emphasized more strongly than in other clinical ethics tools so that, according to the degree of urgency in different situations, different groups of people may be incorporated into the discussion.

Observing the perspectives presented here should also encourage and enable participants to make ethical considerations and urgent decisions in emergency situations. As an extension to the Nimwegen Method of ethical case discussion (Bannert et al. 2005, p. 453), it should be ensured—as in the model introduced here—that the patient and/or the proxy is included in the decision-making process. Special emphasis is placed on knowledge gleamed from experience that neither the clear wishes of the patient nor the individual medical indication should be formed until the physician is able to reflect properly on the situation. Changes in the patient's wishes and the medical indication are also possible. In this circumstance, the prognosis of the affected person's illness must be incorporated into the decision-making process. By including this element of changeability, the chronological dynamics of medical decisions are more clearly emphasized and appropriately considered, thereby complementing methods used in other bioethical paradigms. Through the specification of a clear series of steps and levels, the model creates a procedure based on medical decision-making processes, while at the same time including the caregivers. Furthermore, the decision model also includes other occupational groups, such as physical therapists and occupational therapists; the responsibility for treatment decisions does, however, remain clearly defined. This makes it possible to deal with excessively demanding situations that result from complex decision processes and help overcome the obstacles presented by the "informed consent" standards. "Informed consent" is defined as the conscious consent given by the patient after being sufficiently informed by a physician as to the treatment procedure, its advantages and drawbacks, as well as possible alternatives with its associated advantages and drawbacks (Jonsen et al. 2002, p. 61).

In a survey conducted on patients with amyotrophic lateral sclerosis, 20% of patients strictly refused to make an advance directive (Buchardi et al. 2004). Another survey showed that 73% of patients on dialysis thought their doctors would come to the correct decision on their own about the intensity of treatment needed; 88% expressed the wish that, in the event of their inability to make a decision themselves, they would make a decision in cooperation with their physicians, caregivers, and family members (Eibach and Schäfer 1997). Because patients on dialysis who are chronically ill may have a different relationship of trust with their attending physicians than other patients would have to, for instance, intensive care physicians who are usually not specifically chosen by the patients themselves, these results cannot simply be transferred to other patient groups (Oehmichen 2005). In spite of this, the fact remains that the patient may very well wish *not* to have to make difficult decisions alone. A patient's expressed wish to hand over responsibility must be detected and given due consideration during the decision-making process. The patient's best interests are not served by a simplified version of autonomy. In such situations, it seems necessary to elevate the recognition and enforcement of the patient's authority to the central criterion (Körtner 2005). The expressed wish to hand over responsibility occurs not only in the patients, but also in their advocates, who likewise require appropriate support. For example, a survey conducted on advocates who had agreed to the insertion of a feeding tube revealed that 78.3% felt the decision was a good one; 26.1% felt pressured to agree; and only 45.7% would wish to have this type of nutrition themselves (Mitchell and Lawson 1999).

The suggested model also goes above and beyond the "best interest" standards. "Best interest" corresponds to the wishes that a hypothetically "sensible" patient would express in a particular situation. This standard presupposes a generally accepted agreement with respect to these wishes. Such agreement is, however, not to be found in today's modern society for many questions pertaining to forms of medical treatment, especially with regard to intensive therapy for patients with severe cerebral damage (Oehmichen and Irrgang 2005).

The decision model presented here does not require any general or, so to speak, overall social concurrence; it establishes the decision-making ability under consideration of medical possibilities and with maximum respect given to the patient's wishes. Even minimal reactions on the part of the patient can, when interpreted accordingly as indications, be incorporated into the determination of his/her will and wishes. The model requires—and at the same time enables—the actors to assume responsibility. Viewed in this context, it is comparable to a "best respect" standard. This standard demands respect for the affected person's personality during the decision-making process, under adequate consideration of even the most minor statements currently made by the patient (Tolmein 2004, p. 237). These minimal utterances can only be incorporated into the decision when interpreted in a responsible manner. When the patient's wishes have not been expressed, greater emphasis is placed on the significance of the individual indication. The "best respect" standard and a decision according to the sequence of steps in this model allow respect when a decision places excessive demands on all those participating. Thus, it aims to ease the burden by replacing the wishes not expressed by the patient with greater emphasis on the medical indication or nonindication, as required in the individual situation in decision-making processes, without disregarding or crossing legally established boundaries. In such delicate situations, there is a need not only for medical knowledge, but also for a discerning and keen insight into matters of ethical responsibility (Nacimiento et al. 2007).

◾ Summary

The treatment options available for stroke patients have increased considerably during the past few years. Patients experiencing severe strokes now have greater chances of survival thanks to various advances in emergency and intensive care medicine, as well as through improved medical or interventional therapy. In such cases, the aim of complete recovery is not always achieved; often, severely limited motor function or a reduced level of consciousness is the outcome. Whether keeping a patient alive at any price can or must represent the aim of medical treatment, and whether the patient can or should pay this price, is the subject of individual as well as public discussion. Decisions that balance the alternatives and options are necessary as part of the treatment process—decisions made by patients and physicians alike. This requires not only certain capabilities and a certain amount of willingness in all participants involved in the treatment, but also support and a well-developed moral compass. The need for an ethical approach increases with the number of options available for further action, whether in one individual or on a wider social scale.

Medical decisions are principally made on the basis of a professionally secured indication. After being properly informed, the patient or the patient's proxy either agrees to the treatment procedure suggested by the attending physician or rejects it. Strongly diverging views may be observed in the assessment of neurological damage. These differing points of view are present in physicians as well as in patients and represent an absolute limit in terms of human cognitive abilities. It should therefore come as no surprise that the medical–professional recommendations are equally heterogeneous.

The patient's wishes may dictate further treatment; however, people with severe cerebral damage can communicate their individual wishes only to a limited degree. Although it is true that the patient's wishes can be anticipated and determined accordingly, such a determination still requires confronting the possible existential significance of the decision.

Against this background, it becomes clear that neither a medical indication nor a statement of the patient's wishes can exist without confronting the individual situation or by adapting the theoretical possibilities and general wishes to it. Such an adaptation can only be made by including everyone who is involved in the treatment and medical attendance of the affected patient and on as wide a scale as possible. These individuals must be qualified to make decisions. Only the development of a specific procedure makes it possible to characterize the levels and incorporate perspectives into single steps that are understandable to everyone. Depending on the medical urgency of the situation, the people representing the different perspectives have to be involved directly in the process; in cases of high urgency and acute conditions, these levels (see Decision Model–Levels, p. 160), at least, must be considered. The physician is responsible for the decision, which is also shared by all participating members. This method places a high demand on each participant's ability to communicate. The existence of necessary communication skills cannot always be assumed, however, so graded external support options must also be introduced, if needed. This support system is designed to support the actors in making a responsible decision. The consideration of the treatment decision is therefore understood as a communicative process in which even minimal participation options on the part of the patient are accepted and incorporated. Accordingly, the legal authorization of treatment decisions, or even complete judicial clarification, is necessary only as a last resort in cases of actual dissent. The discussion space that arises from this procedure is sufficiently private for individual decisions, but it also remains transparent enough to prevent misuse.

Patients with severe cerebral damage following stroke require intensive therapy, which may be of a life-prolonging or life-sustaining nature. The treatment of these patients cannot, however, be determined by generally binding guidelines. Patients with severe brain damage are still alive, so life-sustaining therapy may prove necessary. Likewise, such brain-damaged patients can be, or become, dying patients who require palliative care. The difficulties relating to the assessment of the dying process, as well as the associated consequences in the nursing and therapeutic areas, can be discussed in the virtual space for discussion and decision-making.

The use of modern treatment options for stroke patients preserves opportunities; limitations involve the necessary acceptance of a patient's mortality. Here it is not a question of terminating therapeutic measures or even inducing the death process, but, rather, of actively alleviating symptoms and providing moral support.

"I would venture to claim that the entire fate of medicine depends on the ability of physicians to keep a straight course between the deceptive and rocky 'cliffs' of terminal care on the one hand, and deliberate and unnecessary treatment procedures on the other" (Herranz 1994, p. 216).

References

Chapter 1

Ada L, Vattanasilp W, O'Dwyer NJ, Crosbie J. Does spasticity contribute to walking dysfunction after stroke? J Neurol Neurosurg Psychiatry. 1998;64(5):628–635

Anderson CS, Carter KN, Brownlee WJ, Hackett ML, Broad JB, Bonita R. Very long-term outcome after stroke in Auckland, New Zealand. Stroke. 2004;35(8):1920–1924

Appelros P, Nydevik I, Viitanen M. Poor outcome after first-ever stroke: predictors for death, dependency, and recurrent stroke within the first year. Stroke. 2003;34(1):122–126

Barbeau H, Fung J. The role of rehabilitation in the recovery of walking in the neurological population. Curr Opin Neurol. 2001;14(6):735–740

Beck AT, Ward CH, Mendelson M, Mock J, Erbaugh J. An inventory for measuring depression. Arch Gen Psychiatry. 1961;4:561–571

Bobath B. Treatment of adult hemiplegia. Physiotherapy. 1977;63(10):310–313

Bohannon RW, Andrews AW, Smith MB. Rehabilitation goals of patients with hemiplegia. Int J Rehabil Res. 1988;11:181–183

Bonita R, Solomon N, Broad JB. Prevalence of stroke and stroke-related disability. Estimates from the Auckland stroke studies. Stroke. 1997;28(10):1898–1902

Brunnstrom S. Walking Preparation for Adult Patients with Hemiplegia. Phys Ther. 1965;45:17–29

Carandang R, Seshadri S, Beiser A, et al. Trends in incidence, lifetime risk, severity, and 30-day mortality of stroke over the past 50 years. JAMA. 2006;296(24):2939–2946

Carr J, Shepherd R. Neurological Rehabilitation: Optimising Motor Performance. Oxford: Butterworth Heinemann; 1998

Carr J, Shepherd R. Stroke Rehabilitation: Guidelines for Exercises and Training. London: Butterworth Heinemann; 2003

Charlson ME, Pompei P, Ales KL, MacKenzie CR. A new method of classifying prognostic comorbidity in longitudinal studies: development and validation. J Chronic Dis. 1987;40(5):373–383

Counsell C, Dennis M, McDowall M. Predicting functional outcome in acute stroke: comparison of a simple six variable model with other predictive systems and informal clinical prediction. J Neurol Neurosurg Psychiatry. 2004;75(3):401–405

Davidoff GN, Keren O, Ring H, Solzi P. Acute stroke patients: long-term effects of rehabilitation and maintenance of gains. Arch Phys Med Rehabil. 1991;72(11):869–873

Desrosiers J, Bourbonnais D, Noreau L, Rochette A, Bravo G, Bourget A. Participation after stroke compared to normal aging. J Rehabil Med. 2005a;37(6):353–357

Desrosiers J, Rochette A, Corriveau H. Validation of a new lower-extremity motor coordination test. Arch Phys Med Rehabil. 2005b;86(5):993–998

Desrosiers J, Noreau L, Rochette A, Bourbonnais D, Bravo G, Bourget A. Predictors of long-term participation after stroke. Disabil Rehabil. 2006;28(4):221–230

Dobkin BH, Firestine A, West M, Saremi K, Woods R. Ankle dorsiflexion as an fMRI paradigm to assay motor control for walking during rehabilitation. Neuroimage. 2004;23(1):370–381

Duncan PW, Horner RD, Reker DM, et al. Adherence to post-acute rehabilitation guidelines is associated with functional recovery in stroke. Stroke. 2002;33(1):167–177

Eich HJ, Mach H, Werner C, Hesse S. Aerobic treadmill plus Bobath walking training improves walking in subacute stroke: a randomized controlled trial. Clin Rehabil. 2004;18(6):640–651

El-Saed A, Kuller LH, Newman AB, et al. Geographic variations in stroke incidence and mortality among older populations in four US communities. Stroke. 2006;37(8):1975–1979

Foerster O. Die Therapie der Motilitätsstörungen bei den Erkrankungen des Zentralnervensystems. In: Vogt H, ed. Handbuch der Therapie der Nervenkrankheiten. Vol.2. Jena: Gustav Fischer; 1916:860–944

Foley NC, Teasell RW, Bhogal SK, Speechley MR. Stroke rehabilitation evidence-based review: methodology. Top Stroke Rehabil. 2003;10(1):1–7

Goldie PA, Matyas TA, Evans OM. Deficit and change in gait velocity during rehabilitation after stroke. Arch Phys Med Rehabil. 1996;77(10):1074–1082

Goldstein LB, Bertels C, Davis JN. Interrater reliability of the NIH stroke scale. Arch Neurol. 1989;46(6):660–662

Gresham GE, Fitzpatrick TE, Wolf PA, McNamara PM, Kannel WB, Dawber TR. Residual disability in survivors of stroke —the Framingham study. N Engl J Med. 1975;293(19):954–956

Gresham GE, Kelly-Hayes M, Wolf PA, Beiser AS, Kase CS, D'Agostino RB. Survival and functional status 20 or more years after first stroke: the Framingham Study. Stroke. 1998;29(4):793–797

Hackett ML, Duncan JR, Anderson CS, Broad JB, Bonita R. Health-related quality of life among long-term survivors of stroke : results from the Auckland Stroke Study, 1991–1992. Stroke. 2000;31(2):440–447

Hankey GJ, Jamrozik K, Broadhurst RJ, Forbes S, Anderson CS. Long-term disability after first-ever stroke and related prognostic factors in the Perth Community Stroke Study, 1989-1990. Stroke. 2002;33(4):1034–1040

Hardie K, Hankey GJ, Jamrozik K, Broadhurst RJ, Anderson C. Ten-year risk of first recurrent stroke and disability after first-ever stroke in the Perth Community Stroke Study. Stroke. 2004;35(3):731–735

Hendricks HT, van Limbeek J, Geurts AC, Zwarts MJ. Motor recovery after stroke: a systematic review of the literature. Arch Phys Med Rehabil. 2002;83(11):1629–1637

Hesse S, Staats M, Werner C, Bestmann A, Lingnau ML. [Ambulatory rehabilitation exercises for stroke patients at home. Preliminary results of scope, methods and effectiveness]. Nervenarzt. 2001;72(12):950–954

Hesse S, Schmidt H, Werner C, Bardeleben A. Upper and lower extremity robotic devices for rehabilitation and for studying motor control. Curr Opin Neurol. 2003;16 (6):705–710

Hochstenbach J, Prigatano G, Mulder T. Patients' and relatives' reports of disturbances 9 months after stroke: subjective changes in physical functioning, cognition, emotion, and behavior. Arch Phys Med Rehabil. 2005;86 (8):1587–1593

Indredavik B, Bakke F, Slordahl SA, Rokseth R, Hâheim LL. Stroke unit treatment. 10-year follow-up. Stroke. 1999;30(8):1524–1527

Indredavik B, Rohweder G, Naalsund E, Lydersen S. Medical complications in a comprehensive stroke unit and an early supported discharge service. Stroke. 2008;39 (2):414–420

Jönsson AC, Lindgren I, Hallström B, Norrving B, Lindgren A. Prevalence and intensity of pain after stroke: a population based study focusing on patients' perspectives. J Neurol Neurosurg Psychiatry. 2006;77(5):590–595

Jørgensen HS, Nakayama H, Raaschou HO, Olsen TS. Recovery of walking function in stroke patients: the Copenhagen Stroke Study. Arch Phys Med Rehabil. 1995;76 (1):27–32

Kauhanen M, Korpelainen JT, Hiltunen P, et al. Poststroke depression correlates with cognitive impairment and neurological deficits. Stroke. 1999;30(9):1875–1880

Kollen B, van de Port I, Lindeman E, Twisk J, Kwakkel G. Predicting improvement in gait after stroke: a longitudinal prospective study. Stroke. 2005;36(12):2676–2680

Kollen B, Kwakkel G, Lindeman E. Longitudinal robustness of variables predicting independent gait following severe middle cerebral artery stroke: a prospective cohort study. Clin Rehabil. 2006;20(3):262–268

Kolominsky-Rabas PL, Heuschmann PU. Incidence, etiology and long-term prognosis of stroke. [Article in German] Fortschr Neurol Psychiatr. 2002;70(12):657–662

Kolominsky-Rabas PL, Heuschmann PU, Marschall D, et al. Lifetime cost of ischemic stroke in Germany: results and national projections from a population-based stroke registry: the Erlangen Stroke Project. Stroke. 2006;37 (5):1179–1183

Kosak MC, Reding MJ. Comparison of partial body weight-supported treadmill gait training versus aggressive bracing assisted walking post stroke. Neurorehabil Neural Repair. 2000;14(1):13–19

Kuo HK, Leveille SG, Yen CJ, et al. Exploring how peak leg power and usual gait speed are linked to late-life disability: data from the National Health and Nutrition Examination Survey (NHANES), 1999-2002. Am J Phys Med Rehabil. 2006;85(8):650–658

Kwakkel G, Wagenaar RC, Twisk JW, Lankhorst GJ, Koetsier JC. Intensity of leg and arm training after primary middle-cerebral-artery stroke: a randomised trial. Lancet. 1999;354(9174):191–196

Kwakkel G, Kollen BJ, Wagenaar RC. Long term effects of intensity of upper and lower limb training after stroke: a randomised trial. J Neurol Neurosurg Psychiatry. 2002;72(4):473–479

Kwakkel G, Kollen B, Lindeman E. Understanding the pattern of functional recovery after stroke: facts and theories. Restor Neurol Neurosci. 2004;22(3-5):281–299

Langhammer B, Stanghelle JK. Bobath or motor relearning programme? A comparison of two different approaches of physiotherapy in stroke rehabilitation: a randomized controlled study. Clin Rehabil. 2000;14(4):361–369

Langhammer B, Stanghelle JK. Bobath or motor relearning programme? A follow-up one and four years post stroke. Clin Rehabil. 2003;17(7):731–734

Langhorne P, Taylor G, Murray G, et al. Early supported discharge services for stroke patients: a meta-analysis of individual patients' data. Lancet. 2005;365 (9458):501–506

Larsen T, Olsen TS, Sorensen J. Early home-supported discharge of stroke patients: a health technology assessment. Int J Technol Assess Health Care. 2006;22 (3):313–320

Lichtenstein AH, Appel LJ, Brands M, et al; American Heart Association Nutrition Committee. Diet and lifestyle recommendations revision 2006: a scientific statement from the American Heart Association Nutrition Committee. Circulation. 2006;114(1):82–96

Lierse M, Breckenkamp J, Wingendorf I, Laaser U. Morbiditäts- und Mortalitätsraten des Schlaganfalls in Deutschland: Eine bevölkerungsbezogene Szenarioanalyse. Akt Neurol. 2005;32:136–142

Lindmark B, Hamrin E. A five-year follow-up of stroke survivors: motor function and activities of daily living. Clin Rehabil. 1995;9:1–9

Lloyd-Jones D, Adams RJ, Brown TM, et al; Writing Group Members; American Heart Association Statistics Committee and Stroke Statistics Subcommittee. Heart disease and stroke statistics—2010 update: a report from the American Heart Association. Circulation. 2010;121(7):e46–e215

Luft AR, Waller S, Forrester L, et al. Lesion location alters brain activation in chronically impaired stroke survivors. Neuroimage. 2004;21(3):924–935

Luft AR, Forrester L, Macko RF, et al. Brain activation of lower extremity movement in chronically impaired stroke survivors. Neuroimage. 2005;26(1):184–194

MacKay-Lyons M. Central pattern generation of locomotion: a review of the evidence. Phys Ther. 2002;82 (1):69–83

Macko RF, Ivey FM, Forrester LW. Task-oriented aerobic exercise in chronic hemiparetic stroke: training protocols and treatment effects. Top Stroke Rehabil. 2005a;12 (1):45–57

Macko RF, Ivey FM, Forrester LW, et al. Treadmill exercise rehabilitation improves ambulatory function and cardiovascular fitness in patients with chronic stroke: a randomized, controlled trial. Stroke. 2005b;36(10):2206–2211

Meek C, Pollock A, Potter J, Langhorne P. A systematic review of exercise trials post stroke. Clin Rehabil. 2003;17 (1):6–13

Mehrholz J, Pohl M. Aktuelle Konzepte zur Gangrehabilitation nach Schlaganfall. Z Physiother. 2005;57:2–9

Mehrholz J. Dissertationsschrift: Gehfähigkeit, Alltagskompetenz und Lebensqualität von Patienten nach Schlaganfall: Langzeitergebnisse einer randomisierten und kontrollierten Studie. Medizinische Fakultät; TU Dresden; 2007

Meijer R, Ihnenfeldt DS, de Groot IJ, van Limbeek J, Vermeulen M, de Haan RJ. Prognostic factors for ambulation and activities of daily living in the subacute phase after stroke. A systematic review of the literature. Clin Rehabil. 2003a;17(2):119–129

Meijer R, Ihnenfeldt DS, van Limbeek J, Vermeulen M, de Haan RJ. Prognostic factors in the subacute phase after stroke for the future residence after six months to one year. A systematic review of the literature. Clin Rehabil. 2003b;17(5):512–520

Moseley AM, Stark A, Cameron ID, Pollock A. Treadmill training and body weight support for walking after stroke. Cochrane Database Syst Rev. 2005;CD002840

Mumenthaler M. Zerebrovaskuläre Durchblutungsstörungen. In: Mattle H, ed. Neurologie. Vol.11. Stuttgart–New York: Thieme; 2002;131–219

Naess H, Waje-Andreassen U, Thomassen L, Nyland H, Myhr KM. Health-related quality of life among young adults with ischemic stroke on long-term follow-up. Stroke. 2006;37(5):1232–1236

National Center for Health Statistics. Health Data Interactive File, 1981–2006. Hyattsville, Md: National Center for Health Statistics. Available at: http://205207175.93/hdi/ReportFolders/ReportFolders

Newman AB, Simonsick EM, Naydeck BL, et al. Association of long-distance corridor walk performance with mortality, cardiovascular disease, mobility limitation, and disability. JAMA. 2006;295(17):2018–2026

Nilsson L, Carlsson J, Danielsson A, et al. Walking training of patients with hemiparesis at an early stage after stroke: a comparison of walking training on a treadmill with body weight support and walking training on the ground. Clin Rehabil. 2001;15(5):515–527

Norrving B, Adams RJ. Organized stroke care. Stroke. 2006;37(2):326–328

O'Mahony PG, Thomson RG, Dobson R, Rodgers H, James OF. The prevalence of stroke and associated disability. J Public Health Med. 1999;21(2):166–171

Patel MD, Tilling K, Lawrence E, Rudd AG, Wolfe CD, McKevitt C. Relationships between long-term stroke disability, handicap and health-related quality of life. Age Ageing. 2006;35(3):273–279

Paul SL, Sturm JW, Dewey HM, Donnan GA, Macdonell RA, Thrift AG. Long-term outcome in the North East Melbourne Stroke Incidence Study: predictors of quality of life at 5 years after stroke. Stroke. 2005;36(10):2082–2086

Pearson TA, Blair SN, Daniels SR, et al; American Heart Association Science Advisory and Coordinating Committee. AHA Guidelines for Primary Prevention of Cardiovascular Disease and Stroke: 2002 Update: Consensus Panel Guide to Comprehensive Risk Reduction for Adult Patients Without Coronary or Other Atherosclerotic Vascular Diseases. Circulation. 2002;106(3):388–391

Perry J, Garrett M, Gronley JK, Mulroy SJ. Classification of walking handicap in the stroke population. Stroke. 1995;26(6):982–989

Pettersen R, Dahl T, Wyller TB. Prediction of long-term functional outcome after stroke rehabilitation. Clin Rehabil. 2002;16(2):149–159

Pohl M, Mehrholz J, Rutte K, et al. Vergleich der aeroben Übungsintensität bei Patienten nach Schlaganfall—Gangtrainer versus konventionelle Therapie. Eine randomsierte und kontrollierte Longitudinalstudie: Erste Ergebnisse. Neurol Rehabil. 2003;9:S6–S7

Pohl M, Mehrholz J, Werner C. Hesse P. Vergleich der aeroben Übungsintensität bei Patienten nach Schlaganfall—Gangtrainer versus konventionelle Physiotherapie. Eine randomisierte und kontrollierte Longitudinalstudie. Neurol Rehabil. 2004;10:S27

Pohl M, Werner C, Holzgraefe M, et al. Repetitive locomotor training and physiotherapy improve walking and basic activities of daily living after stroke: a single-blind, randomized multicentre trial (DEutsche GAngtrainerStudie, DEGAS). Clin Rehabil. 2007;21(1):17–27

Prencipe M, Culasso F, Rasura M, et al. Long-term prognosis after a minor stroke: 10-year mortality and major stroke recurrence rates in a hospital-based cohort. Stroke. 1998;29(1):126–132

Rosamond WD, Folsom AR, Chambless LE, et al. Stroke incidence and survival among middle-aged adults: 9-year follow-up of the Atherosclerosis Risk in Communities (ARIC) cohort. Stroke. 1999;30(4):736–743

Rossouw JE, Prentice RL, Manson JE, et al. Postmenopausal hormone therapy and risk of cardiovascular disease by age and years since menopause. JAMA. 2007;297(13):1465–1477

Schiemanck SK, Kwakkel G, Post MW, Kappelle LJ, Prevo AJ. Predicting long-term independency in activities of daily living after middle cerebral artery stroke: does information from MRI have added predictive value compared with clinical information? Stroke. 2006;37(4):1050–1054

Scmidt EV, Smirnov VE, Ryabova VS. Results of the seven-year prospective study of stroke patients. Stroke. 1988;19(8):942–949

Seshadri S, Beiser A, Kelly-Hayes M, et al. The lifetime risk of stroke: estimates from the Framingham Study. Stroke. 2006;37(2):345–350

Singh R, Hunter J, Philip A, Todd I. Predicting those who will walk after rehabilitation in a specialist stroke unit. Clin Rehabil. 2006;20(2):149–152

Smith PM, Ottenbacher KJ, Cranley M, Dittmar SS, Illig SB, Granger CV. Predicting follow-up living setting in patients with stroke. Arch Phys Med Rehabil. 2002;83(6):764–770

Spieler JF, Amarenco P. [Socio-economic aspects of stroke management]. [Article in French] Rev Neurol (Paris). 2004;160(11):1023–1028

Spieler JF, Lanoë JL, Amarenco P. Costs of stroke care according to handicap levels and stroke subtypes. Cerebrovasc Dis. 2004;17(2-3):134–142

Steiner T, Mendoza G, De Georgia M, Schellinger P, Holle R, Hacke W. Prognosis of stroke patients requiring mechanical ventilation in a neurological critical care unit. Stroke. 1997;28(4):711–715

Stroke Unit Trialists' Collaboration. Organised in patient (stroke unit) care for stroke. Cochrane Database Syst Rev. 2007 Oct17;(4):CD 000197.

Sturm JW, Dewey HM, Donnan GA, Macdonell RA, McNeil JJ, Thrift AG. Handicap after stroke: how does it relate to disability, perception of recovery, and stroke subtype?: the north North East Melbourne Stroke Incidence Study (NEMESIS). Stroke. 2002;33(3):762–768

Sturm JW, Donnan GA, Dewey HM, et al. Quality of life after stroke: the North East Melbourne Stroke Incidence Study (NEMESIS). Stroke. 2004a;35(10):2340–2345

Sturm JW, Donnan GA, Dewey HM, Macdonell RA, Gilligan AK, Thrift AG. Determinants of handicap after stroke: the North East Melbourne Stroke Incidence Study (NEMESIS). Stroke. 2004b;35(3):715–720

Taylor TN, Davis PH, Torner JC, Holmes J, Meyer JW, Jacobson MF. Lifetime cost of stroke in the United States. Stroke. 1996;27(9):1459–1466

Teasdale TW, Engberg AW. Psychosocial consequences of stroke: a long-term population-based follow-up. Brain Inj. 2005;19(12):1049–1058

Thom T, Haase N, Rosamond W, et al; American Heart Association Statistics Committee and Stroke Statistics Subcommittee. Heart disease and stroke statistics—2006 update: a report from the American Heart Association Statistics Committee and Stroke Statistics Subcommittee. Circulation. 2006;113(6):e85–e151

Thorngren M, Westling B, Norrving B. Outcome after stroke in patients discharged to independent living. Stroke. 1990;21(2):236–240

Truelsen T, Mähönen M, Tolonen H, Asplund K, Bonita R, Vanuzzo D; WHO MONICA Project. Trends in stroke and coronary heart disease in the WHO MONICA Project. Stroke. 2003;34(6):1346–1352

Tuomilehto J, Nuottimäki T, Salmi K, et al. Psychosocial and health status in stroke survivors after 14 years. Stroke. 1995;26(6):971–975

Twitchell TE. The restoration of motor function following hemiplegia in man. Brain. 1951;74(4):443–480

Ungern-Sternberg AV, Küthmann M, Weimann G. Stroke: evaluation of long-term rehabilitation effects. J Neural Transm Suppl. 1991;33:149–155

Van Peppen RP, Kwakkel G, Wood-Dauphinee S, Hendriks HJ, Van der Wees PJ, Dekker J. The impact of physical therapy on functional outcomes after stroke: what's the evidence? Clin Rehabil. 2004;18(8):833–862

van Swieten JC, Koudstaal PJ, Visser MC, Schouten HJ, van Gijn J. Interobserver agreement for the assessment of handicap in stroke patients. Stroke. 1988;19(5):604–607

van Vliet PM, Lincoln NB, Robinson E. Comparison of the content of two physiotherapy approaches for stroke. Clin Rehabil. 2001;15(4):398–414

van Wijk I, Kappelle LJ, van Gijn J, et al; LiLAC study group. Long-term survival and vascular event risk after transient ischaemic attack or minor ischaemic stroke: a cohort study. Lancet. 2005;365(9477):2098–2104

Viitanen M, Eriksson S, Asplund K. Risk of recurrent stroke, myocardial infarction and epilepsy during long-term follow-up after stroke. Eur Neurol. 1988;28(4):227–231

Visintin M, Barbeau H, Korner-Bitensky N, Mayo NE. A new approach to retrain gait in stroke patients through body weight support and treadmill stimulation. Stroke. 1998;29(6):1122–1128

Vogel J. [5 years follow-up study of stroke patients over 65 years of age]. [Article in German] Rehabilitation (Stuttg). 1994;33(3):155–157

Wade DT. Neurologic rehabilitation. Curr Opin Neurol. 1993;6(5):753–755

Werner C, Von Frankenberg S, Treig T, Konrad M, Hesse S. Treadmill training with partial body weight support and an electromechanical gait trainer for restoration of gait in subacute stroke patients: a randomized crossover study. Stroke. 2002;33(12):2895–2901

Wilkinson PR, Wolfe CD, Warburton FG, et al. A long-term follow-up of stroke patients. Stroke. 1997;28(3):507–512

Further Reading

Diener H, Hacke W. Leitlinien für Diagnostik und Therapie in der Neurologie. Stuttgart: Thieme; 2002

Kolominsky-Rabas P, Heuschmann P, Neundörfer B. Epidemiologie des Schlaganfalls. ZFA. 2002;78:494–500

Langhorne P, Duncan P. Does the organization of postacute stroke care really matter? Stroke. 2001;32(1):268–274

Mehrholz J, Werner C, Hesse S, Pohl M. Immediate and long-term functional impact of repetitive locomotor training as an adjunct to conventional physiotherapy for non-ambulatory patients after stroke. Disabil Rehabil. 2008;30(11):830–836

Rosamond W, Flegal K, Friday G, et al; American Heart Association Statistics Committee and Stroke Statistics Subcommittee. Heart disease and stroke statistics—2007 update: a report from the American Heart Association Statistics Committee and Stroke Statistics Subcommittee. Circulation. 2007;115(5):e69–e171

Chapter 2

Dressel A, Kessler C. Primärversorgung von Schlaganfallpatienten. Der Notarzt. 2003;19:1–6

Koennecke H, Brandt T, Bjarnason-Wehrens B, Willemsen D, Witt T, Gysan D. Umsetzungsempfehlungen von Leitlinien nach TIA/Schlaganfall für die kardiologische Rehabilitation. Deutsche Gesellschaft für Prävention und Rehabilitation von Herz-Kreislauferkrankungen, 2005

Chapter 3

Albers GW, Amarenco P, Easton JD, Sacco RL, Teal P. Antithrombotic and thrombolytic therapy for ischemic stroke: the Seventh ACCP Conference on Antithrombotic and Thrombolytic Therapy. Chest. 2004;126(3, Suppl) 483S–512S

Alexandrov AV, Molina CA, Grotta JC, et al; CLOTBUST Investigators. Ultrasound-enhanced systemic thrombolysis for acute ischemic stroke. N Engl J Med. 2004;351 (21):2170–2178

Audebert HJ, Schenkel J, Heuschmann PU, Bogdahn U, Haberl RL; Telemedic Pilot Project for Integrative Stroke Care Group. Effects of the implementation of a telemedical stroke network: the telemedic pilot project for integrative stroke care (TEMPiS) in Bavaria, Germany. Lancet Neurol. 2006;5(9):742–748

Barber PA, Zhang J, Demchuk AM, Hill MD, Buchan AM. Why are stroke patients excluded from TPA therapy? An analysis of patient eligibility. Neurology. 2001;56 (8):1015–1020

Broderick JP, Brott TG, Duldner JE, Tomsick T, Huster G. Volume of intracerebral hemorrhage. A powerful and easy-to-use predictor of 30-day mortality. Stroke. 1993;24 (7):987–993

Brott T, Broderick J, Kothari R, et al. Early hemorrhage growth in patients with intracerebral hemorrhage. Stroke. 1997;28(1):1–5

Bruno A, Biller J, Adams HP Jr, et al, for the Trial of ORG in Acute Stroke Treatment (TOAST) Investigators. Acute blood glucose level and outcome from ischemic stroke. Trial of ORG 10172 in Acute Stroke Treatment (TOAST) Investigators. Neurology. 1999;52(2):280–284

California Acute Stroke Pilot Registry (CASPR) Investigators. Prioritizing interventions to improve rates of thrombolysis for ischemic stroke. Neurology. 2005;64:654–659

Candelise L, Gattinoni M, Bersano A, Micieli G, Sterzi R, Morabito A; PROSIT Study Group. Stroke-unit care for acute stroke patients: an observational follow-up study. Lancet. 2007;369(9558):299–305

Capes SE, Hunt D, Malmberg K, Pathak P, Gerstein HC. Stress hyperglycemia and prognosis of stroke in nondiabetic and diabetic patients: a systematic overview. Stroke. 2001;32(10):2426–2432

Chimowitz MI, Lynn MJ, Howlett-Smith H, et al; Warfarin-Aspirin Symptomatic Intracranial Disease Trial Investigators. Comparison of warfarin and aspirin for symptomatic intracranial arterial stenosis. N Engl J Med. 2005;352 (13):1305–1316

del Zoppo GJ, Higashida RT, Furlan AJ, Pessin MS, Rowley HA, Gent M. PROACT: a phase II randomized trial of recombinant pro-urokinase by direct arterial delivery in acute middle cerebral artery stroke. PROACT Investigators. Prolyse in Acute Cerebral Thromboembolism. Stroke. 1998;29(1):4–11

Diener HC, Aichner F, Bode C, et al. Primär und Sekundärprävention der zerebralen Ischämie. In: Diener HC, Putzki N; Kommission Leitlinien der Deutschen Gesellschaft für Neurologie (ed). Leitlinien für Diagnostik und Therapie in der Neurologie. Stuttgart–New York: Thieme; 2008

Eames PJ, Blake MJ, Dawson SL, Panerai RB, Potter JF. Dynamic cerebral autoregulation and beat to beat blood pressure control are impaired in acute ischaemic stroke. J Neurol Neurosurg Psychiatry. 2002;72(4):467–472

European Stroke Organization (ESO) Executive Committee and the ESO Writing Committee. Guidelines for Management of Ischaemic Stroke and Transient Ischaemic Attack 2008—update January 2009. www.eso-stroke.org

Ferro JM, Correia M, Rosas MJ, Pinto AN, Neves G; Cerebral Venous Thrombosis Portuguese Collaborative Study Group [Venoport]. Seizures in cerebral vein and dural sinus thrombosis. Cerebrovasc Dis. 2003;15(1-2):78–83

Furlan A, Higashida R, Wechsler L, et al, for the PROACT investigators. Intra-arterial prourokinase for acute ischemic stroke. The PROACT II study: a randomized controlled trial. Prolyse in Acute Cerebral Thromboembolism. JAMA. 1999;282(21):2003–2011

Gebel JM Jr, Jauch EC, Brott TG, et al. Relative edema volume is a predictor of outcome in patients with hyperacute spontaneous intracerebral hemorrhage. Stroke. 2002;33 (11):2636–2641

Georgiadis D, Schwarz S, Aschoff A, Schwab S. Hemicraniectomy and moderate hypothermia in patients with severe ischemic stroke. Stroke. 2002;33(6):1584–1588

Georgilis K, Plomaritoglou A, Dafni U, Bassiakos Y, Vemmos K. Aetiology of fever in patients with acute stroke. J Intern Med. 1999;246(2):203–209

Grond M. Spezifische Akuttherapie. In: Diener HC, Busch E, Grond M, Busse O. Stroke Unit Manual. Stuttgart–New York: Thieme; 2005

Haberl R, Aichner F, Baumgartner R, Forsting M, Villringer A. Hirnvenen- und Sinusthrombose. In: Diener HC, Putzki N; Kommission Leitlinien der Deutschen Gesellschaft für Neurologie (ed.). Leitlinien für Diagnostik und Therapie in der Neurologie. Stuttgart, New York: Thieme; 2008

Hacke W, Schwab S, Horn M, Spranger M, De Georgia M, von Kummer R. "Malignant" middle cerebral artery territory infarction: clinical course and prognostic signs. Arch Neurol. 1996;53(4):309–315

Hacke W, Brott T, Caplan L, et al. Thrombolysis in acute ischemic stroke: controlled trials and clinical experience. Neurology. 1999;53(Suppl 4):S3–14

Hacke W, Donnan G, Fieschi C, et al; ATLANTIS Trials Investigators; ECASS Trials Investigators; NINDS rt-PA Study Group Investigators. Association of outcome with early stroke treatment: pooled analysis of ATLANTIS, ECASS, and NINDS rt-PA stroke trials. Lancet. 2004;363 (9411):768–774

Hacke W, Aichner F, Bode C, et al. Akuttherapie des ischämischen Schlaganfalls. In: Diener HC, Putzki N; Kommission Leitlinien der Deutschen Gesellschaft für Neurologie (ed). Leitlinien für Diagnostik und Therapie in der Neurologie. Stuttgart–New York: Thieme; 2008a

Hacke W, Kaste M, Bluhmki E, et al; ECASS Investigators. Thrombolysis with alteplase 3 to 4.5 hours after acute ischemic stroke. N Engl J Med. 2008b;359(13):1317–1329

Hajat C, Hajat S, Sharma P. Effects of poststroke pyrexia on stroke outcome : a meta-analysis of studies in patients. Stroke. 2000;31(2):410–414

Harper G, Castleden CM, Potter JF. Factors affecting changes in blood pressure after acute stroke. Stroke. 1994;25 (9):1726–1729

IMS Study Investigators. Combined intravenous and intra-arterial recanalization for acute ischemic stroke: the Interventional Management of Stroke Study. Stroke. 2004;35(4):904–911

James P, Ellis CJ, Whitlock RML, McNeil AR, Henley J, Anderson NE. Relation between troponin T concentration and mortality in patients presenting with an acute stroke: observational study. BMJ. 2000;320(7248):1502–1504

Jansen PAF, Schulte BPM, Poels EFJ, Gribnau FWJ. Course of blood pressure after cerebral infarction and transient ischemic attack. Clin Neurol Neurosurg. 1987;89 (4):243–246

Kern R, Ringleb PA, Hacke W, Mas JL, Hennerici MG. Stenting for carotid artery stenosis. Nat Clin Pract Neurol. 2007;3(4):212–220

Köhrmann M, Jüttler E, Fiebach JB, et al. MRI versus CT-based thrombolysis treatment within and beyond the 3h time window after stroke onset: a cohort study. Lancet Neurol. 2006;5(8):661–667

Lane RD, Wallace JD, Petrosky PP, Schwartz GE, Gradman AH. Supraventricular tachycardia in patients with right hemisphere strokes. Stroke. 1992;23(3):362–366

Langhorne P; Stroke Unit Trialists Collaboration. How do stroke units improve patient outcomes? A collaborative systematic review of the randomized trials. Stroke. 1997;28(11):2139–2144

Leigh R, Zaidat OO, Suri MF, et al. Predictors of hyperacute clinical worsening in ischemic stroke patients receiving thrombolytic therapy. Stroke. 2004;35(8):1903–1907

Leonardi-Bee J, Bath PMW, Phillips SJ, Sandercock PAG; IST Collaborative Group. Blood pressure and clinical outcomes in the International Stroke Trial. Stroke. 2002;33 (5):1315–1320

Lindsberg PJ, Mattle HP. Therapy of basilar artery occlusion: a systematic analysis comparing intra-arterial and intravenous thrombolysis. Stroke. 2006;37(3):922–928

Lynch JR, Wang H, McGirt MJ, et al. Simvastatin reduces vasospasm after aneurysmal subarachnoid hemorrhage: results of a pilot randomized clinical trial. Stroke. 2005;36(9):2024–2026

Mayer SA, Chong JY. Critical care management of increased intracranial pressure. J Intensive Care Med. 2002;17:55–67

Mayer SA, Brun NC, Begtrup K, et al; Recombinant Activated Factor VII Intracerebral Hemorrhage Trial Investigators. Recombinant activated factor VII for acute intracerebral hemorrhage. N Engl J Med. 2005;352(8):777–785

Mayer SA, Brun NC, Begtrup K, et al; FAST Trial Investigators. Efficacy and safety of recombinant activated factor VII for acute intracerebral hemorrhage. N Engl J Med. 2008;358(20):2127–2137

Mendelow AD, Gregson BA, Fernandes HM, et al; STICH investigators. Early surgery versus initial conservative treatment in patients with spontaneous supratentorial intracerebral haematomas in the International Surgical Trial in Intracerebral Haemorrhage (STICH): a randomised trial. Lancet. 2005;365(9457):387–397

Moraine JJ, Berré J, Mélot C. Is cerebral perfusion pressure a major determinant of cerebral blood flow during head elevation in comatose patients with severe intracranial lesions? J Neurosurg. 2000;92(4):606–614

National Institute of Neurological Disorders and Stroke rt-PA Stroke Study Group. Tissue plasminogen activator for acute ischemic stroke. N Engl J Med. 1995;333(24):1581–1587

Nedeltchev K, Schwegler B, Haefeli T, et al. Outcome of stroke with mild or rapidly improving symptoms. Stroke. 2007;38(9):2531–2535

Nelles G, Busse O. Basistherapie auf der Stroke Unit. In: Diener HC, Busch E, Grond M, Busse O. Stroke Unit Manual. Stuttgart–New York: Thieme; 2005

NIH Stroke Scale [in German]. Ingelheim am Rhein: Boehringer Ingelheim Pharma KG (ed). 1998

Reeves MJ, Arora S, Broderick JP, et al; Paul Coverdell Prototype Registries Writing Group. Acute stroke care in the US: results from 4 pilot prototypes of the Paul Coverdell National Acute Stroke Registry. Stroke. 2005;36(6):1232–1240

Reith J, Jørgensen HS, Pedersen PM, et al. Body temperature in acute stroke: relation to stroke severity, infarct size, mortality, and outcome. Lancet. 1996;347(8999):422–425

Ringelstein EB, Arnold M, Dittrich R, Fazekas F, Sitzer M. Dissektion hirnversorgender supraaortaler Arterien. In: Diener HC, Putzki N; Kommission Leitlinien der Deutschen Gesellschaft für Neurologie (ed). Leitlinien für Diagnostik und Therapie in der Neurologie. Stuttgart–New York: Thieme; 2008

Ringleb PA, Bertram M, Keller E, Hacke W. Hypertension in patients with cerebrovascular accident. To treat or not to treat? Nephrol Dial Transplant. 1998;13(9):2179–2181

Rothwell PM, Eliasziw M, Gutnikov SA, Warlow CP, Barnett HJM; Carotid Endarterectomy Trialists Collaboration. Endarterectomy for symptomatic carotid stenosis in relation to clinical subgroups and timing of surgery. Lancet. 2004;363(9413):915–924

Saver JL. Time is brain—quantified. Stroke. 2006;37(1):263–266

Schellinger PD, Fiebach JB, Hoffmann K, et al. Stroke MRI in intracerebral hemorrhage: is there a perihemorrhagic penumbra? Stroke. 2003;34(7):1674–1679

Schenkel J, Weimar C, Knoll T, et al; German Stroke Data Bank Collaborators. R1—systemic thrombolysis in German stroke units—the experience from the German Stroke data bank. J Neurol. 2003;250(3):320–324

Schwab S, Georgiadis D, Berrouschot J, Schellinger PD, Graffagnino C, Mayer SA. Feasibility and safety of moderate hypothermia after massive hemispheric infarction. Stroke. 2001;32(9):2033–2035

Schwarz S, Georgiadis D, Aschoff A, Schwab S. Effects of body position on intracranial pressure and cerebral perfusion in patients with large hemispheric stroke. Stroke. 2002;33(2):497–501

Scott JF, Robinson GM, French JM, O'Connell JE, Alberti KGMM, Gray CS. Prevalence of admission hyperglycaemia across clinical subtypes of acute stroke. Lancet. 1999;353(9150):376–377

Shaw CM, Alvord EC Jr, Berry RG. Swelling of the brain following ischemic infarction with arterial occlusion. Arch Neurol. 1959;1:161–177

Steiner T, Kaste M, Forsting M, et al; The European Stroke Initiative Writing Committee and the Writing Committee for the EUSI Executive Committee. Recommendations for the management of intracranial haemorrhage—part I: spontaneous intracerebral haemorrhage. Cerebrovasc Dis. 2006;22(4):294–316

Steiner T, Dichgans M, Forsting M, Hamann G, Schwab S. Intrazerebrale Blutungen. In: Diener HC, Putzki N; Kommission Leitlinien der Deutschen Gesellschaft für Neurologie (ed). Leitlinien für Diagnostik und Therapie in der Neurologie. Stuttgart–New York: Thieme; 2008

Steinmetz H, Berkefeld J, Forsting M, et al. Aneurysmale Subarachnoidalblutung. In: Diener HC, Putzki N; Kommission Leitlinien der Deutschen Gesellschaft für Neurologie (ed). Leitlinien für Diagnostik und Therapie in der Neurologie. Stuttgart–New York: Thieme; 2008

Sulter G, Elting JW, Langedijk M, Maurits NM, De Keyser J. Admitting acute ischemic stroke patients to a stroke care monitoring unit versus a conventional stroke unit: a randomized pilot study. Stroke. 2003;34(1):101–104

Szabo K, Lanczik O, Hennerici MG. Vascular diagnosis and acute stroke: what, when and why not? Cerebrovasc Dis. 2005;20(Suppl 2):11–18

Tomura N, Uemura K, Inugami A, Fujita H, Higano S, Shishido F. Early CT finding in cerebral infarction: obscuration of the lentiform nucleus. Radiology. 1988;168(2):463–467

Vahedi K, Hofmeijer J, Juettler E, et al; DECIMAL, DESTINY, and HAMLET investigators. Early decompressive surgery in malignant infarction of the middle cerebral artery: a pooled analysis of three randomised controlled trials. Lancet Neurol. 2007;6(3):215–222

Vespa PM, O'Phelan K, Shah M, et al. Acute seizures after intracerebral hemorrhage: a factor in progressive midline shift and outcome. Neurology. 2003;60(9):1441–1446

Vingerhoets F, Bogousslavsky J, Regli F, Van Melle G. Atrial fibrillation after acute stroke. Stroke. 1993;24(1):26–30

von Kummer R, Meyding-Lamadé U, Forsting M, et al. Sensitivity and prognostic value of early CT in occlusion of the middle cerebral artery trunk. AJNR Am J Neuroradiol. 1994;15(1):9–15, discussion 16–18

von Kummer R, Allen KL, Holle R, et al. Acute stroke: usefulness of early CT findings before thrombolytic therapy. Radiology. 1997;205(2):327–333

Wahlgren N, Ahmed N, Dávalos A, et al; SITS-MOST investigators. Thrombolysis with alteplase for acute ischaemic stroke in the Safe Implementation of Thrombolysis in Stroke-Monitoring Study (SITS-MOST): an observational study. Lancet. 2007;369(9558):275–282

Wardlaw JM, del Zoppo G, Yamaguchi T, Berge E. Thrombolysis for acute ischaemic stroke. Cochrane Database Syst Rev.. 2003: Issue 3

Williams LS, Rotich J, Qi R, et al. Effects of admission hyperglycemia on mortality and costs in acute ischemic stroke. Neurology. 2002;59(1):67–71

www.dsg-info.de

Further Reading

Olsen TS, Langhorne P, Diener HC, et al; European Stroke Initiative Executive Committee; EUSI Writing Committee. European Stroke Initiative Recommendations for Stroke Management—update 2003. Cerebrovasc Dis. 2003;16(4):311–337

www.dgn.org

Chapter 4

Barber M, Stott DJ, Langhorne P. An internationally agreed definition of progressing stroke. Cerebrovasc Dis. 2004;18(3):255–256, author reply 256–257

Bernhardt J, Dewey H, Thrift A, Donnan G. Inactive and alone: physical activity within the first 14 days of acute stroke unit care. Stroke. 2004;35(4):1005–1009

Bernhardt J, Chan J, Nicola I, Collier JM. Little therapy, little physical activity: rehabilitation within the first 14 days of organized stroke unit care. J Rehabil Med. 2007a;39(1):43–48

Bernhardt J, Indredavik B, Dewey H, et al. Mobilisation 'in bed' is not mobilisation. Cerebrovasc Dis. 2007b;24(1):157–158, author reply 159

Bernhardt J, Dewey H, Thrift A, Collier J, Donnan G. A very early rehabilitation trial for stroke (AVERT): phase II safety and feasibility. Stroke. 2008;39(2):390–396

Bernhardt J, Thuy MN, Collier JM, Legg LA. Very early versus delayed mobilisation after stroke. Cochrane Database Syst Rev. 2009; (1):CD006187

Borg G. Perceived exertion as an indicator of somatic stress. Scand J Rehabil Med. 1970;2(2):92–98

Carr JH, Shepherd RB. Stroke Rehabilitation. Guidelines for Exercise and Training to Optimize Motor Skill. Oxford: Butterworth Heinemann; 2003

Carr JH, Shepherd RB. Neurological Rehabilitation Optimizing Motor Performance. 2nd ed. Oxford: Butterworth Heinemann; 2010

de Haan R, Limburg M, Bossuyt P, van der Meulen J, Aaronson N. The clinical meaning of Rankin 'handicap' grades after stroke. Stroke. 1995;26(11):2027–2030

Indredavik B, Bakke F, Solberg R, Rokseth R, Haaheim LL, Holme I. Benefit of a stroke unit: a randomized controlled trial. Stroke. 1991;22(8):1026–1031

Indredavik B, Bakke F, Slørdahl SA, Rokseth R, Håheim LL. Treatment in a combined acute and rehabilitation stroke unit: which aspects are most important? Stroke. 1999;30(5):917–923

Langhorne P, Dennis M. Stroke Units: An Evidence Based Approach. London: BMJ Books; 1998

Lees K. Modified Rankin Scale: a Training and Certification Resource. Glasgow, Scotland: University Department of Medicine and Physics; 2003

Nudo RJ. Functional and structural plasticity in motor cortex: implications for stroke recovery. Phys Med Rehabil Clin N Am. 2003; **14**(1, Suppl)S57–S76

Schädler S, Beer S. Frühphase nach Schlaganfall: So früh wie möglich therapieren. Physiopraxis. 2007;5:24–27

Sinha S, Warburton EA. The evolution of stroke units-towards a more intensive approach? QJM. 2000;93(9):633–638

Stroke Unit Trialists Collaboration. How do stroke units improve patient outcomes? A collaborative systematic review of the randomized trials. Stroke. 1997;28(11):2139–2144

Stroke Unit Trialists' Collaboration. Organised inpatient (stroke unit) care for stroke. Cochrane Database Syst Rev. 2007; (4):CD000197

Chapter 5

Ada L, Foongchomcheay A. Efficacy of electrical stimulation in preventing or reducing subluxation of the shoulder after stroke: a meta-analysis. Aust J Physiother. 2002;48(4):257–267

Ada L, O'Dwyer N, Neilson PD. Improvement in kinematic characteristics and coordination following stroke quantified by linear systems analysis. Hum Mov Sci. 1993;12:137–153

Ada L, Canning C, Dwyer T. Effect of muscle length on strength and dexterity after stroke. Clin Rehabil. 2000;14(1):55–61

Ada L, Canning CG, Low S-L. Stroke patients have selective muscle weakness in shortened range. Brain. 2003;126(Pt 3):724–731

Ada L, Dean C, Mackey FH. Increasing the amount of physical activity undertaken after stroke. Phys Ther Rev. 2006a;11:91–100

Ada L, Dorsch S, Canning CG. Strengthening interventions increase strength and improve activity after stroke: a systematic review. Aust J Physiother. 2006b;52(4):241–248

Agahari I, Shepherd RB, Westwood PA. Comparative evaluation of lower limb forces in two variations of the step exercise in able-bodied subjects. In: Proceedings of 1st Australasian Biomechanics Conference, eds. M Lee, W Gilleard, P Sinclair, et al. Sydney, Australia, 1996; 94–95

Akeson WH, Amiel D, Abel MF, Garfin SR, Woo SL. Effects of immobilization on joints. Clin Orthop Relat Res. 1987;219:28–37

Alberts JL, Butler AJ, Wolf SL. The effects of constraint-induced therapy on precision grip: a preliminary study. Neurorehabil Neural Repair. 2004;18(4):250–258

Alibiglou L, Rymer WZ, Harvey RL, Mirbagheri MM. The relation between Ashworth scores and neuromechanical measurements of spasticity following stroke. J Neuroeng Rehabil. 2008;5:18

American College of Sports Medicine. Guidelines for Exercise Testing and Prescription. Baltimore: Williams and Wilkins; 2000

Anderson C, Laubscher S, Burns R. Validation of the Short Form 36 (SF-36) health survey questionnaire among stroke patients. Stroke. 1996;27(10):1812–1816

Andrews AW, Bohannon RW. Distribution of muscle strength impairments following stroke. Clin Rehabil. 2000;14(1):79–87

Annett J. Acquisition of skill. Br Med Bull. 1971;27(3):266–271

Arbib MA, Iberall T, Lyons D. Coordinated control programs for control of the hand. In: Goodwin AW, Darien-Smith I, eds. Hand Function and the Neocortex (Exp Brain Res Suppl 10), 1985; Berlin: Springer

Arendt-Nielsen L, Gantchev N, Sinkjaer T. The influence of muscle length on muscle fibre conduction velocity and development of muscle fatigue. Electroencephalogr Clin Neurophysiol. 1992;85(3):166–172

Ashworth B. Preliminary trial of carisoprodol in multiple sclerosis. Practitioner. 1964;192:540–542

Barbeau H, Visintin M. Optimal outcomes obtained with body-weight support combined with treadmill training in stroke subjects. Arch Phys Med Rehabil. 2003;84 (10):1458–1465

Barker RN, Brauer SG, Carson RG. Training of reaching in stroke survivors with severe and chronic upper limb paresis using a novel nonrobotic device: a randomized clinical trial. Stroke. 2008;39(6):1800–1807

Barreca S, Sigouin CS, Lambert C, Ansley B. Effects of extra training on the ability of stroke survivors to perform an independent sit-to-stand: a randomized controlled trial. J Geriatr Phys Ther. 2004;27:59–64

Belen'kiĭ VE, Gurfinkel' VS, Pal'tsev EI. [Control elements of voluntary movements]. Biofizika. 1967;12(1):135–141

Bendz P. The functional significance of the fifth metacarpus and hypothenar in two useful grips of the hand. Am J Phys Med Rehabil. 1993;72(4):210–213

Berg K, Wood-Dauphinee S, Williams JI, et al. Measuring balance in the elderly: preliminary development of an instrument. Physiother Can. 1989;41:304–311

Berg KO, Maki BE, Williams JI, Holliday PJ, Wood-Dauphinee SL. Clinical and laboratory measures of postural balance in an elderly population. Arch Phys Med Rehabil. 1992;73 (11):1073–1080

Bernhardt J, Hill K. We only treat what it occurs to us to assess: the importance of knowledge-based assessment. In: Refshauge K, et al, eds. Science-based Rehabilitation Theories in Practice. Oxford: Elsevier; 2005:5–48

Bernhardt J, Dewey H, Thrift A, Donnan G. Inactive and alone: physical activity within the first 14 days of acute stroke unit care. Stroke. 2004;35(4):1005–1009

Bernhardt J, Thuy MN, Collier JM, Legg LA. Very early versus delayed mobilisation after stroke. Cochrane Database Syst Rev. 2009; (1):CD006187

Bernstein N. The Coordination and Regulation of Movements. London: Pergamon Press; 1967

Biernaskie J, Corbett D. Enriched rehabilitative training promotes improved forelimb motor function and enhanced dendritic growth after focal ischemic injury. J Neurosci. 2001;21(14):5272–5280

Blennerhassett J, Dite W. Additional task-related practice improves mobility and upper limb function early after stroke: a randomised controlled trial. Aust J Physiother. 2004;50(4):219–224

Bohannon RW. Muscle strength changes in hemiparetic stroke patients during inpatient rehabilitation. Neurorehabil Neural Repair. 1988;2:163–166

Bohannon RW, Andrews AW. Interrater reliability of handheld dynamometry. Phys Ther. 1987;67(6):931–933

Bohannon RW, Andrews AW. Correlation of knee extensor muscle torque and spasticity with gait speed in patients with stroke. Arch Phys Med Rehabil. 1990;71(5):330–333

Bohannon RW, Smith J, Hull D, Palmeri D, Barnhard R. Deficits in lower extremity muscle and gait performance among renal transplant candidates. Arch Phys Med Rehabil. 1995;76(6):547–551

Boissy P, Bourbonnais D, Carlotti MM, Gravel D, Arsenault BA. Maximal grip force in chronic stroke subjects and its relationship to global upper extremity function. Clin Rehabil. 1999;13(4):354–362

Booth CM, Cortina-Borja MJ, Theologis TN. Collagen accumulation in muscles of children with cerebral palsy and correlation with severity of spasticity. Dev Med Child Neurol. 2001;43(5):314–320

Branch LG, Meyers AR. Assessing physical function in the elderly. Clin Geriatr Med. 1987;3(1):29–51

Brazier JE, Harper R, Jones NMB et al. Validating the SF-36 health survey questionnaire: new outcome measure for primary care. BMJ. 1992;305:158–164

Britton E, Harris N, Turton A. An exploratory randomized controlled trial of assisted practice for improving sit-to-stand in stroke patients in the hospital setting. Clin Rehabil. 2008;22(5):458–468

Brodal A. Self-observations and neuro-anatomical considerations after a stroke. Brain. 1973;96(4):675–694

Brunt D, Greenberg B, Wankadia S, Trimble MA, Shechtman O. The effect of foot placement on sit to stand in healthy young subjects and patients with hemiplegia. Arch Phys Med Rehabil. 2002;83(7):924–929

Buchner DM, Larson EB, Wagner EH, Koepsell TD, de Lateur BJ. Evidence for a non-linear relationship between leg strength and gait speed. Age Ageing. 1996;25(5):386–391

Buonomano DV, Merzenich MM. Cortical plasticity: from synapses to maps. Annu Rev Neurosci. 1998;21:149–186

Burke D, Gandevia SC. Interfering cutaneous stimulation and the muscle afferent contribution to cortical potentials. Electroencephalogr Clin Neurophysiol. 1988;70(2):118–125

Bütefisch C, Hummelsheim H, Denzler P, Mauritz KH. Repetitive training of isolated movements improves the outcome of motor rehabilitation of the centrally paretic hand. J Neurol Sci. 1995;130(1):59–68

Calautti C, Baron JC. Functional neuroimaging studies of motor recovery after stroke in adults: a review. Stroke. 2003;34(6):1553–1566

Canning CG, Ada L, O'Dwyer N. Slowness to develop force contributes to weakness after stroke. Arch Phys Med Rehabil. 1999;80(1):66–70

Carey LM. Somatosensory loss after stroke. Crit Rev Phys Med Rehabil. 1995;7:51–91

Carey LM, Matyas TA, Oke LE. Sensory loss in stroke patients: effective training of tactile and proprioceptive discrimination. Arch Phys Med Rehabil. 1993;74(6):602–611

Carey JR, Burghardt TP. Movement dysfunction following central nervous system lesions: a problem of neurologic or muscular impairment? Phys Ther. 1993;73(8):538–547

Carey JR, Allison JD, Mundale MO. Electromyographic study of muscular overflow during precision handgrip. Phys Ther. 1983;63(4):505–511

Carey JR, Kimberley TJ, Lewis SM, et al. Analysis of fMRI and finger tracking training in subjects with chronic stroke. Brain. 2002;125(Pt 4):773–788

Carlsoo S, Dahlöf AG, Holm J. Kinetic analysis of the gait in patients with hemiparesis and in patients with intermittent claudication. Scand J Rehabil Med. 1974;6(4):166–179

Carr JH, Shepherd RB. Movement Science: Foundations for Physical Therapy in Rehabilitation. 2nd ed; Austin: Pro-Ed; 2000

Carr JH, Shepherd RB. Neurological Rehabilitation Optimizing Motor Performance. 2nd ed. Oxford: Butterworth Heinemann; 2010

Carr JH, Shepherd RB. Stroke Rehabilitation. Guidelines for Exercise and Training to Optimize Motor Skill. Oxford: Butterworth Heinemann; 2003

Carr JH, Shepherd RB, Nordholm L, Lynne D. Investigation of a new motor assessment scale for stroke patients. Phys Ther. 1985;65(2):175–180

Carr JH, Ow JEG, Shepherd RB. Some biomechanical characteristics of standing up at three different speed: implications for functional training. Physiother Theory Pract. 2002;18:47–53

Castiello U, Bennett KMB, Paulignan Y. Does the type of prehension influence the kinematics of reaching? Behav Brain Res. 1992;50(1-2):7–15

Castiello U, Bennett KMB, Stelmach GE. The bilateral reach to grasp movement. Behav Brain Res. 1993;56(1):43–57

Castiello U, Lusher D, Burton C, Glover S, Disler P. Improving left hemispatial neglect using virtual reality. Neurology. 2004;62(11):1958–1962

Chae J, Yang G, Park BK, Labatia I. Muscle weakness and cocontraction in upper limb hemiparesis: relationship to motor impairment and physical disability. Neurorehabil Neural Repair. 2002;16(3):241–248

Chari VR, Kirby RL. Lower-limb influence on sitting balance while reaching forward. Arch Phys Med Rehabil. 1986;67(10):730–733

Cheng PT, Liaw MY, Wong MK, Tang FT, Lee MY, Lin PS. The sit-to-stand movement in stroke patients and its correlation with falling. Arch Phys Med Rehabil. 1998;79(9):1043–1046

Cirstea MC, Levin MF. Compensatory strategies for reaching in stroke. Brain. 2000;123(Pt 5):940–953

National Stroke Foundation. Clinical Guidelines for Stroke Rehabilitation and Recovery. Australia: National Stroke Foundation; 2005

Colebatch JG, Gandevia SC. The distribution of muscular weakness in upper motor neuron lesions affecting the arm. Brain. 1989;112(Pt 3):749–763

Colebatch JG, Rothwell JC, Day BL, Thompson PD, Marsden CD. Cortical outflow to proximal arm muscles in man. Brain. 1990;113(Pt 6):1843–1856

Coote S, Stokes EK. Physiotherapy for upper extremity dysfunction following stroke. Phys Ther Rev. 2001;6:63–69

Cress ME, Schechtman KB, Mulrow CD, Fiatarone MA, Gerety MB, Buchner DM. Relationship between physical performance and self-perceived physical function. J Am Geriatr Soc. 1995;43(2):93–101

Crosbie J, Shepherd RB, Squire TJ. Postural and voluntary movement during reaching in sitting: the role of the lower limbs. Journal of Human Movement Studies. 1995;28:103–126

Davies JM, Mayston MJ, Newham DJ. Electrical and mechanical output of the knee muscles during isometric and isokinetic activity in stroke and healthy adults. Disabil Rehabil. 1996;18(2):83–90

Davis JZ. Task selection and enriched environments: a functional upper extremity training program for stroke survivors. Top Stroke Rehabil. 2006;13(3):1–11

Dean CM, Shepherd RB. Task-related training improves performance of seated reaching tasks after stroke. A randomized controlled trial. Stroke. 1997;28(4):722–728

Dean C, Shepherd R, Adams R. Sitting balance I: trunk-arm coordination and the contribution of the lower limbs during self-paced reaching in sitting. Gait Posture. 1999a;10(2):135–146

Dean CM, Shepherd RB, Adams RD. Sitting balance II: reach direction and thigh support affect the contribution of the lower limbs when reaching beyond arm's length in sitting. Gait Posture. 1999b;10(2):147–153

Dean CM, Richards CL, Malouin F. Task-related circuit training improves performance of locomotor tasks in chronic stroke: a randomized, controlled pilot trial. Arch Phys Med Rehabil. 2000;81(4):409–417

Dean CM, Richards CL, Malouin F. Walking speed over 10 metres overestimates locomotor capacity after stroke. Clin Rehabil. 2001;15(4):415–421

Dean CM, Channon EF, Hall JM. Sitting training early after stroke improves sitting ability and quality and carries over to standing up but not to walking: a randomised trial. Aust J Physiother. 2007;53(2):97–102

De Deyne PG. Application of passive stretch and its implications for muscle fibers. Phys Ther. 2001;81(2):819–827

Deiber MP, Ibañez V, Honda M, Sadato N, Raman R, Hallett M. Cerebral processes related to visuomotor imagery and generation of simple finger movements studied with positron emission tomography. Neuroimage. 1998;7(2):73–85

De Weerdt W, Nuyens G, Feys H, et al. Group physiotherapy improves time use by patients with stroke in rehabilitation. Aust J Physiother. 2001;47(1):53–61

Di Fabio RP. Adaptation of postural stability following stroke. Top Stroke Rehabil. 1997;3:62–75

Di Fabio RP, Badke MB. Stance duration under sensory conflict conditions in patients with hemiplegia. Arch Phys Med Rehabil. 1991;72(5):292–295

Dion L, Malouin F, McFadyen BJ, et al. Assessment of the sit-to-walk capacity after stroke: a validation study. Gait Posture. 1999;1(Suppl):S24

Dion L, Malouin F, McFadyen BJ, Richards CL. Assessing mobility and locomotor coordination after stroke with the rise-to-walk task. Neurorehabil Neural Repair. 2003;17(2):83–92

Driskell JE, Copper C, Moran A. Does mental practice enhance performance? J Appl Psychol. 1994;79:481–492

Dromerick AW, Edwards DF, Hahn M. Does the application of constraint-induced movement therapy during acute rehabilitation reduce arm impairment after ischemic stroke? Stroke. 2000;31(12):2984–2988

Dubost V, Beauchet O, Manckoundia P, Herrmann F, Mourey F. Decreased trunk angular displacement during sitting down: an early feature of aging. Phys Ther. 2005;85(5):404–412

Duchateau J, Enoka RM. Neural adaptations with chronic activity patterns in able-bodied humans. Am J Phys Med Rehabil. 2002; 81(11, Suppl)S17–S27

Duchateau J, Hainaut K. Effects of immobilization on contractile properties, recruitment and firing rates of human motor units. J Physiol. 1990;422:55–65

Duncan PW, Weiner DK, Chandler J, Studenski S. Functional reach: a new clinical measure of balance. J Gerontol. 1990;45(6):M192–M197

Duncan PW, Goldstein LB, Horner RD, Landsman PB, Samsa GP, Matchar DB. Similar motor recovery of upper and lower extremities after stroke. Stroke. 1994;25(6):1181–1188

Duncan P, Studenski S, Richards L, et al. Randomized clinical trial of therapeutic exercise in subacute stroke. Stroke. 2003;34(9):2173–2180

Eastlack ME, Arvidson J, Snyder-Mackler L, Danoff JV, McGarvey CL. Interrater reliability of videotaped observational gait-analysis assessments. Phys Ther. 1991;71(6):465–472

Elbert T, Pantev C, Wienbruch C, Rockstroh B, Taub E. Increased cortical representation of the fingers of the left hand in string players. Science. 1995;270(5234):305–307

Eng JJ, Chu KS. Reliability and comparison of weight-bearing ability during standing tasks for individuals with chronic stroke. Arch Phys Med Rehabil. 2002;83(8):1138–1144

Eng JJ, Winter CD, Patla AE, et al. Role of the torque stabilizer in postural control during rapid voluntary arm movement. In: Woollacott M, Horak F, eds. Posture and Gait: Control Mechanisms. Portland: University of Oregon Books; 1992

Eng JJ, Chu KS, Kim CM, Dawson AS, Carswell A, Hepburn KE. A community-based group exercise program for persons with chronic stroke. Med Sci Sports Exerc. 2003;35(8):1271–1278

Eng JJ, Dawson AS, Chu KS. Submaximal exercise in persons with stroke: test-retest reliability and concurrent validity with maximal oxygen consumption. Arch Phys Med Rehabil. 2004;85(1):113–118

Eng J, Harris J, Dawson A, et al. Grasp guidelines and manual. www.rehab.ubc.ca/jeng/Our_Exercise_Manuals/Grasp.htm; 2009

Engardt M, Olsson E. Body weight-bearing while rising and sitting down in patients with stroke. Scand J Rehabil Med. 1992;24(2):67–74

Engardt M, Ribbe T, Olsson E. Vertical ground reaction force feedback to enhance stroke patients' symmetrical body-weight distribution while rising/sitting down. Scand J Rehabil Med. 1993;25(1):41–48

Engardt M, Knutsson E, Jonsson M, Sternhag M. Dynamic muscle strength training in stroke patients: effects on knee extension torque, electromyographic activity, and motor function. Arch Phys Med Rehabil. 1995;76(5):419–425

Enoka RM. Neural strategies in the control of muscle force. Muscle Nerve Suppl. 1997;5(Suppl 5):S66–S69

Esmonde T, McGinley J, Wittwer J, Goldie P, Martin C. Stroke rehabilitation: patient activity during non-therapy time. Aust J Physiother. 1997;43(1):43–51

Eriksrud O, Bohannon RW. Relationship of knee extension force to independence in sit-to-stand performance in patients receiving acute rehabilitation. Phys Ther. 2003;83(6):544–551

Faghri PD, Rodgers MM, Glaser RM, Bors JG, Ho C, Akuthota P. The effects of functional electrical stimulation on shoulder subluxation, arm function recovery, and shoulder pain in hemiplegic stroke patients. Arch Phys Med Rehabil. 1994;75(1):73–79

Farmer SF, Swash M, Ingram DA, Stephens JA. Changes in motor unit synchronization following central nervous lesions in man. J Physiol. 1993;463:83–105

Foldvari M, Clark M, Laviolette LC, et al. Association of muscle power with functional status in community-dwelling elderly women. J Gerontol A Biol Sci Med Sci. 2000;55(4):M192–M199

Foley NC, Teasell RW, Bhogal SK, Doherty T, Speechley MR. The efficacy of stroke rehabilitation: a qualitative review. Top Stroke Rehabil. 2003;10(2):1–18

Forssberg H. Spinal locomotion functions and descending control. In: Sjolund B, Bjorklund A, eds. Brain Stem Control of Spinal mechanisms, New York, NY: Elsevier Biomedical Press; 1982

Friel KM, Nudo RJ. Restraint of the unimpaired hand is not sufficient to retain spared hand representation after focal cortical injury. Society for Neuroscience Abstracts. 1998;24:405

Frontera WR, Grimby L, Larsson L. Firing rate of the lower motoneuron and contractile properties of its muscle fibers after upper motoneuron lesion in man. Muscle Nerve. 1997;20(8):938–947

Fugl-Meyer AR, Jääskö L, Leyman I, Olsson S, Steglind S. The post-stroke hemiplegic patient. 1. a method for evaluation of physical performance. Scand J Rehabil Med. 1975;7(1):13–31

Fuhr P, Cohen LG, Dang N, et al. Physiological analysis of motor reorganization following lower limb amputation. Electroencephalogr Clin Neurophysiol. 1992;85(1):53–60

Gallichio J, Kluding P. Virtual reality in stroke rehabilitation: Review of the emerging research. Phys Ther Rev. 2004;9:207–212

Gemperline JJ, Allen S, Walk D, Rymer WZ. Characteristics of motor unit discharge in subjects with hemiparesis. Muscle Nerve. 1995;18(10):1101–1114

Gentile AM. Skill Acquisition: Action, Movement, and Neuromotor Processes. In: Carr JH, Shepherd RB, eds. Movement Science Foundations for Physical Therapy in Rehabilitation. Rockville, MD: Aspen Publishers; 2000

Ghez C. Posture. In: Kandel ER, Schwartz JH, Jessell TM, eds. Principles of Neural Science. 3rd ed. Norwalk, CT: Appleton and Lange; 1991

Given JD, Dewald JP, Rymer WZ. Joint dependent passive stiffness in paretic and contralateral limbs of spastic patients with hemiparetic stroke. J Neurol Neurosurg Psychiatry. 1995;59(3):271–279

Goldie PA, Matyas TA, Evans OM, Galea M, Bach TM. Maximum voluntary weight-bearing by the affected and unaffected legs in standing following stroke. Clin Biomech (Bristol, Avon). 1996;11(6):333–342

Gordon NF, Gulanick M, Costa F, et al; American Heart Association Council on Clinical Cardiology, Subcommittee on Exercise, Cardiac Rehabilitation, and Prevention; the Council on Cardiovascular Nursing; the Council on Nutrition, Physical Activity, and Metabolism; and the Stroke Council. Physical activity and exercise recommendations for stroke survivors: an American Heart Association scientific statement from the Council on Clinical Cardiology, Subcommittee on Exercise, Cardiac Rehabilitation, and Prevention; the Council on Cardiovascular Nursing; the Council on Nutrition, Physical Activity, and Metabolism; and the Stroke Council. Stroke. 2004;35(5):1230–1240

Gottlieb GL, Corcos DM, Jaric S, Agarwal GC. Practice improves even the simplest movements. Exp Brain Res. 1988;73(2):436–440

Gracies JM. Pathophysiology of spastic paresis. I: Paresis and soft tissue changes. Muscle Nerve. 2005a;31(5):535–551

Gracies JM. Pathophysiology of spastic paresis. II: Emergence of muscle overactivity. Muscle Nerve. 2005b;31(5):552–571

Gracies J-M, Wilson L, Gandevia SC, et al. Stretched position of spastic muscles aggravates their co-contraction in hemiplegic patients. Ann Neurol. 1997;42:438–439

Gracies J-M, Marosszeky JE, Renton R, Sandanam J, Gandevia SC, Burke D. Short-term effects of dynamic lycra splints on upper limb in hemiplegic patients. Arch Phys Med Rehabil. 2000;81(12):1547–1555

Granger CV, Hamilton BB, Sherwin FS. Guide for the Use of Medical Rehabilitation. New York: Project Office, Buffalo General Hospital; 1986

Gregson JM, Leathley MJ, Moore AP, Smith TL, Sharma AK, Watkins CL. Reliability of measurements of muscle tone and muscle power in stroke patients. Age Ageing. 2000;29(3):223–228

Guadagnoli MA, Lee TD. Challenge point: a framework for conceptualizing the effects of various practice conditions in motor learning. J Mot Behav. 2004;36(2):212–224

Guadagnoli M, McNevin N, Wulf G. Cognitive influences to balance and posture. Orthop Phys Ther Clin N Am. 2002;11:131–141

Guyatt GH, Sullivan MJ, Thompson PJ, et al. The 6-minute walk: a new measure of exercise capacity in patients with chronic heart failure. Can Med Assoc J. 1985;132(8):919–923

Hachisuka K, Umezu Y, Ogata H. Disuse muscle atrophy of lower limbs in hemiplegic patients. Arch Phys Med Rehabil. 1997;78(1):13–18

Häkkinen K, Newton RU, Gordon SE, et al. Changes in muscle morphology, electromyographic activity, and force production characteristics during progressive strength training in young and older men. J Gerontol A Biol Sci Med Sci. 1998;53(6):B415–B423

Halkjaer-Kristensen J, Ingemann-Hansen T. Wasting of the human quadriceps muscle after knee ligament injuries. Scand J Rehabil Med Suppl. 1985;13:5–55

Harridge SDR, Kryger A, Stensgaard A. Knee extensor strength, activation, and size in very elderly people following strength training. Muscle Nerve. 1999;22(7):831–839

Harris JE, Eng JJ, Miller WC, Dawson AS. A self-administered Graded Repetitive Arm Supplementary Program (GRASP) improves arm function during inpatient stroke rehabilitation: a multi-site randomized controlled trial. Stroke. 2009;40(6):2123–2128

Harris ML, Polkey MI, Bath PM, Moxham J. Quadriceps muscle weakness following acute hemiplegic stroke. Clin Rehabil. 2001;15(3):274–281

Harris-Love ML, Macko RF, Whitall J, Forrester LW. Improved hemiparetic muscle activation in treadmill versus overground walking. Neurorehabil Neural Repair. 2004;18(3):154–160

Hebert EP, Landin D. Effects of a learning model and augmented feedback on tennis skill acquisition. Res Q Exerc Sport. 1994;65(3):250–257

Held JM, Gordon J, Gentile AM. Environmental influences on locomotor recovery following cortical lesions in rats. Behav Neurosci. 1985;99(4):678–690

Herbert R. How muscles respond to stretch. In: Refshauge K, Ada L, Ellis E, eds. Science-Based Rehabilitation. Oxford: Butterworth Heinemann; 2005

Hermsdörfer J, Mai N. Disturbed grip-force control following cerebral lesions. J Hand Ther. 1996;9(1):33–40

Herzog W, Koh T, Hasler E, et al. Specificity and plasticity of mammalian skeleton muscles. J Appl Biomech. 1991;16:98–109

Hesse S, Schauer M, Malezic M, Jahnke M, Mauritz KH. Quantitative analysis of rising from a chair in healthy and hemiparetic subjects. Scand J Rehabil Med. 1994;26(3):161–166

Hesse S, Bertelt C, Jahnke MT, et al. Treadmill training with partial body weight support compared with physiotherapy in nonambulatory hemiparetic patients. Stroke. 1995;26(6):976–981

Hesse S, Helm B, Krajnik J, et al. Treadmill training with partial weight support: influence of body weight release on the gait of hemiparetic patients. Neurorehabil Neural Repair. 1997;11:15–20

Hesse S, Konrad M, Uhlenbrock D. Treadmill walking with partial body weight support versus floor walking in hemiparetic subjects. Arch Phys Med Rehabil. 1999;80 (4):421–427

Hesse S, Schulte-Tigges G, Konrad M, Bardeleben A, Werner C. Robot-assisted arm trainer for the passive and active practice of bilateral forearm and wrist movements in hemiparetic subjects. Arch Phys Med Rehabil. 2003;84 (6):915–920

Hesse S, Schmidt H, Werner C. Machines to support motor rehabilitation after stroke: 10 years of experience in Berlin. J Rehabil Res Dev. 2006;43:671–678

Hidler J, Nichols D, Pelliccio M, Brady K. Advances in the understanding and treatment of stroke impairment using robotic devices. Top Stroke Rehabil. 2005;12 (2):22–35

Hill K, Bernhardt J, McGann A, et al. A new test of dynamic standing balance for stroke patients: reliability and comparison with healthy elderly. Physiother Can. 1996;48:257–262

Hill K, Ellis P, Bernhardt J, Maggs P, Hull S. Balance and mobility outcomes for stroke patients: a comprehensive audit. Aust J Physiother. 1997;43(3):173–180

Hill K, Denisenko S, Miller K, et al. Clinical Outcome Measurement in Adult Neurological Physiotherapy. Melbourne: Australian Physiotherapy Association; 2005

Hoff B, Arbib MA. Models of trajectory formation and temporal interaction of reach and grasp. J Mot Behav. 1993;25(3):175–192

Holden M, Dyar T. Virtual training: a new tool for neurorehabilitation. Neurology Report. 2002;26:62–71

Horak FB. Invited commentary. Phys Ther. 1997;77:382–383

Horak FB, Esselman P, Anderson ME, Lynch MK. The effects of movement velocity, mass displaced, and task certainty on associated postural adjustments made by normal and hemiplegic individuals. J Neurol Neurosurg Psychiatry. 1984;47(9):1020–1028

Hummelsheim A, Mauritz K-H. Chronic transformation of muscle in spasticity: a peripheral contribution to increased tone. J Neurol Neurosurg Psychiatry. 1985;48:676–685

Hunt SM, McEwen J, McKenna SP. Measuring health status: a new tool for clinicians and epidemiologists. J R Coll Gen Pract. 1985;35(273):185–188

Huxham FE, Goldie PA, Patla AE. Theoretical considerations in balance assessment. Aust J Physiother. 2001;47(2):89–100

Iberall T, Bingham G, Arbib MA. Opposition space as a structuring concept for the analysis of skilled hand movement. Exp Brain Res. 1986;15:158–173

Ikai T, Tei K, Yoshida K, Miyano S, Yonemoto K. Evaluation and treatment of shoulder subluxation in hemiplegia: relationship between subluxation and pain. Am J Phys Med Rehabil. 1998;77(5):421–426

Indredavik B, Slørdahl SA, Bakke F, Rokseth R, Håheim LL. Stroke unit treatment. Long-term effects. Stroke. 1997;28 (10):1861–1866

Janssen WGM, Bussmann HBJ, Stam HJ. Determinants of the sit-to-stand movement: a review. Phys Ther. 2002;82 (9):866–879

Jeannerod M. Intersegmental coordination during reaching at natural visual objects. In: Long J, Baddeley A, eds. Attention and Performance 9. Hillsdale, NJ: Erlbaum; 1981

Johansson BB. Brain plasticity and stroke rehabilitation. The Willis lecture. Stroke. 2000;31(1):223–230

Johansson BB, Ohlsson A-L. Environment, social interaction, and physical activity as determinants of functional outcome after cerebral infarction in the rat. Exp Neurol. 1996;139(2):322–327

Johansson RS, Westling G. Roles of glabrous skin receptors and sensorimotor memory in automatic control of precision grip when lifting rougher or more slippery objects. Exp Brain Res. 1984;56(3):550–564

Johansson RS, Westling G. Programmed and triggered actions to rapid load changes during precision grip. Exp Brain Res. 1988;71(1):72–86

Johansson RS, Westling G. Tactile afferent signals in the control of precision grip. In: Jeannerod M, ed. Attention and Performance. Hillsdale, NJ: Erlbaum; 1990

Johansson RS, Riso R, Häger C, Bäckström L. Somatosensory control of precision grip during unpredictable pulling loads. I. Changes in load force amplitude. Exp Brain Res. 1992a;89(1):181–191

Johansson RS, Häger C, Riso R. Somatosensory control of precision grip during unpredictable pulling loads. II. Changes in load force rate. Exp Brain Res. 1992b;89 (1):192–203

Johansson RS, Hger C, Bäckström L. Somatosensory control of precision grip during unpredictable pulling loads. III. Impairments during digital anesthesia. Exp Brain Res. 1992c;89(1):204–213

Kamper DG, Rymer WZ. Impairment of voluntary control of finger motion following stroke: role of inappropriate muscle coactivation. Muscle Nerve. 2001;24(5):673–681

Karnath H-O, Ferber S, Dichgans J. The origin of contraversive pushing: evidence for a second graviceptive system in humans. Neurology. 2000;55(9):1298–1304

Kautz SA, Brown DA. Relationships between timing of muscle excitation and impaired motor performance during cyclical lower extremity movement in post-stroke hemiplegia. Brain. 1998;121(Pt 3):515–526

Keith RA. Activity patterns of a stroke rehabilitation unit. Soc Sci Med, Med Psychol Med Sociol. 1980;14A(6):575–580

Kelly JO, Kilbreath SL, Davis GM, Zeman B, Raymond J. Cardiorespiratory fitness and walking ability in subacute stroke patients. Arch Phys Med Rehabil. 2003;84 (12):1780–1785

Khemlani MM, Carr JH, Crosbie WJ. Muscle synergies and joint linkages in sit-to-stand under two initial foot positions. Clin Biomech (Bristol, Avon). 1999;14(4):236–246

Kilbreath SL, Davis GM. Cardiorespiratory fitness after stroke. In: Refshauge K, et al, eds. Science-based Rehabilitation Theories into Practice. Oxford: Elsevier; 2005;131–158

Kilbreath SL, Heard RC. Frequency of hand use in healthy older persons. Aust J Physiother. 2005;51(2):119–122

Kilbreath SL, Perkins S, Crosbie J, McConnell J. Gluteal taping improves hip extension during stance phase of walking following stroke. Aust J Physiother. 2006;52(1):53–56

Kim CM, Eng JJ. The relationship of lower-extremity muscle torque to locomotor performance in people with stroke. Phys Ther. 2003;83(1):49–57

Kirker SGB, Simpson DS, Jenner JR, Wing AM. Stepping before standing: hip muscle function in stepping and standing balance after stroke. J Neurol Neurosurg Psychiatry. 2000;68(4):458–464

Kleim JA, Jones TA, Schallert T. Motor enrichment and the induction of plasticity before or after brain injury. Neurochem Res. 2003;28(11):1757–1769

Koceja DM, Allway D, Earles DR. Age differences in postural sway during volitional head movement. Arch Phys Med Rehabil. 1999;80(12):1537–1541

Kolb B. Brain, Plasticity and Behaviour. Mahwah: Lawrence Erlbaum; 1995

Kolb B. Overview of cortical plasticity and recovery from brain injury. Phys Med Rehabil Clin N Am. 2003; **14**(1, Suppl)S7–S25, viii

Komi PV. The stretch-shortnening cycle and human power output. In: Jones NC, et al, eds. Human Muscle Power. Champaign, Ill: Human Kinetic Publishers; 1986

Kozlowski DA, James DC, Schallert T. Use-dependent exaggeration of neuronal injury after unilateral sensorimotor cortex lesions. J Neurosci. 1996;16(15):4776–4786

Krebs HI, Volpe BT, Ferraro M, et al. Robot-aided neurorehabilitation: from evidence-based to science-based rehabilitation. Top Stroke Rehabil. 2002;8(4):54–70

Kuan TS, Tsou JY, Su FC. Hemiplegic gait of stroke patients: the effect of using a cane. Arch Phys Med Rehabil. 1999;80(7):777–784

Kunkel A, Kopp B, Müller G, et al. Constraint-induced movement therapy for motor recovery in chronic stroke patients. Arch Phys Med Rehabil. 1999;80(6):624–628

Kwakkel G, Wagenaar RC, Twisk JW, Lankhorst GJ, Koetsier JC. Intensity of leg and arm training after primary middle-cerebral-artery stroke: a randomised trial. Lancet. 1999;354(9174):191–196

Kwakkel G, Kollen BJ, van der Grond J, Prevo AJ. Probability of regaining dexterity in the flaccid upper limb: impact of severity of paresis and time since onset in acute stroke. Stroke. 2003;34(9):2181–2186

Kwakkel G, Van Peppen R, Wagenaar RC, et al. Effects of augmented exercise therapy time after stroke: a meta-analysis. Stroke. 2004;35(11):2529–2539

Lam YS, Man DWK, Tam SF, Weiss PL. Virtual reality training for stroke rehabilitation. NeuroRehabilitation. 2006;21(3):245–253

Lamontagne A, Fung J. Faster is better: implications for speed-intensive gait training after stroke. Stroke. 2004;35(11):2543–2548

Lamontagne A, Richards CL, Malouin F. Coactivation during gait as an adaptive behavior after stroke. J Electromyogr Kinesiol. 2000;10(6):407–415

Lance JM. Symposium synopsis. In: Feldman RG, Young RR, Koella WP, eds. Spasticity: Disorder of Motor Control. Chicago, Ill: Year Book Medical Pubs; 1980

Lance JW. What is spasticity? Lancet. 1990;335(8689):606

Lannin NA, Herbert RD. Is hand splinting effective for adults following stroke? A systematic review and methodologic critique of published research. Clin Rehabil. 2003;17(8):807–816

Latash LP, Latash ML. A new book by N. A. Bernstein: "On dexterity and its development". J Mot Behav. 1994;26(1):56–62

Laufer Y, Dickstein R, Resnik S, Marcovitz E. Weight-bearing shifts of hemiparetic and healthy adults upon stepping on stairs of various heights. Clin Rehabil. 2000;14(2):125–129

Lemon RN. Stroke recovery. Curr Biol. 1993;3(7):463–465

Lemon RN, Bennett KM, Werner W. The cortico-motor substrate for skilled movements of the primate hand. In: Requin GE, Stelmark GE, eds. Tutorials in Motor Neuroscience. Dordrecht: Kluwer; 1991

Levin MF, Selles RW, Verheul MH, Meijer OG. Deficits in the coordination of agonist and antagonist muscles in stroke patients: implications for normal motor control. Brain Res. 2000;853(2):352–369

Li Z-M, Latash ML, Newell KM, Zatsiorsky VM. Motor redundancy during maximal voluntary contraction in four-finger tasks. Exp Brain Res. 1998a;122(1):71–78

Li Z-M, Latash ML, Zatsiorsky VM. Force sharing among fingers as a model of the redundancy problem. Exp Brain Res. 1998b;119(3):276–286

Lieber RL. Comparison between animal and human studies of skeletal muscle adaptation to chronic stimulation. Clin Orthop Relat Res. 1988;233(233):19–24

Lieber RL, Fridén JO, Hargens AR, Feringa ER. Long-term effects of spinal cord transection on fast and slow rate skeletal muscle. II. Morphometric properties. Exp Neurol. 1986;91(3):435–448

Lieber RL, Steinman S, Barash IA, Chambers H. Structural and functional changes in spastic skeletal muscle. Muscle Nerve. 2004;29(5):615–627

Liepert J, Tegenthoff M, Malin JP. Changes of cortical motor area size during immobilization. Electroencephalogr Clin Neurophysiol. 1995;97(6):382–386

Liepert J, Miltner WHR, Bauder H, et al. Motor cortex plasticity during constraint-induced movement therapy in stroke patients. Neurosci Lett. 1998;250(1):5–8

Liepert J, Bauder H, Wolfgang HR, Miltner WH, Taub E, Weiller C. Treatment-induced cortical reorganization after stroke in humans. Stroke. 2000;31(6):1210–1216

Liepert J, Uhde I, Gräf S, Leidner O, Weiller C. Motor cortex plasticity during forced-use therapy in stroke patients: a preliminary study. J Neurol. 2001;248(4):315–321

Lin K-C, Wu C-Y, Trombly CA. Effects of task goal on movement kinematics and line bisection performance in adults without disabilities. Am J Occup Ther. 1998;52(3):179–187

Lincoln NB, Gamlen R, Thomason H. Behavioural mapping of patients on a stroke unit. Int Disabil Stud. 1989;11(4):149–154

Lincoln NB, Jackson JM, Adams SA. Reliability and revision of the Nottingham Sensory Assessment for stroke patients. Physiotherapy. 1998;84:358–365

Lincoln NB, Parry RH, Vass CD. Randomized, controlled trial to evaluate increased intensity of physiotherapy treatment of arm function after stroke. Stroke. 1999;30(3):573–579

Lindboe CF, Platou CS. Effect of immobilization of short duration on the muscle fibre size. Clin Physiol. 1984;4 (2):183–188

Loewen SC, Anderson BA. Predictors of stroke outcome using objective measurement scales. Stroke. 1990;21 (1):78–81

Lord S, Sherrington C, Menz H, et al. Falls in Older People, 2nd ed. Cambridge: Cambridge University Press; 2007

Lord SE, McPherson K, McNaughton HK, Rochester L, Weatherall M. Community ambulation after stroke: how important and obtainable is it and what measures appear predictive? Arch Phys Med Rehabil. 2004;85 (2):234–239

Lord SR, Murray SM, Chapman K, Munro B, Tiedemann A. Sit-to-stand performance depends on sensation, speed, balance, and psychological status in addition to strength in older people. J Gerontol A Biol Sci Med Sci. 2002;57 (8):M539–M543

Lum PS, Burgar CG, Shor PC, Majmundar M, Van der Loos M. Robot-assisted movement training compared with conventional therapy techniques for the rehabilitation of upper-limb motor function after stroke. Arch Phys Med Rehabil. 2002;83(7):952–959

Mackey F, Ada L, Heard R, Adams R. Stroke rehabilitation: are highly structured units more conducive to physical activity than less structured units? Arch Phys Med Rehabil. 1996;77(10):1066–1070

Mackay-Lyons MJ, Howlett J. Exercise capacity and cardiovascular adaptations to aerobic training early after stroke. Top Stroke Rehabil. 2005;12(1):31–44

Mackay-Lyons MJ, Makrides L. Cardiovascular stress during a contemporary stroke rehabilitation program: is the intensity adequate to induce a training effect? Arch Phys Med Rehabil. 2002;83(10):1378–1383

Mackay-Lyons MJ, Makrides L. Longitudinal changes in exercise capacity after stroke. Arch Phys Med Rehabil. 2004;85(10):1608–1612

Macko RF, De Souza CA, Tretter LD, et al. Treadmill aerobic exercise training reduces the energy and cardiovascular demands of hemiparetic gait in chronic stroke patients. A preliminary report. Stroke. 1997;28:326–330

Magill RA. Motor Learning Concepts and Applications, 6th ed. New York: McGraw-Hill; 2001

Magnan A, McFadyen BJ, St-Vincent G. Modification of the sit-to-stand task with the addition of gait initiation. Gait Posture. 1996;4:232–241

Mahoney FI, Barthel DW. Functional evaluation: the Barthel Index. Md State Med J. 1965;14:61–65

Malouin F, Richard CL. Assessment and Training of Locomotion after Stroke: Evolving Concepts. In: Refshauge K, Ada L, Ellis E, eds. Science-Based Rehabilitation. Oxford: Butterworth Heinemann; 2005

Malouin F, Pichard L, Bonneau C, Durand A, Corriveau D. Evaluating motor recovery early after stroke: comparison of the Fugl-Meyer Assessment and the Motor Assessment Scale. Arch Phys Med Rehabil. 1994;75(11):1206–1212

Malouin F, Bonneau C, Pichard L, Corriveau D. Non-reflex mediated changes in plantarflexor muscles early after stroke. Scand J Rehabil Med. 1997;29(3):147–153

Malouin F, McFadyen B, Dion L, Richards CL. A fluidity scale for evaluating the motor strategy of the rise-to-walk task after stroke. Clin Rehabil. 2003;17(6):674–684

Malouin F, Belleville S, Richards CL, Desrosiers J, Doyon J. Working memory and mental practice outcomes after stroke. Arch Phys Med Rehabil. 2004a;85(2):177–183

Malouin F, Richards CL, Doyon J, Desrosiers J, Belleville S. Training mobility tasks after stroke with combined mental and physical practice: a feasibility study. Neurorehabil Neural Repair. 2004b;18(2):66–75

Marigold DS, Eng JJ, Tokuno CD, Donnelly CA. Contribution of muscle strength and integration of afferent input to postural instability in persons with stroke. Neurorehabil Neural Repair. 2004;18(4):222–229

Marteniuk RB, Leavitt JL, MacKenzie CL, MacKenzie S. Functional relationships between grasp and transport components in a prehension task. Hum Mov Sci. 1990;9:149–176

Mayo NE, Wood-Dauphinee S, Ahmed S, et al. Disablement following stroke. Disabil Rehabil. 2005;27:258–268

McComas AJ. Human neuromuscular adaptations that accompany changes in activity. Med Sci Sports Exerc. 1994;26(12):1498–1509

McConnell J. Recalcitrant chronic low back and leg pain—a new theory and different approach to management. Man Ther. 2002;7(4):183–192

McCrea PH, Eng JJ, Hodgson AJ. Time and magnitude of torque generation is impaired in both arms following stroke. Muscle Nerve. 2003;28(1):46–53

McNevin NH, Wulf G, Carlson C. Effects of attentional focus, self-control, and dyad training on motor learning: implications for physical rehabilitation. Phys Ther. 2000;80 (4):373–385

Means KM, Rodell DE, O'Sullivan PS. Use of an obstacle course to assess balance and mobility in the elderly. A validation study. Am J Phys Med Rehabil. 1996;75(2):88–95

Mehrholz J, Wagner K, Meissner D, et al. Reliability of the Modified Tardieu Scale and the Modified Ashworth Scale in adult patients with severe brain injury: a comparison study. Clin Rehabil. 2005;19(7):751–759

Mehrholz J, Werner C, Kugler J, Pohl M. Electromechanical-assisted training for walking after stroke. Cochrane Database Syst Rev. 2007; (4):CD006185

Mercer VS, Sahrmann SA. Postural synergies associated with a stepping task. Phys Ther. 1999;79(12):1142–1152

Merians AS, Jack D, Boian R, et al. Virtual reality-augmented rehabilitation for patients following stroke. Phys Ther. 2002;82(9):898–915

Miller GJT, Light KE. Strength training in spastic hemiparesis: should it be avoided? Neurorehabilitation. 1997;9:17–28

Miltner WH, Bauder H, Sommer M, Dettmers C, Taub E. Effects of constraint-induced movement therapy on patients with chronic motor deficits after stroke: a replication. Stroke. 1999;30(3):586–592

Mirbagheri MM, Barbeau H, Kearney RE. Intrinsic and reflex contributions to human ankle stiffness: variation with activation level and position. Exp Brain Res. 2000;135 (4):423–436

Morrissey MC, Harman EA, Johnson MJ. Resistance training modes: specificity and effectiveness. Med Sci Sports Exerc. 1995;27(5):648–660

Moseley AM, Adams R. Measurement of passive ankle dorsiflexion: procedures and reliability. Aust J Physiother. 1991;37:175–181

Moseley AM, Stark A, Cameron ID, Pollock A. Treadmill training and body weight support for walking after stroke. Cochrane Database Syst Rev. 2005; (4):CD002840

Mudie MH, Matyas TA. Can simultaneous bilateral movement involve the undamaged hemisphere in reconstruction of neural networks damaged by stroke? Disabil Rehabil. 2000;22(1-2):23–37

Nakayama H, Jørgensen HS, Raaschou HO, Olsen TS. Recovery of upper extremity function in stroke patients: the Copenhagen Stroke Study. Arch Phys Med Rehabil. 1994;75(4):394–398

Nashner LM. Analysis of movement control in man using the movable platform. In: Desmedt JE, ed. Motor Control Mechanisms in Disease and Health. New York: Raven Press; 1983

Nelles G. Cortical reorganization—effects of intensive therapy. Restor Neurol Neurosci. 2004;22(3-5):239–244

Nelles G, Jentzen W, Jueptner M, Müller S, Diener HC. Arm training induced brain plasticity in stroke studied with serial positron emission tomography. Neuroimage. 2001;13(6 Pt 1):1146–1154

Newham DJ. Muscle performance after stroke. In: Refshauge K, Ada L, Ellis E, eds. Science-Based Rehabilitation. Oxford: Elsevier; 2005

Newham DJ, Hsiao S-F. Knee muscle isometric strength, voluntary activation and antagonist co-contraction in the first six months after stroke. Disabil Rehabil. 2001;23 (9):379–386

Newham DJ, Mayston MJ, Davies JM. Quadriceps isometric force, voluntary activation and relaxation speed in stroke. Muscle Nerve. 1996;(Suppl 4):S53

Nielsen JB, Crone C, Hultborn H. The spinal pathophysiology of spasticity—from a basic science point of view. Acta Physiol (Oxf). 2007;189(2):171–180

Ng S, Shepherd RB. Weakness in patients with stroke: implications for strength training in neurorehabilitation. Phys Ther Rev. 2000;5:227–238

Nudo RJ. Functional and structural plasticity in motor cortex: implications for stroke recovery. Phys Med Rehabil Clin N Am. 2003; 14(1, Suppl)S57–S76

Nudo RJ, Milliken GW. Reorganization of movement representations in primary motor cortex following focal ischemic infarcts in adult squirrel monkeys. J Neurophysiol. 1996;75(5):2144–2149

Nudo RJ, Wise BM, SiFuentes F, Milliken GW. Neural substrates for the effects of rehabilitative training on motor recovery after ischemic infarct. Science. 1996;272 (5269):1791–1794

Nudo RJ, Plautz EJ, Frost SB. Role of adaptive plasticity in recovery of function after damage to motor cortex. Muscle Nerve. 2001;24(8):1000–1019

Nyberg L, Gustafson Y. Patient falls in stroke rehabilitation. A challenge to rehabilitation strategies. Stroke. 1995;26 (5):838–842

O'Dwyer NJ, Ada L, Neilson PD. Spasticity and muscle contracture following stroke. Brain. 1996;119(Pt 5):1737–1749

Ohlsson A-L, Johansson BB. Environment influences functional outcome of cerebral infarction in rats. Stroke. 1995;26(4):644–649

Olney SJ. Training gait after stroke: a biomechanical perspective. In: Refshauge K, Ada L, Ellis E, eds. Science-Based Rehabilitation. Oxford: Butterworth Heinemann; 2005

Olney SJ, Richards C. Hemiparetic gait following stroke. Pt 1: Characteristics. Gait Posture. 1996;4:136–148

Olney SJ, Monga TN, Costigan PA. Mechanical energy of walking of stroke patients. Arch Phys Med Rehabil. 1986;67(2):92–98

Olney SJ, Jackson VG, George SR. Gait re-education guidelines for stroke patients with hemiplegia using mechanical energy and power analyses. Physiother Can. 1988;40:242–248

Olney SJ, Griffin MP, Monga TN, McBride ID. Work and power in gait of stroke patients. Arch Phys Med Rehabil. 1991;72(5):309–314

Paci M. Physiotherapy based on the Bobath concept for adults with post-stroke hemiplegia: a review of effectiveness studies. J Rehabil Med. 2003;35(1):2–7

Page SJ, Levine P, Sisto SA, Johnston MV. Mental practice combined with physical practice for upper-limb motor deficit in subacute stroke. Phys Ther. 2001;81(8):1455–1462

Page SJ, Sisto S, Levine P, et al. Efficacy of modified constraint-induced movement therapy in chronic stroke: a single-blinded randomized controlled trial. Arch Phys Med Rehabil. 2004;85:1377–1381

Pai Y-C, Rogers MW, Hedman LD, Hanke TA. Alterations in weight-transfer capabilities in adults with hemiparesis. Phys Ther. 1994;74(7):647–657, discussion 657–659

Pandyan AD, Price CI, Rodgers H, Barnes MP, Johnson GR. Biomechanical examination of a commonly used measure of spasticity. Clin Biomech (Bristol, Avon). 2001;16 (10):859–865

Pandyan AD, Gregoric M, Barnes MP, et al. Spasticity: clinical perceptions, neurological realities and meaningful measurement. Disabil Rehabil. 2005;27(1-2):2–6

Pang MY, Eng JJ, Dawson AS, McKay HA, Harris JE. A community-based fitness and mobility exercise program for older adults with chronic stroke: a randomized, controlled trial. J Am Geriatr Soc. 2005;53(10):1667–1674

Pang MYC, Eng JJ, Dawson AS, Gylfadóttir S. The use of aerobic exercise training in improving aerobic capacity in individuals with stroke: a meta-analysis. Clin Rehabil. 2006;20(2):97–111

Pang MY, Harris JE, Eng JJ. A community-based upper-extremity group exercise program improves motor function and performance of functional activities in chronic stroke: a randomized controlled trial. Arch Phys Med Rehabil. 2006;87(1):1–9

Paolucci S, Grasso MG, Antonucci G, et al. Mobility status after inpatient stroke rehabilitation: 1-year follow-up and prognostic factors. Arch Phys Med Rehabil. 2001;82 (1):2–8

Partridge C, Mackenzie M, Edwards S, et al. Is dosage of physiotherapy a critical factor in deciding patterns of recovery from stroke: a pragmatic randomized controlled trial. Physiother Res Int. 2000;5(4):230–240

Pascual-Leone A, Cammarota A, Wassermann EM, Brasil-Neto JP, Cohen LG, Hallett M. Modulation of motor cortical outputs to the reading hand of Braille readers. Ann Neurol. 1993;34(1):33–37

Patla AE. A Framework for Understanding Mobility Problems in the Elderly. In: Craik RL, Oatis CA, eds. Gait Analysis: Theory and Application. St Louis: Mosby; 1995

Peat M. Functional anatomy of the shoulder complex. Phys Ther. 1986;66(12):1855–1865

Pennisi G, Rapisarda G, Bella R, Calabrese V, Maertens De Noordhout A, Delwaide PJ. Absence of response to early transcranial magnetic stimulation in ischemic stroke patients: prognostic value for hand motor recovery. Stroke. 1999;30(12):2666–2670

Pinniger GJ, Steele JR, Thorstensson A, Cresswell AG. Tension regulation during lengthening and shortening actions of the human soleus muscle. Eur J Appl Physiol. 2000;81(5):375–383

Platz T. Impairment-oriented training (IOT)—scientific concept and evidence-based treatment strategies. Restor Neurol Neurosci. 2004;22(3-5):301–315

Plautz EJ, Milliken GW, Nudo RJ. Effects of repetitive motor training on movement representations in adult squirrel monkeys: role of use versus learning. Neurobiol Learn Mem. 2000;74(1):27–55

Podsiadlo D, Richardson S. The timed 'up and go': a test of functional mobility for frail elderly persons. Journal of the American Geriatrics. 1991;39:142–148

Pohl M, Mehrholz J, Ritschel C, Rückriem S. Speed-dependent treadmill training in ambulatory hemiparetic stroke patients: a randomized controlled trial. Stroke. 2002;33 (2):553–558

Pomeroy VM, Dean D, Sykes L, et al. The unreliability of clinical measures of muscle tone: implications for stroke therapy. Age Ageing. 2000;29(3):229–233

Potempa K, Lopez M, Braun LT, Szidon JP, Fogg L, Tincknell T. Physiological outcomes of aerobic exercise training in hemiparetic stroke patients. Stroke. 1995;26(1):101–105

Potempa K, Braun LT, Tinknell T, Popovich J. Benefits of aerobic exercise after stroke. Sports Med. 1996;21 (5):337–346

Potter JM, Evans AL, Duncan G. Gait speed and activities of daily living function in geriatric patients. Arch Phys Med Rehabil. 1995;76(11):997–999

Rajaratnam BS, Venketasubramanian N, Kumar PV, Goh JC, Chan YH. Predictability of simple clinical tests to identify shoulder pain after stroke. Arch Phys Med Rehabil. 2007;88(8):1016–1021

Richards CL, Malouin F, Wood-Dauphinee S, Williams JI, Bouchard JP, Brunet D. Task-specific physical therapy for optimization of gait recovery in acute stroke patients. Arch Phys Med Rehabil. 1993;74(6):612–620

Richards CL, Malouin F, Dean C. Gait in stroke: assessment and rehabilitation. Clin Geriatr Med. 1999;15(4):833–855

Riddle DL, Stratford PW. Interpreting validity indexes for diagnostic tests: an illustration using the Berg balance test. Phys Ther. 1999;79(10):939–948

Rimmer JH, Braunschweig C, Silverman K, Riley B, Creviston T, Nicola T. Effects of a short-term health promotion intervention for a predominantly African-American group of stroke survivors. Am J Prev Med. 2000;18(4):332–338

Risedal A, Mattsson B, Dahlqvist P, Nordborg C, Olsson T, Johansson BB. Environmental influences on functional outcome after a cortical infarct in the rat. Brain Res Bull. 2002;58(3):315–321

Rodgers H, Mackintosh J, Price C, et al. Does an early increased-intensity interdisciplinary upper limb therapy programme following acute stroke improve outcome? Clin Rehabil. 2003;17(6):579–589

Roy G, Nadeau S, Gravel D, Malouin F, McFadyen BJ, Piotte F. The effect of foot position and chair height on the asymmetry of vertical forces during sit-to-stand and stand-to-sit tasks in individuals with hemiparesis. Clin Biomech (Bristol, Avon). 2006;21(6):585–593

Rushworth G. Spasticity and rigidity: an experimental study and review. J Neurol Neurosurg Psychiatry. 1960;23:99–118

Rutherford OM. Muscular coordination and strength training. Implications for injury rehabilitation. Sports Med. 1988;5(3):196–202

Sahrmann SA, Norton BJ. The relationship of voluntary movement to spasticity in the upper motor neuron syndrome. Ann Neurol. 1977;2(6):460–465

Said CM, Goldie PA, Patla AE, Sparrow WA, Martin KE. Obstacle crossing in subjects with stroke. Arch Phys Med Rehabil. 1999;80(9):1054–1059

Said CM, Goldie PA, Culham E, Sparrow WA, Patla AE, Morris ME. Control of lead and trail limbs during obstacle crossing following stroke. Phys Ther. 2005;85(5):413–427

Salazar-Torres J de J, Pandyan AD, Price CI, Davidson RI, Barnes MP, Johnson GR. Does spasticity result from hyperactive stretch reflexes? Preliminary findings from a stretch reflex characterization study. Disabil Rehabil. 2004;26(12):756–760

Salbach NM, Mayo NE, Wood-Dauphinee S, Hanley JA, Richards CL, Côté R. A task-orientated intervention enhances walking distance and speed in the first year post stroke: a randomized controlled trial. Clin Rehabil. 2004;18(5):509–519

Schenkman M, Berger RA, Riley PO, Mann RW, Hodge WA. Whole-body movements during rising to standing from sitting. Phys Ther. 1990;70(10):638–648, discussion 648–651

Schenkman M, Hughes MA, Samsa G, Studenski S. The relative importance of strength and balance in chair rise by functionally impaired older individuals. J Am Geriatr Soc. 1996;44(12):1441–1446

Schmidt RA. Motor Control and Learning. Champaign, Il: Human Kinetic Pubs; 1988

Seidler RD, Stelmach GE. Trunk-assisted prehension: specification of body segments with imposed temporal constraints. J Mot Behav. 2000;32(4):379–389

Sharp SA, Brouwer BJ. Isokinetic strength training of the hemiparetic knee: effects on function and spasticity. Arch Phys Med Rehabil. 1997;78(11):1231–1236

Shea CH, Wulf G, Whitacre C. Enhancing training efficiency and effectiveness through the use of dyad training. J Mot Behav. 1999;31(2):119–125

Shea CH, Wright DL, Wulf G, Whitacre C. Physical and observational practice afford unique learning opportunities. J Mot Behav. 2000;32(1):27–36

Sheean G. The pathophysiology of spasticity. Eur J Neurol. 2002;9(Suppl 1):3–9, 53–61

Shepherd RB, Carr JH. Response to discussion paper: new aspects for the physiotherapy of pushing behaviour by D. Broetz and H-O Karnath. Neurorehabilitation. 2005;20:343–345

Shepherd RB, Gentile AM. Sit-to-stand: functional relationships between upper body and lower limb segments. Hum Mov Sci. 1994;13:817–840

Shepherd RB, Koh HP. Some biomechanical consequences of varying foot placement in sit-to-stand in young women. Scand J Rehabil Med. 1996;28(2):79–88

Sherrington C, Lord SR. Home exercise to improve strength and walking velocity after hip fracture: a randomized controlled trial. Arch Phys Med Rehabil. 1997;78 (2):208–212

Sherrington C, Whitney JC, Lord SR, Herbert RD, Cumming RG, Close JC. Effective exercise for the prevention of falls: a systematic review and meta-analysis. J Am Geriatr Soc. 2008;56(12):2234–2243

Shumway-Cook A, Horak FB. Assessing the influence of sensory interaction of balance. Suggestion from the field. Phys Ther. 1986;66(10):1548–1550

Shumway-Cook A, Woollacott MH. Motor Control: Translating Research into Clinical Practice, 3rd ed. Philadelphia: Lippincott Williams and Wilkins; 2007

Singer BJ, Dunne JW, Singer KP, Allison GT. Velocity dependent passive plantarflexor resistive torque in patients with acquired brain injury. Clin Biomech (Bristol, Avon). 2003;18(2):157–165

Sinkjaer T, Magnussen I. Passive, intrinsic and reflex-mediated stiffness in the ankle extensors of hemiparetic patients. Brain. 1994;117(Pt 2):355–363

Smeets JBJ, Brenner EA. A new view on grasping. Mot Contr. 1999;3(3):237–271

Stroke Trialists' Collaboration. Organised inpatient (stroke unit) care for stroke. Cochrane Database Syst Rev. 2001: Issue 3

Sunderland A, Tinson D, Bradley L, Hewer RL. Arm function after stroke. An evaluation of grip strength as a measure of recovery and a prognostic indicator. J Neurol Neurosurg Psychiatry. 1989;52(11):1267–1272

Sunnerhagen KS, Svantesson U, Lönn L, Krotkiewski M, Grimby G. Upper motor neuron lesions: their effect on muscle performance and appearance in stroke patients with minor motor impairment. Arch Phys Med Rehabil. 1999;80(2):155–161

Svantesson U, Sunnerhagen KS. Stretch-shortening cycle in patients with upper motor neuron lesion due to stroke. Eur J Appl Physiol. 1997;75:312–318

Svantesson U, Takahashi H, Carlsson U, Danielsson A, Sunnerhagen KS. Muscle and tendon stiffness in patients with upper motor neuron lesion following a stroke. Eur J Appl Physiol. 2000;82(4):275–279

Talvitie U. Socio-affective characteristics and properties of extrinsic feedback in physiotherapy. Physiother Res Int. 2000;5(3):173–189

Taub E. Somatosensory Deafferentation Research with Monkey: Implications for Rehabilitation Medicine. In: Ince LP, ed. Behavioral Psychology in Rehabilitation Medicine: Clinical Applications. New York. Williams Wilkins; 1980

Taub E, Wolf SL. Constraint induced movement techniques to facilitate upper extremity use in stroke patients. Top Stroke Rehabil. 1997;3:38–61

Taub E, Miller NE, Novack TA, et al. Technique to improve chronic motor deficit after stroke. Arch Phys Med Rehabil. 1993;74(4):347–354

Tax AAM, Denier van der Gon JJ, Erkelens CJ. Differences in coordination of elbow flexor muscles in force tasks and in movement tasks. Exp Brain Res. 1990;81(3):567–572

Teasell R, Bitensky J, Foley N, Bayona NA. Training and stimulation in post stroke recovery brain reorganization. Top Stroke Rehabil. 2005;12(3):37–45

Teixeira-Salmela LF, Olney SJ, Nadeau S, Brouwer B. Muscle strengthening and physical conditioning to reduce impairment and disability in chronic stroke survivors. Arch Phys Med Rehabil. 1999;80(10):1211–1218

Teixeira-Salmela LF, Nadeau S, Mcbride I, Olney SJ. Effects of muscle strengthening and physical conditioning training on temporal, kinematic and kinetic variables during gait in chronic stroke survivors. J Rehabil Med. 2001;33 (2):53–60

Thielman GT, Dean CM, Gentile AM. Rehabilitation of reaching after stroke: task-related training versus progressive resistive exercise. Arch Phys Med Rehabil. 2004;85 (10):1613–1618

Thilmann AF, Fellows SJ, Garms E. The mechanism of spastic muscle hypertonus. Variation in reflex gain over the time course of spasticity. Brain. 1991;114(Pt 1A):233–244

Tinson DJ. How stroke patients spend their days. An observational study of the treatment regime offered to patients in hospital with movement disorders following stroke. Int Disabil Stud. 1989;11(1):45–49

Toffola ED, Sparpaglione D, Pistorio A, Buonocore M. Myoelectric manifestations of muscle changes in stroke patients. Arch Phys Med Rehabil. 2001;82(5):661–665

Trombly CA. Deficits of reaching in subjects with left hemiparesis: a pilot study. Am J Occup Ther. 1992;46 (10):887–897

Tyson S, Selley A. A content analysis of physiotherapy for postural control in people with stroke: an observational study. Disabil Rehabil. 2006;28(13-14):865–872

Tyson S, Turner G. Discharge and follow-up for people with stroke: what happens and why. Clin Rehabil. 2000;14 (4):381–392

Vander Linden DW, Brunt D, McCulloch MU. Variant and invariant characteristics of the sit-to-stand task in healthy elderly adults. Arch Phys Med Rehabil. 1994;75:653–660

Van Peppen RPS, Kwakkel G, Wood-Dauphinee S, Hendriks HJ, Van der Wees PJ, Dekker J. The impact of physical therapy on functional outcomes after stroke: what's the evidence? Clin Rehabil. 2004;18(8):833–862

van Vliet P. An investigation of the task-specificity of reaching: implications for retraining. Physiother Theory Pract. 1993;9:69–76

van Vliet P, Kerwin DG, Sheridan M, et al. The influence of functional goals on the kinematics of reaching following stroke. Neurol Rep. 1995;19:11–16

van Vliet PM, Lincoln NB, Foxall A. Comparison of Bobath based and movement science based treatment for stroke: a randomized controlled trial. Neurol Neurosurg Psychiatry. 2005;76:504–508

Vandervoort AA, Chesworth BM, Cunningham DA, Paterson DH, Rechnitzer PA, Koval JJ. Age and sex effects on mobility of the human ankle. J Gerontol. 1992;47(1):M17–M21

Verkerk PH, Schouten JP, Oosterhuis HJGH. Measurement of the handcoordination. Clin Neurol Neurosurg. 1990;92(2):105–109

Volpe BT, Krebs HI, Hogan N, Edelstein OTR L, Diels C, Aisen M. A novel approach to stroke rehabilitation: robot-aided sensorimotor stimulation. Neurology. 2000;54(10):1938–1944

von Schroeder HP, Coutts RD, Lyden PD, Billings E Jr, Nickel VL. Gait parameters following stroke: a practical assessment. J Rehabil Res Dev. 1995;32(1):25–31

Wade DT. Measurement in Stroke Rehabilitation. Oxford: Oxford University Press; 1992

Wagenaar RC. Functional Recovery After Stroke. Amsterdam: VU University Press; 1990

Walker-Batson D, Smith P, Curtis S, Unwin DH. Neuromodulation paired with learning dependent practice to enhance post stroke recovery? Restor Neurol Neurosci. 2004;22(3-5):387–392

Wanklyn P, Forster A, Young J. Hemiplegic shoulder pain (HSP): natural history and investigation of associated features. Disabil Rehabil. 1996;18(10):497–501

Weiss A, Suzuki T, Bean J, Fielding RA. High intensity strength training improves strength and functional performance after stroke. Am J Phys Med Rehabil. 2000;79(4):369–376, quiz 391–394

Weiller C. Imaging recovery from stroke. Exp Brain Res. 1998;123(1-2):13–17

Whitall J, McCombe Waller S, Silver KH, Macko RF. Repetitive bilateral arm training with rhythmic auditory cueing improves motor function in chronic hemiparetic stroke. Stroke. 2000;31(10):2390–2395

Whiting HTA. Dimensions of control in motor learning. In: Stelmach GE, Requin J, eds. Tutorials in Motor Behavior. New York: North Holland; 1980, 537–550

Wiesendangar M, Kazennikov O, Perrig S et al. Two hands–one action. In: Hand and Brain. Neurophysiology and Psychology of Hand Movements. Orlando: Academic Press; 1996, 283–300

Wilson LR, Gandevia SC, Inglis JT, Gracies J, Burke D. Muscle spindle activity in the affected upper limb after a unilateral stroke. Brain. 1999;122(Pt 11):2079–2088

Wing AM, Fraser C. The contribution of the thumb to reaching movements. Q J Exp Psychol A. 1983;35(Pt 2):297–309

Wing AM, Goodrich S, Virji-Babul N, Jenner JR, Clapp S. Balance evaluation in hemiparetic stroke patients using lateral forces applied to the hip. Arch Phys Med Rehabil. 1993;74(3):292–299

Winstein CJ, Rose DK, Tan SM, Lewthwaite R, Chui HC, Azen SP. A randomized controlled comparison of upper-extremity rehabilitation strategies in acute stroke: A pilot study of immediate and long-term outcomes. Arch Phys Med Rehabil. 2004;85(4):620–628

Winter DA. Concerning the scientific basis for the diagnosis of pathological gait and for rehabilitation protocols. Physiother Can. 1985;37:245–252

Winter DA. The Biomechanics and Motor Control of Human Gait. Waterloo, Ont: University of Waterloo Press; 1987

Winter DA. ABC of Balance During Standing and Walking. Waterloo, Ont: University of Waterloo Press; 1995

Winter DA, Patla AE, Frank JS, Walt SE. Biomechanical walking pattern changes in the fit and healthy elderly. Phys Ther. 1990;70(6):340–347

Winters JM, Kleweno DG. Effect of initial upper-limb alignment on muscle contributions to isometric strength curves. J Biomech. 1993;26(2):143–153

Wolf SL, Catlin PA, Ellis M, Archer AL, Morgan B, Piacentino A. Assessing Wolf motor function test as outcome measure for research in patients after stroke. Stroke. 2001;32(7):1635–1639

Wolf SL, Blanton S, Baer H, Breshears J, Butler AJ. Repetitive task practice: a critical review of constraint-induced movement therapy in stroke. Neurologist. 2002;8(6):325–338

Wolf SL, Winstein CJ, Miller JP, et al; EXCITE Investigators. Effect of constraint-induced movement therapy on upper extremity function 3 to 9 months after stroke: the EXCITE randomized clinical trial. JAMA. 2006;296(17):2095–2104

Wu C, Trombly CA, Lin K, Tickle-Degnen L. A kinematic study of contextual effects on reaching performance in persons with and without stroke: influences of object availability. Arch Phys Med Rehabil. 2000;81(1):95–101

Wulf G, Weigelt C. Instructions about physical principles in learning a complex motor skill: to tell or not to tell .... Res Q Exerc Sport. 1997;68(4):362–367

Wulf G, Höß M, Prinz W. Instructions for Motor Learning: Differential Effects of Internal Versus External Focus of Attention. J Mot Behav. 1998;30(2):169–179

Wulf G, McNevin N, Shea C. Learning phenomena: future challenges for the dynamical systems approach to understanding the learning of complex motor skills. Int J Psychol. 1999a;30:531–557

Wulf G, Lauterbach B, Toole T. The learning advantages of an external focus of attention in golf. Res Q Exerc Sport. 1999b;70(2):120–126

Zajac FE. Muscle and tendon: properties, models, scaling, and application to biomechanics and motor control. Crit Rev Biomed Eng. 1989;17(4):359–411

Zattara M, Bouisset S. Chronometric analysis of the posturokinetic programming of voluntary movement. J Motor Behav. 1988;18:215–225

Zorowitz RD. Recovery patterns of shoulder subluxation after stroke: a six-month follow-up study. Top Stroke Rehabil. 2001;8(2):1–9

Further Reading

Ada L, O'Dwyer N. Do associated reactions in the upper limp after stroke contribute to contracture formation? Clin Rehabil. 2001;15(2):186–194

Chapter 6

Bienstein C, Fröhlich A. Basale Stimulation in der Pflege. Seelze-Velber: Kallmyer; 2003

Conzelmann A, Manz P. Schlaganfall Pflege in der Akutphase. Stuttgart: Kohlhammer; 2003

Kellnhauser E, Schewior-Popp S, Sitzmann F, Geißner U, Gümmer M, Ullrich L. Thiemes Pflege. Stuttgart: Thieme; 2000

Thranberend T. Pflegende sind Partner in der Rehabilitation. Die Schwester/Der Pfleger 2007;2:104

Nydahl P, Bartoszek G. Basale Stimulation. Neue Wege in der Intensivpflege. Munich: Urban & Fischer; 2000

Further Reading

Fisching R, Synowitz H-J, Wolf F. Professionelle neurologische und neurochirurgische Pflege. Bern: Hans Huber; 2003

Gliem U. Stroke-Unit-Aufgabenvielfalt in der Pflege. Die Schwester/Der Pfleger 2002;8:648

Korthgassner C, Schönbock S, Jung J. Stroke Unit, Intermediate Care und Video-EEG. Osterr Pflegezeitschrift 2003;3:19

Schulz J, Enders H. Pflege nach Schlaganfall. Heilberufe. 2005;9:18

Seel M. Die Pflege des Menschen. Hagen: Brigitte Kunz; 1994

Spieß-Koch G. Schlaganfall-Akutstation-SAS-Stroke Unit. Pflege Aktuell 2000;1:18

Chapter 7

American Medical Association 1981. Uniform Determination of Death Act 1981. Drafted by the National Conference of Commissioners on Uniform State Laws. American Medical Association 1981.

Anschütz F. Indikation zum ärztlichen Handeln. Berlin, Heidelberg, New York: Springer; 1982

Anschütz F. Stichwort Indikation. In: Eser A, Luterotti M, Sporken P (eds). Lexikon Medizin, Ethik, Recht. Freiburg: Herder; 1989

Bannert R, Fink U, Heimermann G, Lätzsch G. Werkbuch Medizinethik I. Münster: Lit Verlag; 2005

Beauchamp TL, Childress JF. Principles of Biomedical Ethics. New York: Oxford University Press; 2001

British Medical Association 2007. Advance decisions and proxy decision-making in medical treatment and research. Guidance from the BMA's Medical Ethics Department. June 2007.

British Medical Association 2009. End-of-life decisions. Views of the BMA. August 2009.

Buchardi N, Rauprich O, Vollmann J. Patientenselbstbestimmung und Patientenverfügungen aus der Sicht von Patienten mit amyotropher Lateralsklerose. Ethik Med 2004;16:7–21

Bundesärztekammer 1979: Richtlinien für die Sterbehilfe. Dtsch Arztebl 1979;76:957–960

Bundesärztekammer 1998: Grundsätze der Bundesärztekammer zur ärztlichen Sterbebegleitung. Dtsch Arztebl 1998;95:B1851–1853

Christakis NA, Lamont EB. Extent and determinants of error in doctors' prognoses in terminally ill patients: prospective cohort study. BMJ. 2000;320(7233):469–472

Delbrück H. Stichwort Rehabilitation. In: Korff W, Beck L, Mikat P (eds). Lexikon der Bioethik. Gütersloh: Gütersloher Verlagshaus; 1998:179

Eibach U. Künstliche Ernährung um jeden Preis? MedR. 2002;20:123–131

Eibach U, Schäfer K. Autonomie von Patienten und Patientenwünsche bei Dialysepatienten. Zschr Med Ethik. 1997;43:261–272

Gahl K. Indication—reasoning structure for medical actions. [Article in German] Dtsch Med Wochenschr. 2005;130 (18):1155–1158

Herranz G. [Euthanasia—prescriptions and proscriptions of assistance in dying]. Med Klin (Munich). 1994;89 (4):216–221

Holloway RG, Benesch CG, Burgin WS, Zentner JB. Prognosis and decision making in severe stroke. JAMA. 2005;294 (6):725–733

Hunold GW. Stichwort Palliative Therapie. In: Korff W, Beck L, Mikat P (eds). Lexikon der Bioethik. Gütersloh: Gütersloher Verlagshaus; 1998

Jonsen AR, Sieler M, Winslade WJ. Klinische Ethik. Cologne: Deutscher Ärzte-Verlag; 2002

Kirchhoff P. Das Recht auf Leben und Gesundheit für alle Generationen. Z Med Ethik. 2005;51:229–241

Körtner UHJ. Mit Krankheit leben. Theol Literaturz. 2005;130:1273–1290

Merz JF. An empirical analysis of the medical informed consent Doctrine: the search for a "standard" of disclosure. Risk: Issues in Health & Safety 1991;2:27-76.

Mitchell SL, Lawson FME. Decision-making for long-term tube-feeding in cognitively impaired elderly people. CMAJ 1999;160(12):1705–1709

Nacimiento W, Nolden-Koch M, Schröer W, Papke K, Borasio GD. Schlaganfall: Medizinischer Sachverstand und ethisches Gespür. Dtsch Ärztebl. 2007;104: A708–711

Oehmichen F. [Article in German] Wien Klin Wochenschr. 2005;117(Suppl 6):17–23

Oehmichen F. Ethischer Diskurs im interdisziplinären Kontext in der Palliative Care und Intensivmedizin. In: Knipping C, ed. Lehrbuch der Palliativpflege. Bern: Huber; 2006

Oehmichen F, Irrgang B. Ethische Fragen der künstlichen Ernährung. Ethica. 2005;13:69–91

Plenter C. Ethische Aspekte in der Pflege von Wachkoma-Patienten. Hannover: Schlütersche; 2001

Schäfer A, Noack T, Fangerau H. Stichwort: Prognose. In: Jagow B, Steger F (eds). Literatur und Medizin—Ein Lexikon. Göttingen: Vandenhoeck & Ruprecht; 2005

Schneider W. „Death Telling" im medizinischen Kontext aus soziologischer Sicht. Notfall Hausarztmed. 2004;30:534–540

Spittler JF. Disorders of consciousness: the basis for ethical assessment. [Article in German] Fortschr Neurol Psychiatr 1999;67(1):37–47

Sporken P. Stichwort: Sterbebeistand/Sterbebegleitung. In: Eser A, Luterotti M, Sporken P (eds). Lexikon Medizin, Ethik, Recht. Freiburg: Herder; 1989

Stedman's Medical Dictionary. 25th ed. Baltomire: Williams & Wilkins; 1990.

Steinkamp N, Gordijn B. Ethik in der Klinik—ein Arbeitsbuch. Neuwied, Cologne, Munich: Luchterhand; 2003

Strätling M, Scharf VE. Medical rights review tables. Definitions, criteria, statutes, checklists for everyday clinical use. [Article in German] Anaesthesist 2000;49(7):669–674

Strätling M, Schmucker P. Entscheidungen am Lebensende in der Intensivmedizin. Anasthesiol Intensivmed Notfallmed Schmerzther 2004;39:1–20

Tolle P. Erwachsene im Wachkoma. Frankfurt am Main: Peter Lang; 2005

Tolmein O. Selbstbestimmungsrecht und Einwilligungsfähigkeit. Frankfurt am Main: Mabuse; 2004

van Oorschot B, Lipp V, Tietze A, Nickel N, Simon A. Attitudes on euthanasia and medical advance directives. [Article in German] Dtsch Med Wochenschr 2005;130 (6):261–265

Wedekind C, Klug N. Frühe Prognose nach schwerer Schädel-Hirn-Verletzung. Dtsch Ärztebl. 2005;102:A503–508

World Health Organization (WHO)1990. Cancer pain relief and palliative care. Report of a WHO Expert Committee (Technical Report Series No.804). Geneva: World Health Organization.

Index